2022

福建省肿瘤登记年报

FUJIAN CANCER REGISTRY ANNUAL REPORT 2022

主 编　陈传本

Editor in Chief　Chen Chuanben

福建省肿瘤防治办公室

福 建 省 肿 瘤 医 院

Fujian Provincial Office for Cancer Prevention and Control

Fujian Cancer Hospital

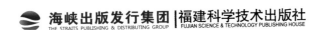

海峡出版发行集团 | 福建科学技术出版社
THE STRAITS PUBLISHING & DISTRIBUTING GROUP | FUJIAN SCIENCE & TECHNOLOGY PUBLISHING HOUSE

图书在版编目（CIP）数据

2022 福建省肿瘤登记年报 / 陈传本主编 . —福州：
福建科学技术出版社，2023.7
ISBN 978-7-5335-7012-5

Ⅰ . ① 2… Ⅱ . ①陈… Ⅲ . ①肿瘤 – 卫生统计 – 福建 –
2022 – 年报 Ⅳ . ① R73-54

中国国家版本馆 CIP 数据核字（2023）第 065975 号

书　　名	2022 福建省肿瘤登记年报	
主　　编	陈传本	
出版发行	福建科学技术出版社	
社　　址	福州市东水路 76 号（邮编 350001）	
网　　址	www.fjstp.com	
经　　销	福建新华发行（集团）有限责任公司	
印　　刷	福建东南彩色印刷有限公司	
开　　本	889 毫米 ×1194 毫米　1/16	
印　　张	11.75	
字　　数	356 千字	
版　　次	2023 年 7 月第 1 版	
印　　次	2023 年 7 月第 1 次印刷	
书　　号	ISBN 978-7-5335-7012-5	
定　　价	93.00 元	

书中如有印装质量问题，可直接向本社调换

编委会

Editorial Board

前　言

　　肿瘤登记资料为肿瘤防治策略与措施制定、肿瘤病因学研究及肿瘤预防效果评价等提供科学依据，肿瘤登记是肿瘤防控中最基础、最重要的一项工作。福建省最早于1986年在胃癌高发现场长乐县开展人群肿瘤登记工作；2009年起在"国家重大公共卫生服务项目"的推动下，肿瘤登记工作覆盖的地区逐步扩大；2022年福建省肿瘤防治办公室按照《健康中国行动——癌症防治实施方案（2019-2022年）》的要求，在全省所有县区开展人群肿瘤登记工作，把此项工作推向人群全覆盖的新阶段。

　　福建省2014年起每年编撰《福建省肿瘤登记年报》，旨在分析福建省肿瘤流行特征，将最新数据提供给卫生行政部门及专业科研人员。2022年福建省肿瘤防治办公室经严格质控、筛选2019年肿瘤登记数据，将长乐区、厦门市区、涵江区、新罗区、永安市、蕉城区等24个质量较好的登记处数据合并分析，撰写《2022福建省肿瘤登记年报》。24个登记处覆盖9个市15427160户籍人口，占全省户籍人口数的39.6%，数据更加具有代表性。年报首次采用中英文编写，希望能为更多的肿瘤防治专业人员提供重要的研究线索。

　　本年报是在国家癌症中心、福建省卫生健康委员会的指导和支持下完成的，凝结着全省肿瘤登记工作人员的辛勤劳动，在此表示衷心的感谢！希望本年报的出版能促进全省肿瘤防治和研究事业的发展！

福建省肿瘤防治办公室　主任
福 建 省 肿 瘤 医 院　院长
福 建 省 肿 瘤 研 究 所　所长

陈 传 本

Foreword

Population-based cancer registration data provides the scientific basis for the formulation of cancer prevention and control strategies and measures, cancer etiology research and cancer prevention effect evaluation, which is the most basic and important work in cancer prevention and control. In Fujian Province, the program of cancer registration started in 1986 in Changle County, a site with a high incidence of stomach cancer. Since 2009, the coverage of cancer registration has been gradually expanded under the promotion of the "National Major Public Health Services Project". In 2022, in accordance with the requirements of the *Healthy China Initiative-Implementation Plan for Cancer Prevention and Control (2019-2022)*, Fujian Provincial Office for Cancer Prevention and Control carried out population-based cancer registration in all regions of the province, bringing this work to a new stage of full population coverage.

The *Fujian Cancer Registry Annual Report* has been compiling every year since 2014, aiming to analyze the epidemiological characteristics of cancer in the province and provide the latest data to health administration departments and professional researchers. In 2022, after strict quality control and screening of cancer registration data in 2019, the Fujian Provincial Office for Cancer Prevention and Control combined and analyzed the high-quality data of 24 cancer registries, including Changle District, Xiamen City, Hanjiang District, Xinluo District, Yong'an County and Jiaocheng District, to write the *Fujian Cancer Registry Annual Report 2022*. The 24 cancer registries included in this annual report covered 15,427,160 household registered populations in 9 prefectures, accounting for 39.6% of the household registered population in the province, making the data more representative. This annual report was compiled in both Chinese and English for the first time, hoping to provide important research clues for more cancer prevention and control professionals.

This annual report is completed under the guidance and support of the National Cancer Center and Health Commission of Fujian Province, which condenses the hard work of all the cancer registry staff in the province. It is hoped that the publication of this annual report can promote the development of cancer prevention and research in the province.

Director of Fujian Provincial Office for Cancer Prevention and Control
President of Fujian Cancer Hospital
Director of Fujian Institute of Cancer Research

Chen Chuanben

目 录

Contents

第一章 概述
Chapter 1 Introduction

自 20 世纪 70 年代福建省开展第一次死因回顾性调查以来，恶性肿瘤一直是居民首位死因，占死因构成随时间呈明显上升趋势，对国民经济、社会发展、卫生服务等造成极大影响。目前肿瘤预防与控制已成为卫生战略的重点。肿瘤登记是一项系统经常性的收集、储存、整理、统计分析和评价肿瘤发病、死亡和生存资料的统计报告制度。全面、准确和及时掌握人群恶性肿瘤发病、死亡及其相关信息是肿瘤预防与控制工作的基础，是制订卫生事业发展规划、肿瘤防治策略与措施的重要参考依据。

Since the first retrospective survey of death causes in Fujian Province in the 1970s, cancer has been the leading cause of death in the population, accounting for a significant increase in the composition of death causes over time, which has had a great impact on the national economy, social development and health services. Cancer prevention and control have now become a priority in health strategies. Population-based cancer registration is a statistical reporting system for the collection, storage, sorting, analysis and evaluation of cancer incidence, mortality and survival data. Comprehensive, accurate and timely understanding of cancer incidence, mortality and its related information is the foundation of cancer prevention and control, and is an important reference basis for formulating health development plans, cancer prevention and control strategies and measures.

第一节 背景

福建省人群肿瘤登记工作最早开始于 20 世纪 80 年代，1986 年长乐县被原省科委和省卫生厅确定为胃癌高发现场，同年长乐县成立肿瘤登记处，开展人群肿瘤发病与死亡登记报告工作。长乐县早期肿瘤发病、死亡资料被《五大洲癌症发病率》第八卷，《中国试点市、县恶性肿瘤发病与死亡》第一卷（1988-1992）、第二卷（1993-1997）、第三卷（1998-2002），

Section 1 Background

The provincial program of cancer registration in Fujian began in the 1980s. In 1986, Changle County was identified by the former Provincial Science Committee and Provincial Department of Health as a site with a high incidence of stomach cancer, and in the same year, Changle County Cancer Registry was established to carry out the registration of cancer incidence and mortality. The data on cancer incidence and mortality in Changle were included in *Cancer Incidence in Five Continents*, Volume VIII, *Cancer Incidence and Mortality in Chinese Pilot*

《中国癌症发病与死亡 2003–2007》收录。长乐肿瘤登记数据为肿瘤防治研究提供了重要的基础数据。

福建省卫生健康委员会十分重视肿瘤防治及基础数据的收集工作，为了掌握福建省恶性肿瘤流行情况及分布特征，早在 2007 年原福建省卫生厅下发《关于开展恶性肿瘤发病登记报告工作的通知》（闽卫函〔2007〕571 号），制订《福建省恶性肿瘤发病登记报告工作方案（试行）》，由省肿瘤防治办公室和省疾病预防控制中心牵头，开展全省二级及以上的医院恶性肿瘤住院患者发病登记报告工作，委托省肿瘤防治办公室开发肿瘤登记报告软件，拨出专项经费定期举办全省肿瘤登记技术培训班，对全省各级疾病预防控制中心及二级以上医院肿瘤登记工作人员进行技术培训。此项工作为福建省人群肿瘤登记工作奠定了坚实的基础。

2009 年以来，在"国家重大公共卫生服务项目"支持下，福建省人群肿瘤登记报告工作进入快速发展阶段，在长乐肿瘤登记处基础上，陆续新增加了厦门市区（包含思明区、湖里区、集美区、海沧区）、南平建瓯市、泉州惠安县、莆田涵江区、龙岩永定区、厦门同安区、三明永安市、漳州长泰县、福州福清市、龙岩新罗区、厦门翔安区和宁德古田县等国家级登记处。截至 2021 年福建省国家级肿瘤登记处达 30 个，覆盖 33 个县（市、

Cities or Counties, Volume I (1988–1992), Volume II (1993–1997), Volume III (1998–2002), and *Cancer Incidence and Mortality in China, 2003–2007*. The cancer registration data of Changle District provides important basic data for cancer prevention and control research.

The Health Commission of Fujian Province attaches great importance to cancer prevention and control and the collection of basic data. In order to grasp the prevalence and distribution characteristics of cancer in Fujian Province, the Provincial Health Commission issued the administrative document of *Registration and Reporting of Cancer Incidence* and formulated the administrative document of *Work Plan of Cancer Incidence Registration and Reporting in Fujian Province (for trial implementation)* in 2007. Cancer registration was led by the Fujian Provincial Office for Cancer Prevention and Control and the Provincial Center for Disease Control and Prevention to carry out the incidence registration of cancer inpatients in secondary and above hospitals. The Provincial Office for Cancer Prevention and Control was entrusted to develop the corresponding software, and dedicated funds were allocated to hold regular training courses on cancer registration technology in the whole province. Technical training was provided to the cancer registration staff of the Centers for Disease Control and Prevention and the secondary and above–level hospitals in the province. This work has laid a solid foundation for population–based cancer registration in Fujian Province.

Since 2009, with the support of the "National Major Public Health Services Project", the population–based cancer registration work in Fujian Province has gone through a stage of rapid development. Based on the cancer registry in Changle District, national registries have been added in Xiamen City (including Siming District, Huli District, Jimei District and Haicang District), Jian'ou County of Nanping City, Hui'an County of Quanzhou City, Hanjiang District of Putian City, Yongding District of Longyan City, Tong'an District

区）的 1873.99 万人口。2022 年福建省卫生健康委员会下发"关于进一步加强'以人群为基础'肿瘤登记报告工作的通知（闽卫疾控函〔2022〕66 号）"，落实"健康中国行动 – 癌症防治实施方案（2019–2022）"要求，在全省所有县（市、区）开展人群肿瘤登记工作，为福建省全面开展肿瘤登记工作提供了政策保障。

自 2014 年以来，福建省肿瘤防治办公室每年选取质量较好的登记处数据编撰《福建省肿瘤登记年报》，已连续 8 年出版省级年报，及时将掌握的恶性肿瘤流行数据提供给业内专家及卫生行政部门。《2022 福建省肿瘤登记年报》收录 24 个登记处的数据，覆盖全省 39.6% 户籍人口，首次采用中英文编写，数据更加具有代表性，希望能为肿瘤防治研究提供重要线索，为各级卫生行政部门制订防治策略和措施提供科学依据。

of Xiamen City, Yong'an County of Sanming City, Changtai County of Zhangzhou City, Fuqing County of Fuzhou City, Xinluo District of Longyan City, Xiang'an District of Xiamen City and Gutian County of Ningde City. By 2021, there were 30 national cancer registries in Fujian province, covering 33 counties (cities, districts) with a population of 18.7399 million. In 2022, the Health Commission of Fujian Province issued the administrative document of *Further Strengthening Population–based Cancer Registration* to implement the requirements of the *Healthy China Initiative–Implementation Plan for Cancer Prevention and Control(2019–2022)* to carry out population–based cancer registration in all regions of Fujian Province. It provides a policy guarantee for the comprehensive development of cancer registration in the province.

Since 2014, Fujian Provincial Office for Cancer Prevention and Control has selected registry data of good quality to compile the *Fujian Cancer Registry Annual Report* each year, which has been published for 8 consecutive years, providing the epidemiological data of cancer to experts and health administration departments in time. *Fujian Cancer Registry Annual Report 2022* contains data from 24 registries, covering 39.6% of the province's household population, which makes the data more representative. The annual report is compiled in both Chinese and English for the first time, it is expected to provide clues for the research of cancer prevention and control and a scientific basis for the health administrative departments to formulate prevention and control strategies and measures.

第二节 肿瘤登记方法

一、开展人群肿瘤登记报告的基本条件

1. 建立肿瘤登记报告制度，制订相应法规或政策

在新开展肿瘤登记报告的地区，首先要由当地政府或卫生行政部门制订和颁布实行肿瘤登记报告制度的法规或规范性文件，建立肿瘤登记处。

2. 制订肿瘤登记报告实施细则

新建立的肿瘤登记处根据《中国肿瘤登记工作指导手册》要求和当地的实际情况，制订符合当地具体情况的肿瘤新病例登记报告实施细则，以保证此项工作建立和长期正常运行。

3. 健全的基层医疗保健网、死亡统计制度和人口学资料

建立肿瘤新发病例和死亡病例发现途径，与基层医疗保健网络和有肿瘤诊疗能力的医疗机构建立工作关系，开展病例核实和随访工作，保证数据的准确性。以死亡统计资料为基础开展死亡补充登记工作，并定期从公安、户籍等相关部门取得人口资料。

4. 开展人员培训

肿瘤登记处的工作人员必须定期接受专业

Section 2　Registration methods

1. Basic conditions for cancer registration

1.1 Establish a cancer registration report system and formulate corresponding regulations or policies

In the newly launched areas of cancer registration, the local government or the health administration department should formulate and promulgate regulations or normative documents on cancer registration, and establish a cancer registry.

1.2 Formulate implementation rules for cancer registration

In accordance with the requirements of the *Chinese Guideline for Cancer Registration* and the actual local conditions, the newly established cancer registry shall formulate the implementation rules for the registration in line with the specific local conditions, so as to ensure the establishment and long-term operation of this work.

1.3 Robust primary health care network, mortality statistics system and demographic information

Establish a method to discover new cancer cases and death cases, establish a working relationship with primary health care networks and medical institutions capable of cancer diagnosis and treatment, and carry out case verification and follow-up to ensure the accuracy of data. Supplementary registration of deaths is carried out on the basis of death statistics, and population data are regularly obtained from Public Security Bureau, Household Registration Bureau and other relevant departments.

1.4 Conduct personnel training

Cancer registry staff must receive regular

技术培训。培训内容包括肿瘤新发病例、死亡病例、人口资料的收集技术与方法、肿瘤分类与编码、登记资料的统计和分析、登记软件使用等。

technical training. It includes techniques and methods of data collection, cancer classification and coding, statistics and analysis of registration data, application of registration software, etc.

二、肿瘤登记工作流程

按福建省卫生健康委员会要求，全省二级及以上医院需指定工作人员，定期通过"福建省肿瘤登记信息直报平台"（简称"平台"）报告肿瘤新发病例资料，平台根据病例户籍地址自动将病例信息推送到户籍地登记处。

登记处定期对病例进行查重，整合重复报告病例信息，定期从城镇居民、职工医疗保险数据库及新型农村合作医疗保险数据库获取肿瘤病例就医诊断信息，与平台肿瘤发病信息比对，补充漏报病例。登记处从辖区生命统计部门获取人群死因信息，定期与平台肿瘤病例进行关联匹配，匹配病例补充死亡信息；未匹配的肿瘤死亡病例进行补充发病报告。

登记处定期通过平台将肿瘤病例信息推送到户籍所属的乡镇（社区）卫生服务部门进行核实和随访，并将结果通过平台上报。登记处多渠道获得的信息形成肿瘤数据库，根据公安或统计部门获取的人口资料，定期进行辖区肿瘤发病、死亡分析。

福建省肿瘤防治办公室日常维护平台运行，实时动态监测全省肿瘤登记地区工作进度，定期向全国肿瘤登记中心提交本省肿瘤登记数据。

2. Cancer registration workflow

According to the requirements of the Health Commission of Fujian Province, secondary and above hospitals in the province were required to designate staff to regularly report the data of new cancer cases through the Fujian Provincial Cancer Registration Information Reporting Platform (referred to as "Platform"), which will automatically push the case information to the registry of the home place according to the household registration address of the cases.

The registry regularly checks cases, consolidates information of duplicate reported cases, obtains medical diagnosis information of cancer cases from the database of medical insurance for urban residents and employees and the database of the new rural cooperative medical system, and compares it with the cancer incidence information in the Platform to supplement under-reported cases. The registry obtains information on the cause of death of the population from the vital statistics department of the district, and regularly matches it with the cancer cases in the platform to supplement the death information of the matched cases. The cancer death cases that are not matched are supplemented with the incidence report.

The registry regularly pushes the cancer case information to the township (community) health service department of the registered residence for verification and follow-up through the Platform, and reports the results through the Platform. The information obtained by the registry through multiple departments is formed into a cancer database, and the incidence and mortality of cancer in the jurisdiction are analyzed regularly according to the

三、肿瘤登记资料收集内容

肿瘤登记处收集辖区范围内全部恶性肿瘤和中枢神经系统良性及其动态未定肿瘤的发病、死亡和生存信息，以及辖区的人口资料。

1. 人口资料

人口资料来源于人口普查资料或公安、统计部门逐年提供相应的人口资料。人口资料包括户籍居民人口总数及其性别、年龄构成。年龄按 0~ 岁、1~4 岁、5~9 岁、10~14 岁……75~79 岁、80~84 岁、85 岁及以上分组。

2. 新发病例资料

新发病例收集个人基本信息、诊断信息和报告单位信息，个人基本信息包括姓名、性别、出生日期、身份证号、年龄、民族、婚姻状况、职业、联系电话、户籍地址等；诊断信息包括发病部位、病理类型、分期、诊断依据、诊断日期、ICD10 编码、治疗信息等；报告单位信息包括报告日期、诊断单位、报告医师等。

3. 死亡病例资料

肿瘤登记处通过本地区负责生命统计的专业机构（如疾病预防控制中心等）获得肿瘤死亡资料，主要收集死亡日期、死亡原因、死亡地点等。

4. 生存资料

肿瘤登记处以被动随访和主动随访相结合的方式获取肿瘤病例的生存信息。被动随访，即定期通过肿瘤发病资料与全死因资料进行关

population data obtained by the Public Security Bureau or Statistics Bureau.

Fujian Provincial Office for Cancer Prevention and Control regularly maintains the operation of the Platform, monitors the work progress of cancer registration areas in the province dynamically, and submits cancer registration data of the province to the national cancer registration center regularly.

3. Contents of data collection

The registry collects all cancers information on incidence, mortality and survival, including neoplasms of central nerve systems with benign or uncertain behaviors. The data on population coverage should also be collected.

3.1 Population data

The population data originate from census data, bureaus of statistics or public security. The detailed population data should cover the overall population with age-specific data by age groups of 5- years and gender-specific data.

3.2 Incidence

Basic information, diagnosis information and reporting unit information of newly diagnosed cases were collected. Basic information including name, gender, date of birth, identity card number, age, race, marital status, career, contact number, and address. The diagnostic information included the site of disease, pathological type, stage, diagnostic basis, date of diagnosis, ICD-10 code, and treatment information. The reporting unit information included reporting date, clinics of diagnosis, and reporting doctors.

3.3 Mortality

The data on cancer mortality were obtained from the local professional institutions responsible for vital statistics (such as the Centers for Disease Control and Prevention, etc.), mainly including the

联匹配，获得肿瘤病例的生存结局信息。主动随访，即经基层医疗部门定期通过电话、访视等方式获得病人的生存状况（存活、死亡、移居、失访等）和生存时间等信息。

四、肿瘤登记数据质量控制

肿瘤登记工作的质量控制要从发病报告、数据随访、重复报告病例整合、定期考核等各个环节制订工作规范并严格执行。资料要满足完整性、有效性和时效性等评价标准。

登记资料的完整性是指登记处覆盖地区的目标人群中发现所有肿瘤发病病例的程度。常用死亡发病比（M/I）、仅有死亡医学证明书比例（DCO%）、相邻年份发病（死亡）率的稳定性等指标评价。

有效性指登记病例中具有给定特征（例如部位、年龄、性别、诊断、编码）的真正属性的病例所占的比例。常用组织学诊断比例（MV%）、部位不明的比例（O&U%）等指标评价。平台参考工具软件"IARCcrgTools"设置一致性和有效性审核功能。校验的逻辑关系包括：性别和部位、身份证号与出生日期、部位和病理类型、病理类型与行为、病理类型和分级、病理类型与诊断依据等。逻辑关系正确的病例才能够通过校验上报。

时效性是指肿瘤登记处收集、处理、报告足够可靠和完整的肿瘤资料的及时性。按照福

date of death, cause of death, and place of death.

3.4 Survival

The cancer registry used the ways of passive and active follow-up to obtain the survival information of cancer cases. Passive follow-up was to obtain the survival outcome information of cancer cases by regularly linking and matching the data of cancer incidence and all death cases. Active follow-up was to obtain the survival status (survival, death, migration, loss of follow-up, etc.) and survival time of patients through regular telephone calls and visits by primary medical departments.

4. Quality control

The quality control of cancer registration should be standardized and strictly implemented from the aspects of incidence report, data follow-up, integration of repeated cases and regular assessment. The data should meet the evaluation criteria of completeness, validity and timeliness.

The completeness of cancer registration data concerns to what extent the new cases that occurred in a defined population were registered in the cancer registration database. The indicators to evaluate the completeness includes the mortality/incidence(M/I) ratio, percentage of death certificate only(DCO%), and stability of incidence (mortality) in adjacent years.

The validity refers to the proportion of registered cases with real attributes of a given characteristic (such as the site of disease, age, gender, diagnosis, and code). Commonly used evaluation indicators are percentage of morphological verification of diagnosis(MV%) and the percentage of cases of other or unspecified sites(O&U%). Platform refers to software "IARCcrgTools" to set up consistency and validity audit functions. The logical relations of verification include gender and site of disease, ID number and date of birth, site of disease and pathological type,

建省肿瘤登记实施方案，患者出院后需要上报发病资料，最晚不得超过次月 25 日。

登记处每年对辖区报告单位至少进行一次考核，内容包括数据完整性（漏报情况）、报告信息准确性（平台填报项目和病案首页信息一致程度）和报告及时性等。登记处每年对乡镇（社区）卫生部门的随访核实工作进行质控，抽取部分病例调查，评估随访资料的真实性。

pathological type and behavior, pathological type and grade, pathological type and diagnostic basis. Only cases with correct logical relationships can be reported through verification.

Timeliness refers to the rapidity of the cancer registry to collect, process and report sufficiently reliable and complete cancer data. According to the implementation plan of cancer registration in Fujian Province, patients are required to report the onset data after discharge, no later than the 25th day of the following month.

The registry evaluated the reporting units under the jurisdiction at least once a year, including data integrity (under-reported), the accuracy of reporting information (consistency between the items filled in the Platform and the information on the front page of medical records), and timeliness of reporting. The registry conducts annual quality control on the follow-up verification work of township (community) health departments, takes some cases for investigation, and evaluates the authenticity of the follow-up information.

第三节　肿瘤登记资料的统计分析

一、常用统计分析指标

1. 年平均人口数

人口数是计算当年当地肿瘤发病（死亡）率的分母，由于人口受出生、死亡、迁移等因素影响，每日人口总数都有所变动，因此通常使用年平均人口数作为代表。

$$年平均人口数 = \frac{年初（上年末）人口数 + 年末人口数}{2}$$

2. 性别、年龄别人口数

性别、年龄别人口数是指按男、女性别和不同年龄分组的人口数，年龄的分组一般以 5 岁为组间距，分为：0~ 岁、1~4 岁、5~9 岁、10~14 岁……75~79 岁、80~84 岁和 85 岁及以上年龄组。

3. 发病（死亡）率

发病（死亡）率又称为粗发病（死亡）率，是指某年某地登记的每 10 万人口恶性肿瘤新发（死亡）病例数，是反映人群肿瘤发病（死亡）情况最基本的指标，常以 10 万分率（1/10 万）表示。

$$发病（死亡）率 = \frac{某年某地恶性肿瘤新发病（死亡）例数}{某年某地年平均人口数}$$

$$\times 100000（1/10 万）$$

Section 3　Statistical analysis

1. Statistical indicators

1.1 Average annual population

The population is the denominator to calculate the incidence (mortality) rate in that year. Because the population is affected by birth, death, migration and other factors, the total number of people varies from day to day, so the average annual population is usually used as a representative.

Average annual population=

$$\frac{\text{population in the beginning of the year(or at the end of the last year)}}{2}$$

$$+ \frac{\text{population at the end of the year}}{2}$$

1.2 Gender–and age–specific population

Gender– and age–specific population is the population by gender and different age groups. The age group is generally divided into 0 ~ , 1~4, 5~9, 10~14...75~79, 80~84, 85+years.

1.3 Incidence (mortality) rate

The incidence (mortality) rate is a measure of the frequency with which an event, such as a new case of cancer (cancer death), occurs in a population over a period of time, often expressed as a 100,000 rate (1/100,000).

Incidence (mortality) rate=

$$\frac{\text{new cases (new cancer deaths)occurring during a given time period}}{\text{population at risk during the same time period}}$$

$$\times 100,000$$

4. 性别、年龄别发病（死亡）率

人口的性别、年龄结构是影响恶性肿瘤发病(死亡)水平的重要因素,性别、年龄别发病(死亡)率是按男女性别、不同年龄组分别计算的发病（死亡）率。

男（女）某年龄别发病（死亡）率 =

$$\frac{男（女）性某年龄别新发病（死亡）例数}{男（女）性同年龄别年平均人口数}$$

$\times 100000$（1/10 万）

5. 年龄标准化发病（死亡）率

由于恶性肿瘤发病（死亡）率在各年龄组间差别较大，在比较不同地区或者同一地区人群不同时期的肿瘤发病（死亡）率时，不能直接用肿瘤粗发病（死亡）率进行比较，需要计算年龄标准化发病（死亡）率，即按照某一标准人口的年龄结构所计算的发病（死亡）率。常用 2000 年全国人口普查的人口年龄构成计算中国人口标准化率，用 Segi's 世界人口年龄构成计算世界人口标准化率。

标化发病（死亡）率的计算（直接法）：

（1）计算年龄组发病（死亡）率。

（2）以各年龄组发病（死亡）率乘以相应的标准人口年龄构成百分比，得到各年龄组相应的分配发病（死亡）率。

（3）将各年龄组的分配发病（死亡）率相加，即为标准化的发病（死亡）率。

标准化发病（死亡）率 =

$$\frac{\sum 标准人口年龄构成 \times 年龄别发病（死亡）率}{\sum 标准人口年龄构成}$$

1.4 Gender- and age-specific incidence (mortality) rate

Gender and age structure are important factors affecting the incidence and mortality of cancer. Gender-specific and age-specific incidence and mortality are calculated by gender and age groups.

Age-specific incidence (mortality) rate=

$$\frac{cases\ (cancer\ deaths)\ in\ a\ specific\ age\ group}{population\ in\ the\ age\ group} \times 100,000$$

1.5 Age-standardized rates (ASR)

Because the crude incidence(mortality) rate would be substantially affected by the age structure of the population, when comparing the incidence(mortality) rate in different regions or in the same region but at different periods of time, in order to eliminate the influence of the population's age structure on the incidence or mortality, it is necessary to calculate the age-standardized incidence(mortality) rate (ASIR or ASMR). In other words, the ASIR or ASMR represents the incidence or mortality rate after adjusting age by a standardized age structure of a certain population. In this annual report, the population standards we used are the world Segi's population and the fifth Chinese national census of 2000.

Direct method calculating incidence (mortality) rate:

（1） Calculating the rates for subjects in a specific age category in a study population.

（2） Calculating the weighted age-specific rates. The weights applied represent the relative age distribution of the standard population.

（3） Adding up each weighted age-specific rate. The summary rates reflect the adjusted rates.

Adjusted rate=

$$\frac{\sum standard\ population\ in\ corresponding\ age\ group \times age\text{-}specific\ rate}{\sum standard\ population}$$

6. 分类构成

恶性肿瘤发病（死亡）构成百分比反映各类恶性肿瘤对居民健康危害的情况。恶性肿瘤发病（死亡）分类构成百分比的计算公式如下：

$$某恶性肿瘤发病（死亡）构成 = \frac{某恶性肿瘤发病（死亡）人数}{总恶性肿瘤发病（死亡）人数} \times 100\%$$

7. 累积发病（死亡）率

累积发病（死亡）率是指某病在某一年龄阶段内按年龄（岁）的发病（死亡）率进行累积相加。累积发病（死亡）率消除了年龄构成不同的影响，故不需要标准化便可以用于不同地区直接进行比较。恶性肿瘤一般是计算 0~74 岁的累积发病（死亡）率。

$$累积率 = [\sum（年龄组发病[死亡]率 \times 年龄组距）] \times 100\%$$

二、数据统计分析

年报选取数据质量较好的登记处资料进行合并分析，计算粗率、中国人口标准化率（中标率）、世界人口标准化率（世标率）、年龄别率和累积率等指标。根据登记地区发病（死亡）情况及各地区年龄、性别人口构成，估算 2019 年福建全省总体恶性肿瘤和各部位恶性肿瘤的发病和死亡病例数。常用恶性肿瘤分类统计（大类、细分类）见表 1-1、表 1-2。中标率按 2000 年全国人口普查年龄构成计算，世标率按 Segi's 世界人口年龄构成计算（表 1-3）。

本年报在计算各部位男女合计发病（死亡）

1.6 Proportion

The proportional distribution indicates the site-specific percentage level of incident cases and deaths compared with the total cases recorded. The formula is:

$$\text{The proportion of a certain type of cancer} = \frac{\text{No. of cases (deaths) of a particular cancer}}{\text{No. of cases (deaths) of all cancers}} \times 100\%$$

1.7 Cumulative incidence (mortality) rate

A cumulative rate expresses the probability of onset of cancer between birth and a specific age. The rate can be compared without age standardization as it is not affected by age structures. This is often expressed at risk between age 0 and 74 years for cancer.

$$\text{Cumulative rate} = [\sum（\text{age-specific rate} \times \text{width of the age group}）] \times 100\%$$

2. Statistical analysis of data

Data from cancer registries with good data quality were selected for combined analysis. Crude rate, ASR China, ASR World, age-specific rate and cumulative rate were calculated. According to the incidence (mortality) in the registration areas and the age and gender population composition of each area, the number of new cases and death cases of all cancer sites and each cancer site in Fujian province in 2019 was estimated. The statistics of common cancer classification are shown in Table 1-1 and Table 1-2. The ASR China is calculated based on the Chinese national census of 2000, and the ASR World is calculated based on the world Segi's population(Table1-3).

In this annual report, when calculating the incidence (mortality) rates of all sites for both males and females, for cancers that can occur

率时，对于男性和女性均可发生的恶性肿瘤：如口腔、鼻咽、食管、胃、肺等恶性肿瘤，将男性和女性人口合并作为分母进行计算；对于男性特有的恶性肿瘤：如阴茎、前列腺、睾丸和其他男性生殖器等恶性肿瘤，以男性人口作为分母进行计算；对于女性特有或男性罕见的恶性肿瘤：如乳房、外阴、阴道、子宫颈、子宫体、卵巢、其他女性生殖器和胎盘等恶性肿瘤，以女性人口作为分母进行计算。

in both males and females, such as oral cancer, nasopharyngeal cancer, esophageal cancer, stomach cancer and lung cancer, the combined population of males and females was used as the denominator for calculation. For male-specific cancers, such as penile cancer, prostate cancer, testicular cancer and other male cancers, the male population was used as the denominator. For cancers that are specific to women or rare to men, such as breast cancer, vulvar cancer, vaginal cancer, cervix cancer, corpus uterus cancer, ovarian cancer, other cancers of female genitalia, and placental cancer, the female population was used as the denominator.

表 1-1　常用恶性肿瘤分类统计表（大类）
Table 1-1　Cancer categories by ICD-10

部位 Sites	ICD-10	部位 Sites	ICD-10
口腔和咽喉（除外鼻咽）Oral Cavity & Pharynx but Nasopharynx	C00-C10, C12-C14	子宫颈 Cervix Uteri	C53
鼻咽 Nasopharynx	C11	子宫体及子宫部位不明 Uterus & Unspecified	C54-C55
食管 Esophagus	C15	卵巢 Ovary	C56
胃 Stomach	C16	前列腺 Prostate	C61
结直肠肛门 Colon, Rectum & Anus	C18-C21	睾丸 Testis	C62
肝脏 Liver	C22	肾及泌尿系统不明 Kidney & Unspecified Urinary Organs	C64-C66,C68
胆囊及其他 Gallbladder, etc.	C23-C24	膀胱 Bladder	C67
胰腺 Pancreas	C25	脑及中枢神经系统 Brain & Central Nervous System	C70-C72,D32-D33, D42-D43
喉 Larynx	C32	甲状腺 Thyroid	C73
气管，支气管，肺 Traches, Bronchus & Lung	C33-C34	淋巴瘤 Lymphoma	C81-C85,C88,C90,C96
其他胸腔器官 Other Thoracic Organs	C37-C38	白血病 Leukaemia	C91-C95,D45-D47
骨和关节软骨 Bone	C40-C41	其他 Unspecified and All Others	Other（除以上外）
皮肤黑色素瘤 Melanoma of Skin	C43	所有部位合计 All Sites in Total	ALL
乳房 Breast	C50		

表 1-2 常用恶性肿瘤分类统计表（细分类）

Table 1-2 Cancer classification of ICD-10

部位 Sites	ICD-10	部位 Sites	ICD-10
唇 Lip	C00	子宫颈 Cervix Uteri	C53
舌 Tongue	C01-C02	子宫体 Corpus Uteri	C54
口 Mouth	C03-C06	子宫，部位不明 Uterus Unspecified	C55
唾液腺 Salivary Gland	C07-C08	卵巢 Ovary	C56
扁桃体 Tonsil	C09	其他女性生殖器 Other Female Genital Organs	C57
其他口咽 Other Oropharynx	C10	胎盘 Placenta	C58
鼻咽 Nasopharynx	C11	阴茎 Penis	C60
喉咽 Hypopharynx	C12-C13	前列腺 Prostate	C61
咽，部位不明 Pharynx Unspecified	C14	睾丸 Testis	C62
食管 Esophagus	C15	其他男性生殖器 Other Male Genital Organs	C63
胃 Stomach	C16	肾 Kidney	C64
小肠 Small Intestine	C17	肾盂 Renal Pelvis	C65
结肠 Colon	C18	输尿管 Ureter	C66
直肠 Rectum	C19-C20	膀胱 Bladder	C67
肛门 Anus	C21	其他泌尿器官 Other Urinary Organs	C68
肝脏 Liver	C22	眼 Eye	C69
胆囊及其他 Gallbladder, ete.	C23-C24	脑及中枢神经系统 Brain & Central Nervous System	C70-C72,D32-33, D42-D43
胰腺 Pancreas	C25	甲状腺 Thyroid	C73
鼻，鼻窦及其他 Nose, Sinuses etc.	C30-C31	肾上腺 Adrenal Gland	C74
喉 Larynx	C32	其他内分泌腺 Other Endocrine	C75
气管，支气管，肺 Trachea, Bronchus and Lung	C33-C34	霍奇金病 Hodgkin Disease	C81
其他胸腔器官 Other Thoracic Organs	C37-C38	非霍奇金病淋巴瘤 Non-Hodgkin Lymphoma	C82-C85,C96
骨和关节软骨 Bone	C40-C41	免疫增生性疾病 Immunoproliferative Disease	C88
皮肤黑色素瘤 Melanoma of Skin	C43	多发性骨髓瘤 Multiple Myeloma	C90
其他皮肤 Other Skin	C44	淋巴样白血病 . Lymphoid Leukaemia	C91
间皮瘤 Mesothelioma	C45	髓样白血病 Myeloid Leukaemia	C92-C94,D45-D47
卡波西肉瘤 Kaposi Sarcoma	C46	白血病，未特指 Leukaemia Unspecified	C95
周围神经，其他结缔组织、软组织 Connective and Soft Tissue	C47,C49	其他或未指明部位 Unspecified and All Others	O&U
乳房 Breast	C50	所有部位合计 All Sites in Total	ALL
外阴 Vulva	C51	所有部位除 C44 外 All Sites but C44	ALLbC44
阴道 Vagina	C52		

表 1-3 中国和世界标准人口构成

Table 1-3 Standard population construction

年龄组 Age group	中国人口构成（2000年） China population(2000)	世界人口构成（Segi's） Segi's population
0~	13793799	2400
1~	55184575	9600
5~	90152587	10000
10~	125396633	9000
15~	103031165	9000
20~	94573174	8000
25~	117602265	8000
30~	127314298	6000
35~	109147295	6000
40~	81242945	6000
45~	85521045	6000
50~	63304200	5000
55~	46370375	4000
60~	41703848	4000
65~	34780460	3000
70~	25574149	2000
75~	15928330	1000
80~	7989158	500
85+	4001925	500
合计 Total	1242612226	100000

第二章 肿瘤登记数据收集和质量评价
Chapter 2 Data collection and quality assessment

第一节 数据收集情况

一、时间范围

年报收集通过质控审核的登记处数据，包括发病日期为 2019 年 1 月 1 日至 2019 年 12 月 31 日的新发恶性肿瘤病例数据和同期恶性肿瘤死亡病例。

二、覆盖地区

年报数据来自 24 个肿瘤登记处，覆盖 9 个地市的 27 个县（市、区）。按照国家最新行政区划，将长乐区、思明区、湖里区、海沧区、集美区、翔安区、涵江区、泉港区、芗城区、长泰区、延平区、新罗区、永定区和蕉城区归为城市地区；将福清市、永泰县、仙游县、宁化县、大田县、永安市、安溪县、晋江市、南靖县、平和县、浦城县、建瓯市和上杭县归为农村地区（图 2-1，表 2-1）。

Section 1 Data collection

1. Time range

This annual report collects data from registries that have passed quality control audits, including data on new cases of cancer with onset dates from January 1, 2019 to December 31, 2019, and deaths from cancer during the same period.

2. Area coverage

Data for this annual report came from 24 cancer registries covering 27 counties (cities and districts) in 9 prefectures. According to the administrative divisions, Changle District, Siming District, Huli District, Haicang District, Jimei District, Xiang'an District, Hanjiang District, Quangang District, Xiangcheng District, Changtai District, Yanping District, Xinluo District, Yongding District and Jiaocheng District are classified as urban areas. Fuqing County, Yongtai County, Xianyou County, Ninghua County, Datian County, Yong'an County, Anxi County, Jinjiang County, Nanjing County, Pinghe County, Pucheng County, Jian'ou County and Shanghang County are classified as rural areas (Figure 2-1, Table 2-1).

表 2-1　《年报》收录的肿瘤登记地区分布情况

Table 2-1　Distribution of cancer registration areas included in the annual report

设区市 District city	登记地区覆盖人口 Population covered by the registration areas	占当地人口比例 Proportion of the local population	登记地区 Registration Areas	登记机构 Registry
福州 Fuzhou	2530045	35.77%	长乐区 Changle District	长乐区肿瘤防治研究所 Changle Cancer Prevention and Control Institute
			永泰县 Yongtai County	永泰县疾病预防控制中心 Yongtai Center for Disease Control and Prevention
			福清市 Fuqing County	福清市疾病预防控制中心 Fuqing Center for Disease Control and Prevention
厦门 Xiamen	2120190	84.20%	思明区、湖里区、集美区、海沧区 Siming District, Huli District, Jimei District, Haicang District	厦门市疾病预防控制中心 Xiamen Center for Disease Control and Prevention
			翔安区 Xiang'an District	翔安区疾病预防控制中心 Xiang'an Center for Disease Control and Prevention
莆田 Putian	1624997	44.86%	涵江区 Hanjiang District	涵江区疾病预防控制中心 Hanjiang Center for Disease Control and Prevention
			仙游县 Xianyou County	仙游县疾病预防控制中心 Xianyou Center for Disease Control and Prevention
三明 Sanming	1122709	38.87%	宁化县 Ninghua County	宁化县疾病预防控制中心 Ninghua Center for Disease Control and Prevention
			大田县 Datian County	大田县疾病预防控制中心 Datian Center for Disease Control and Prevention
			永安市 Yong'an County	永安市疾病预防控制中心 Yong'an Center for Disease Control and Prevention

续表

设区市 District city	登记地区覆盖人口 Population covered by the registration areas	占当地人口比例 Proportion of the local population	登记地区 Registration Areas	登记机构 Registry
泉州 Quanzhou	2824491	37.22%	泉港区 Quangang District	泉港区疾病预防控制中心 Quangang Center for Disease Control and Prevention
			安溪县 Anxi County	安溪县疾病预防控制中心 Anxi Center for Disease Control and Prevention
			晋江市 Jinjiang County	晋江市疾病预防控制中心 Jinjiang Center for Disease Control and Prevention
漳州 Zhangzhou	1667794	31.96%	芗城区 Xiangcheng District	芗城区疾病预防控制中心 Xiangcheng Center for Disease Control and Prevention
			长泰区 Changtai District	长泰区疾病预防控制中心 Changtai Center for Disease Control and Prevention
			南靖县 Nanjing County	南靖县疾病预防控制中心 Nanjing Center for Disease Control and Prevention
			平和县 Pinghe County	平和县疾病预防控制中心 Pinghe Center for Disease Control and Prevention
南平 Nanping	1477561	46.31%	延平区 Yanping District	延平区疾病预防控制中心 Yanping Center for Disease Control and Prevention
			浦城县 Pucheng County	浦城县疾病预防控制中心 Pucheng Center for Disease Control and Prevention
			建瓯市 Jian'ou County	建瓯市疾病预防控制中心 Jian'ou Center for Disease Control and Prevention
龙岩 Longyan	1592794	49.99%	新罗区 Xinluo District	新罗区疾病预防控制中心 Xinluo Center for Disease Control and Prevention
			永定区 Yongding District	永定区疾病预防控制中心 Yongding Center for Disease Control and Prevention
			上杭县 Shanghang County	上杭县疾病预防控制中心 Shanghang Center for Disease Control and Prevention
宁德 Ningde	466579	13.13%	蕉城区 Jiaocheng District	蕉城区疾病预防控制中心 Jiaocheng Center for Disease Control and Prevention

三、覆盖人口

24个肿瘤登记处覆盖15427160户籍人口，占全省户籍人口数的39.6%。其中男性7921758人，女性7505402人。城市地区6464030人（男性3255006人，女性3209024人），占覆盖人口数的41.9%；农村地区8963130人（男性4666752人，女性4296378人），占覆盖人口数的58.1%。分性别、分城乡各年龄组人口数及占比详见表2-2和图2-2~图2-4。

3. Population coverage

The population covered by 24 Fujian cancer registries was 15,427,160 (7,921,758 males and 7,505,402 females), which comprised 39.6% of Fujian's household registered population. Among them, the population in urban areas was 6,464,030 (3,255,006 males and 3,209,024 females) and the population in rural areas was 8,963,130 (4,666,752 males and 4,296,378 females), accounting for 41.9% and 58.1% respectively. The number and percentage of population in each age group by gender and by urban and rural areas are detailed in Table 2-2 and Figures 2-2~2-4.

表 2-2　2019 年福建省肿瘤登记地区覆盖人口

Table 2-2　Population in Fujian cancer registration areas, 2019

年龄组 Age group	全省 Total			城市地区 Urban areas			农村地区 Rural areas		
	合计 ALL	男性 Male	女性 Female	合计 ALL	男性 Male	女性 Female	合计 ALL	男性 Male	女性 Female
0~	123867	67333	56534	63047	33891	29156	60820	33442	27378
1~	866663	473899	392764	398900	215337	183563	467763	258562	209201
5~	1119812	611146	508666	459859	246559	213300	659953	364587	295366
10~	944660	511637	433023	360152	191303	168849	584508	320334	264174
15~	716131	385160	330971	270123	142339	127784	446008	242821	203187
20~	750606	405172	345434	278707	146153	132554	471899	259019	212880
25~	1216180	634009	582171	490865	246853	244012	725315	387156	338159
30~	1411384	709987	701397	608594	295288	313306	802790	414699	388091
35~	1177557	593756	583801	545575	266637	278938	631982	327119	304863
40~	1179097	599739	579358	505135	251102	254033	673962	348637	325325
45~	1301240	654093	647147	540205	268905	271300	761035	385188	375847
50~	1202471	601881	600590	488078	244291	243787	714393	357590	356803
55~	911685	454443	457242	386117	191790	194327	525568	262653	262915
60~	817453	409645	407808	346743	172127	174616	470710	237518	233192
65~	645032	318637	326395	272513	132269	140244	372519	186368	186151
70~	399689	200271	199418	173613	85761	87852	226076	114510	111566
75~	270299	132757	137542	115539	56336	59203	154760	76421	78339
80~	207680	94142	113538	89292	40810	48482	118388	53332	65056
85+	165654	64051	101603	70973	27255	43718	94681	36796	57885
合计 Total	15427160	7921758	7505402	6464030	3255006	3209024	8963130	4666752	4296378

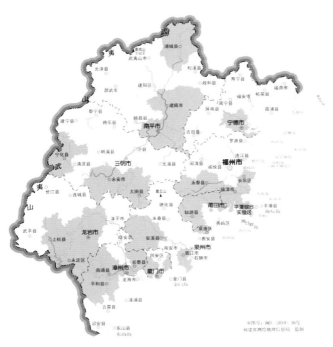

图 2-1　福建省人群肿瘤登记地区地理分布

Figure 2-1　Geographical distribution of cancer registration areas

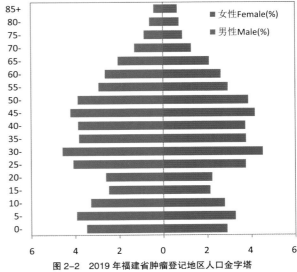

图 2-2　2019 年福建省肿瘤登记地区人口金字塔

Figure 2-2　Population pyramid in Fujian cancer registration areas, 2019

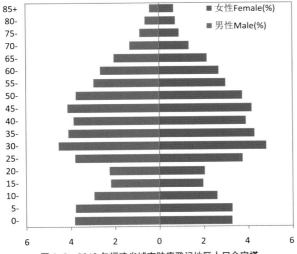

图 2-3　2019 年福建省城市肿瘤登记地区人口金字塔

Figure 2-3　Population pyramid in urban areas of Fujian cancer registries, 2019

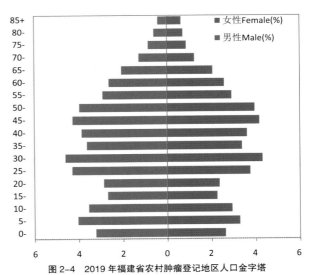

图 2-4　2019 年福建省农村肿瘤登记地区人口金字塔

Figure 2-4　Population pyramid in rural areas of Fujian cancer registries, 2019

第二节　数据质量评价

福建省肿瘤防治办公室根据《中国肿瘤登记工作指导手册》和国际癌症研究署/国际癌症登记协会（IARC/IACR）制定的数据审核规则进行质量控制，2022 年对各登记处上报的 2019 年肿瘤发病、死亡数据的资料进行综合审核与评价，选取质量符合标准的 24 个登记处资料进行合并分析。

福建省肿瘤登记地区 2019 年新发病例组织学诊断比例（MV%）为 77.74%，城市地区和农村地区分别为 78.56% 和 77.03%；合计死亡发病比（M/I）为 0.53，城市地区和农村地区分别为 0.48 和 0.58；仅有死亡医学证明书比例（DCO%）为 0.20%，城市地区和农村地区分别为 0.14% 和 0.26%（表 2-3）。

福建省各登记处数据评价指标见表 2-4，芗城区 MV% 值偏高，为 91.22%，浦城县 MV% 值偏低，为 50.17%；新罗区 M/I 为 0.38，偏低的原因是甲状腺癌、乳腺癌占比较大，历年该指标均较低；各登记处 DCO% 值偏低，在 0.00%~1.32% 区间，可能与部分登记处在收集肿瘤死因数据的同时要求登记发病日期有关。

Section 2　Data quality evaluation

Fujian Provincial Office for Cancer Prevention and Control conducted quality control based on the *Chinese Guideline for Cancer Registration* and the guidelines of International Agency for Research on Cancer/International Association of Cancer Registries (IARC/IACR). The cancer incidence and mortality data in 2019 from all cancer registries were comprehensively reviewed and evaluated by Fujian Provincial Office for Cancer Prevention and Control in 2022. Data from 24 registries that met the standards were selected for combined analysis.

The overall MV% in Fujian cancer registration areas in 2019 was 77.74%, with 78.56% in urban areas and 77.03% in rural areas. The overall M/I was 0.53, with 0.48 and 0.58 in urban and rural areas, respectively. The DCO% was 0.20%, with 0.14% in urban areas and 0.26% in rural areas (Table 2-3).

The data evaluation indexes of each registry in Fujian Province are shown in Table 2-4. The MV% of Xiangcheng District was relatively high (91.22%), and the MV% of Pucheng County was relatively low (50.17%). The M/I of Xinluo District was 0.38, which was relatively low and might be due to the large proportion of thyroid cancer and breast cancer, and the index was always low over the years. The DCO% of each cancer registry was low, ranging from 0.00% to 1.32%, which might be related to the requirement to register the date of cancer onset while collecting the data on cancer death in some registries.

表 2-3　2019 年福建省肿瘤登记数据质量评价指标

Table 2-3　Quality evaluation indicators of data in Fujian cancer registration areas, 2019

部位 Sites	全省 Total			城市地区 Urban areas			农村地区 Rural areas		
	MV%	DCO%	M/I	MV%	DCO%	M/I	MV%	DCO%	M/I
口腔和咽喉（除外鼻咽）Oral Cavity & Pharynx but Nasopharynx	85.08	0.00	0.51	81.39	0.00	0.54	88.59	0.00	0.49
鼻咽 Nasopharynx	74.78	0.00	0.52	74.39	0.00	0.61	75.00	0.00	0.47
食管 Esophagus	78.19	0.30	0.90	76.16	0.09	0.79	79.70	0.46	0.98
胃 Stomach	79.40	0.23	0.74	79.49	0.16	0.70	79.32	0.28	0.77
结直肠肛门 Colon, Rectum & Anus	82.46	0.09	0.43	82.78	0.08	0.41	82.18	0.10	0.45
肝脏 Liver	48.57	0.62	0.92	56.08	0.46	0.84	42.47	0.75	1.00
胆囊及其他 Gallbladder etc.	53.41	0.00	0.76	60.12	0.00	0.80	48.52	0.00	0.73
胰腺 Pancreas	49.74	1.03	0.98	54.04	1.10	0.93	45.95	0.97	1.03
喉 Larynx	83.40	0.00	0.62	85.83	0.00	0.51	81.29	0.00	0.71
气管，支气管，肺 Traches, Bronchus & Lung	77.33	0.20	0.72	78.85	0.15	0.63	75.96	0.25	0.79
其他胸腔器官 Other Thoracic Organs	77.30	0.00	0.54	78.87	0.00	0.62	75.71	0.00	0.46
骨和关节软骨 Bone	52.94	0.00	1.15	53.33	0.00	1.08	52.63	0.00	1.20
皮肤黑色素瘤 Melanoma of Skin	94.03	0.00	0.63	87.50	0.00	0.81	100.00	0.00	0.46
乳房 Breast	88.14	0.03	0.18	87.47	0.00	0.17	88.78	0.07	0.18
子宫颈 Cervix Uteri	87.34	0.20	0.28	86.11	0.17	0.24	88.12	0.22	0.29
子宫体及子宫部位不明 Uterus & Unspecified	86.45	0.13	0.23	84.81	0.00	0.19	87.83	0.24	0.26
卵巢 Ovary	77.04	0.22	0.45	78.16	0.49	0.45	76.52	0.00	0.45
前列腺 Prostate	70.54	0.00	0.39	74.16	0.00	0.37	66.89	0.00	0.41
睾丸 Testis	92.31	0.00	0.13	92.59	0.00	0.11	92.00	0.00	0.16
肾及泌尿系统不明 Kidney & Unspecified Urinary Organs	79.79	0.26	0.31	78.91	0.26	0.36	80.66	0.25	0.27
膀胱 Bladder	84.19	0.14	0.32	85.33	0.00	0.33	83.15	0.27	0.32
脑及中枢神经系统 Brain & Central Nervous System	66.87	0.15	0.43	66.41	0.00	0.35	67.29	0.29	0.50
甲状腺 Thyroid	89.68	0.00	0.02	86.34	0.00	0.02	93.70	0.00	0.02
淋巴瘤 Lymphoma	94.35	0.09	0.47	89.13	0.18	0.47	99.47	0.00	0.47
白血病 Leukaemia	93.63	0.13	0.68	87.50	0.28	0.67	98.85	0.00	0.68
不明及其他恶性肿瘤 Unspecified and All Others	67.25	0.53	0.56	72.12	0.30	0.59	63.84	0.70	0.55
所有部位合计 All Sites in Total	77.74	0.20	0.53	78.56	0.14	0.48	77.03	0.26	0.58

表 2–4　福建省各肿瘤登记处数据质量评价指标

Table 2–4　Data quality evaluation indicators of each cancer registry in Fujian Province

登记地区 Registration Areas	地区 Areas	人口数 Population	MV%	DCO%	M/I
福州市长乐区 Changle District, Fuzhou City	城市 Urban	756979	74.77	0.79	0.48
永泰县 Yongtai County	农村 Rural	385762	74.19	0.00	0.50
福清市 Fuqing County	农村 Rural	1387304	79.53	0.86	0.48
厦门市区（思明、湖里、集美、海沧） Xiamen City (Siming, Huli, Jimei, Haicang)	城市 Urban	1750826	79.25	0.08	0.42
厦门市翔安区 Xiang'an District, Xiamen City	城市 Urban	369364	75.34	0.00	0.50
莆田市涵江区 Hanjiang District, Putian City	城市 Urban	449996	83.87	0.00	0.49
仙游县 Xianyou County	农村 Rural	1175001	85.39	0.00	0.61
宁化县 Ninghua County	农村 Rural	376388	59.50	0.00	0.69
大田县 Datian County	农村 Rural	415985	67.80	0.20	0.52
永安市 Yong'an County	农村 Rural	330336	74.55	0.00	0.54
泉州市泉港区 Quangang District, Quanzhou City	城市 Urban	421740	73.93	0.00	0.66
安溪县 Anxi County	农村 Rural	1215224	83.59	0.00	0.70
晋江市 Jinjiang County	农村 Rural	1187527	76.64	0.00	0.55
漳州市芗城区 Xiangcheng District, Zhangzhou City	城市 Urban	472261	91.22	0.00	0.56
漳州市长泰区 Changtai District, Zhangzhou City	城市 Urban	212501	88.17	0.00	0.62
南靖县 Nanjing County	农村 Rural	361360	87.63	0.00	0.64
平和县 Pinghe County	农村 Rural	621672	87.67	0.00	0.72
南平市延平区 Yanping District, Nanping City	城市 Urban	498956	61.65	0.00	0.44
浦城县 Pucheng County	农村 Rural	427705	50.17	0.00	0.53
建瓯市 Jian'ou County	农村 Rural	550900	65.67	1.32	0.62
龙岩市新罗区 Xinluo District, Longyan City	城市 Urban	568083	79.19	0.10	0.38
龙岩市永定区 Yongding District, Longyan City	城市 Urban	496745	79.64	0.35	0.55
上杭县 Shanghang County	农村 Rural	527966	77.90	0.00	0.54
宁德市蕉城区 Jiaocheng District, Ningde City	城市 Urban	466579	84.35	0.00	0.54

第三章　福建省肿瘤登记地区恶性肿瘤的发病与死亡
Chapter 3　Incidence and mortality of all cancer sites in Fujian cancer registration areas

第一节　全部恶性肿瘤

一、全部恶性肿瘤发病情况

福建省肿瘤登记地区 2019 年新发恶性肿瘤病例 46975 例（男性 25255 例，女性 21720 例）。其中城市地区 21939 例，占新发病例数的 46.70%；农村地区 25036 例，占新发病例数的 53.30%。全省肿瘤登记地区粗发病率为 304.50/10 万（男性 318.81/10 万，女性 289.39/10 万），中标率为 221.59/10 万，世标率为 213.81/10 万，累积率（0~74 岁）为 24.63%。根据登记地区发病情况及年龄、性别人口构成，估计福建省 2019 年新发恶性肿瘤病例 118483 例。

城市肿瘤登记地区粗发病率为 339.40/10 万（男性 352.50/10 万，女性 326.11/10 万），中标率为 244.36/10 万，世标率为 235.16/10 万，累积率（0~74 岁）为 26.82%，估计福建省城市地区 2019 年新发恶性肿瘤病例 44269 例。

农村肿瘤登记地区粗发病率为 279.32/10 万（男性 295.30/10 万，女性 261.96/10 万），中标率为 204.80/10 万，世标率为 198.17/10 万，

Section 1　All cancer sites

1. Incidence of all cancer sites

There were 46,975 new cases (25,255 males and 21,720 females) in Fujian cancer registration areas in 2019. Among all new cases, 21,939 (46.70%) came from urban areas, and 25,036 (53.30%) came from rural areas. The incidence rate of all cancer sites was 304.50 per 100,000 (318.81 per 100,000 for males and 289.39 per 100,000 for females), with an ASR China of 221.59 per 100,000, an ASR World of 213.81 per 100,000, and a cumulative rate (0−74 years old) of 24.63%. According to the incidence stratified by age and sex groups of the registration areas, there were an estimated 118,483 new cases of cancer in Fujian Province in 2019.

The incidence rate of all cancer sites in urban areas was 339.40 per 100,000 (352.50 per 100,000 for males and 326.11 per 100,000 for females), with an ASR China of 244.36 per 100,000, an ASR World of 235.16 per 100,000, and a cumulative rate (0−74 years old) of 26.82%. There were an estimated 44,269 new cases of cancer in urban areas of Fujian Province in 2019.

The incidence rate of all cancer sites in rural areas was 279.32 per 100,000 (295.30 per 100,000 for males and 261.96 per 100,000 for females), with an ASR China of 204.80 per 100,000, an ASR World of 198.17 per 100,000, and a cumulative rate (0−74 years old) of

累积率（0~74 岁）为 23.02%，估计福建省农村地区 2019 年新发恶性肿瘤病例 74214 例。

不论男女，城市肿瘤登记地区的粗发病率、中标率、世标率、累积率均高于农村肿瘤登记地区（表 3-1）。

23.02%. There were an estimated 74,214 new cases of cancer in rural areas of Fujian Province in 2019.

The crude incidence rate, ASRs China for incidence, ASRs World for incidence and cumulative incidence rate of all cancer sites were all higher in urban areas than those in rural areas for both sexes (Table 3-1).

表 3-1　2019 年福建省肿瘤登记地区全部恶性肿瘤发病主要指标
Table 3-1　Incidence of all cancer sites in Fujian cancer registration areas, 2019

地区 Areas	性别 Sex	全省估计发病数 Estimated cases in Fujian province	登记地区发病数 Cases	发病率 Crude rate （1/10^5）	中国人口标化率 ASR China （1/10^5）	世界人口标化率 ASR World （1/10^5）	累积率 Cum. rate （0~74，%）
全省 All	合计 Both	118483	46975	304.50	221.59	213.81	24.63
	男性 Male	64169	25255	318.81	232.99	229.78	27.49
	女性 Female	54314	21720	289.39	211.99	199.68	21.84
城市地区 Urban areas	合计 Both	44269	21939	339.40	244.36	235.16	26.82
	男性 Male	23145	11474	352.50	251.86	248.08	29.41
	女性 Female	21124	10465	326.11	238.50	224.27	24.34
农村地区 Rural areas	合计 Both	74214	25036	279.32	204.80	198.17	23.02
	男性 Male	41024	13781	295.30	219.37	216.62	26.09
	女性 Female	33190	11255	261.96	191.92	181.22	19.95

二、全部恶性肿瘤年龄别发病率

福建省肿瘤登记地区全部恶性肿瘤年龄别发病率随着年龄的增长而上升，0~34 岁发病率处于较低水平，呈缓慢上升，35 岁以后上升速度加快，在 75~79 岁年龄组达到最高，80 岁以后有所下降。

城市肿瘤登记地区和农村肿瘤登记地区年龄别发病率变化趋势基本相同，发病高峰均出

2. Age-specific incidence rates of all cancer sites

The age-specific incidence rates of all cancer sites in Fujian cancer registration areas increased with age. The age-specific incidence rates were relatively low from age 0 to 34 years old, showing a slow increase, but sharply increased after 35 years old, reached the peak at the age group of 75-79 years, and decreased slightly after the age group of 80+ years.

The overall trend of age-specific incidence rates in urban areas was similar to that in rural areas, and reached the peak at the age group of 75-79

现在 75~79 岁年龄组。城市地区男性在 1~4 岁年龄组略低于农村地区，在其他年龄组均高于农村地区；城市地区女性在 0~ 岁和 10~14 岁年龄组略低于农村地区，其他年龄组均高于农村地区（表 3-2，图 3-1a~ 图 3-1d）。

years. Urban areas had slightly lower incidence rates for males at the age group of 1–4 years and higher incidence rates for the other age groups, compared to rural areas. Urban areas had slightly lower incidence rates for females at the age groups of 0– and 10–14 years and higher incidence rates for the other age groups, compared to rural areas (Table 3–2, Figure 3–1a~3–1d).

表 3-2　2019 年福建省肿瘤登记地区恶性肿瘤年龄别发病率（1/10 万）

Table 3-2　Age-specific incidence of all cancer sites in Fujian registration areas, 2019 (1/10⁵)

年龄组 Age group (years)	全省 All			城市地区 Urban areas			农村地区 Rural areas		
	合计 Both	男性 Male	女性 Female	合计 Both	男性 Male	女性 Female	合计 Both	男性 Male	女性 Female
0~	24.22	29.70	17.69	23.79	29.51	17.15	24.66	29.90	18.26
1~	13.38	14.14	12.48	11.28	9.75	13.07	15.18	17.79	11.95
5~	7.86	8.51	7.08	8.70	8.92	8.44	7.27	8.23	6.09
10~	11.01	12.90	8.78	10.55	13.59	7.11	11.29	12.49	9.84
15~	16.20	18.17	13.90	17.40	18.97	15.65	15.47	17.71	12.80
20~	31.04	21.97	41.69	40.90	30.11	52.81	25.22	17.37	34.76
25~	65.37	47.79	84.51	78.23	53.88	102.86	56.67	43.91	71.27
30~	90.97	60.00	122.33	105.00	66.04	141.71	80.34	55.70	106.68
35~	144.62	97.18	192.87	165.70	107.64	221.20	126.43	88.65	166.96
40~	224.15	152.40	298.43	250.23	171.25	328.30	204.61	138.83	275.11
45~	329.99	255.47	405.32	370.60	282.26	458.16	301.17	236.77	367.17
50~	446.33	412.37	480.36	479.02	422.45	535.71	424.00	405.49	442.54
55~	612.27	668.73	556.16	666.90	717.97	616.49	572.14	632.77	511.57
60~	788.55	955.71	620.64	860.87	1034.12	690.09	735.27	898.88	568.63
65~	967.55	1247.19	694.56	1030.41	1315.50	761.53	921.56	1198.70	644.10
70~	1175.16	1521.44	827.41	1266.03	1626.61	914.04	1105.38	1442.67	759.19
75~	1274.14	1692.57	870.28	1378.76	1787.49	989.81	1196.05	1622.59	779.94
80~	1144.07	1580.59	782.12	1330.47	1862.29	882.80	1003.48	1365.03	707.08
85+	854.79	1261.49	598.41	1073.65	1574.02	761.70	690.74	1030.00	475.08

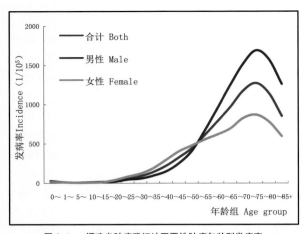

图 3-1a 福建省肿瘤登记地区恶性肿瘤年龄别发病率
Figure 3-1a Age-specific incidence of all cancer sites in Fujian cancer registration areas

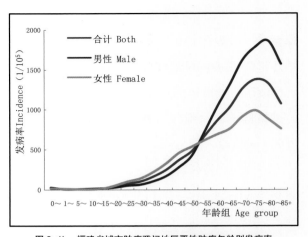

图 3-1b 福建省城市肿瘤登记地区恶性肿瘤年龄别发病率
Figure 3-1b Age-specific incidence of all cancer sites in urban areas of Fujian cancer registries

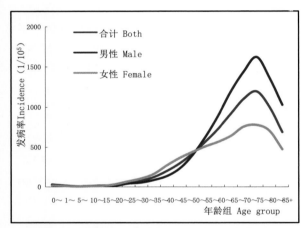

图 3-1c 福建省农村地肿瘤登记区恶性肿瘤年龄别发病率
Figure 3-1c Age-specific incidence of all cancer sites in rural areas of Fujian cancer registries

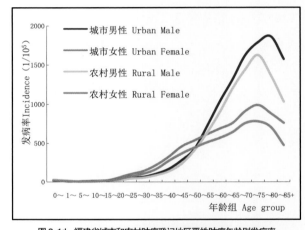

图 3-1d 福建省城市和农村肿瘤登记地区恶性肿瘤年龄别发病率
Figure 3-1d Age-specific incidence of all cancer sites in urban and rural areas of Fujian cancer registries

三、全部恶性肿瘤死亡情况

福建省肿瘤登记地区 2019 年恶性肿瘤死亡报告病例 24953 例（其中男性 16575 例，女性 8378 例）。其中城市地区 10524 例，占死亡例数的 42.18%；农村地区 14429 例，占死亡例数的 57.82%。全省肿瘤登记地区粗死亡率为 161.75/10 万（其中男性 209.23/10 万，女性 111.63/10 万），中标率为 107.18/10 万，世标率为 105.99/10 万，累积率（0~74 岁）为 12.30%。

3. Mortality of all cancer sites

There were 24,953 cancer deaths (16,575 males and 8,378 females) in Fujian cancer registration areas in 2019. Among all cancer deaths, 10,524 (42.18%) came from urban areas, and 14,429 (57.82%) came from rural areas. The mortality rate of all cancer sites was 161.75 per 100,000 (209.23 per 100,000 for males and 111.63 per 100,000 for females), with an ASR China of 107.18 per 100,000, an ASR World of 105.99 per 100,000, and a cumulative rate (0-74 years old) of 12.30%. According to the mortality stratified by age

根据登记地区死亡情况及年龄、性别人口构成，估计福建省 2019 年恶性肿瘤死亡 64767 例。

城市肿瘤登记地区粗死亡率为 162.81/10 万（其中男性 214.35/10 万，女性 110.53/10 万），中标率为 105.57/10 万，世标率为 104.62/10 万，累积率（0~74 岁）为 12.00%，估计福建省城市地区 2019 年恶性肿瘤死亡 21663 例。

农村肿瘤登记地区粗死亡率为 160.98/10 万（其中男性 205.67/10 万，女性 112.44/10 万），中标率为 108.39/10 万，世标率为 107.03/10 万，累积率（0~74 岁）为 12.53%，估计福建省农村地区 2019 年恶性肿瘤死亡 43104 例。

城市肿瘤登记地区合计及男性粗死亡率均高于农村地区，中标率和世标率低于农村肿瘤登记地区；城市肿瘤登记地区女性粗死亡率、中标率和世标率均低于农村肿瘤登记地区（表 3-3）。

and sex groups of the registration areas, there were an estimated 64,767 death cases of cancer in Fujian Province in 2019.

The mortality rate of all cancer sites in urban areas was 162.81 per 100,000 (214.35 per 100,000 for males and 110.53 per 100,000 for females), with an ASR China of 105.57 per 100,000, an ASR World of 104.62 per 100,000, and a cumulative rate (0–74 years old) of 12.00%. There were an estimated 21,663 death cases of cancer in urban areas of Fujian Province in 2019.

The mortality rate of all cancer sites in rural areas was 160.98 per 100,000 (205.67 per 100,000 for males and 112.44 per 100,000 for females), with an ASR China of 108.39 per 100,000, an ASR World of 107.03 per 100,000, and a cumulative rate (0–74 years old) of 12.53%. There were an estimated 43,104 death cases of cancer in rural areas of Fujian Province in 2019.

The total and male crude mortality rates in urban areas were higher than those in rural areas, the ASRs China for mortality and ASRs World for mortality were lower than those in rural areas. The female crude mortality rate, ASRs China for mortality and ASRs World for mortality in urban areas were lower than those in rural areas (Table 3–3).

表 3-3　2019 年福建省肿瘤登记地区全部恶性肿瘤死亡主要指标
Table 3–3　Mortality of all cancer sites in Fujian cancer registration areas, 2019

地区 Areas	性别 Sex	全省估计死亡数 Estimated cases in Fujian province	登记地区 死亡数 Cases	死亡率 Crude rate （1/10⁵）	中国人口 标化率 ASR China （1/10⁵）	世界人口 标化率 ASR World （1/10⁵）	累积率 Cum. rate （0~74，%）
全省 All	合计 Both	64767	24953	161.75	107.18	105.99	12.30
	男性 Male	43002	16575	209.23	145.81	144.83	16.90
	女性 Female	21765	8378	111.63	69.90	68.68	7.73
城市地区 Urban areas	合计 Both	21663	10524	162.81	105.57	104.62	12.00
	男性 Male	14289	6977	214.35	144.37	143.98	16.63
	女性 Female	7374	3547	110.53	69.05	67.80	7.51
农村地区 Rural areas	合计 Both	43104	14429	160.98	108.39	107.03	12.53
	男性 Male	28713	9598	205.67	146.80	145.40	17.10
	女性 Female	14391	4831	112.44	70.57	69.41	7.90

四、全部恶性肿瘤年龄别死亡率

福建省肿瘤登记地区全部恶性肿瘤年龄别死亡率随着年龄的增长而上升，0~49 岁死亡率处于较低水平，50 岁以后快速上升，在 80~84 岁年龄组达到最高，85 岁以后有所下降。

城市肿瘤登记地区和农村肿瘤登记地区年龄别死亡率变化趋势基本相同，高峰均出现在 80~84 岁年龄组。城市地区男性 75 岁之前年龄别死亡率与农村地区差别不大，75 岁以后高于农村地区；城市地区女性 80 岁之前年龄别死亡率与农村地区差别不大（表 3-4, 图 3-2a~ 图 3-2d）。

4. Age-specific mortality rates of all cancer sites

The age-specific mortality rates of all cancer sites in Fujian cancer registration areas increased with age. The age-specific mortality rates were relatively low from age 0 to 49 years old, but sharply increased after 50 years old, reached the peak at the age group of 80–84 years, and decreased slightly after the age group of 85+ years.

The overall trend of age-specific mortality rate in urban areas was similar to that in rural areas, and reached the peak at the age group of 80–84 years. The age-specific mortality rates for males in urban areas were similar to those in rural areas before 75 years old, and were higher than that in rural areas after 75 years old. The age-specific mortality rates for females in urban areas were similar to those in rural areas before 80 years old (Table 3-4, Figures 3-2a~3-2d).

表 3-4 2019 年福建省肿瘤登记地区恶性肿瘤年龄别死亡率（1/10 万）
Table 3-4 Age-specific mortality of all cancer sites in Fujian registration areas, 2019 (1/10^5)

年龄组 Age group (years)	全省 All			城市地区 Urban areas			农村地区 Rural areas		
	合计 Both	男性 Male	女性 Female	合计 Both	男性 Male	女性 Female	合计 Both	男性 Male	女性 Female
0~	11.30	11.88	10.61	9.52	11.80	6.86	13.15	11.96	14.61
1~	4.38	4.64	4.07	3.51	3.25	3.81	5.13	5.80	4.30
5~	2.86	3.27	2.36	3.70	4.06	3.28	2.27	2.74	1.69
10~	4.45	4.69	4.16	6.11	6.27	5.92	3.42	3.75	3.03
15~	5.45	5.71	5.14	4.81	3.51	6.26	5.83	7.00	4.43
20~	4.26	5.18	3.18	3.23	3.42	3.02	4.87	6.18	3.29
25~	7.56	8.83	6.18	6.72	7.70	5.74	8.13	9.56	6.51
30~	15.87	17.89	13.83	14.95	14.90	15.00	16.57	20.01	12.88
35~	26.07	28.97	23.12	24.19	23.63	24.74	27.69	33.32	21.65
40~	54.62	65.20	43.67	56.42	63.72	49.21	53.27	66.26	39.35
45~	88.30	115.73	60.57	83.67	107.84	59.71	91.59	121.24	61.20
50~	156.93	208.85	104.90	153.87	196.90	110.75	159.02	217.01	100.90
55~	249.21	349.44	149.59	242.15	342.04	143.57	254.39	354.84	154.04
60~	403.57	569.03	237.37	400.30	573.99	229.07	405.98	565.43	243.58
65~	584.62	839.20	336.10	571.35	842.22	315.88	594.33	837.05	351.33
70~	851.16	1151.44	549.60	823.67	1129.88	524.75	872.27	1167.58	569.17
75~	1087.68	1512.54	677.61	1081.89	1523.00	662.13	1092.01	1504.82	689.31
80~	1343.89	1807.91	959.15	1351.74	1881.89	905.49	1337.97	1751.29	999.14
85+	1194.06	1700.21	874.97	1313.18	1922.58	933.25	1104.76	1535.49	830.96

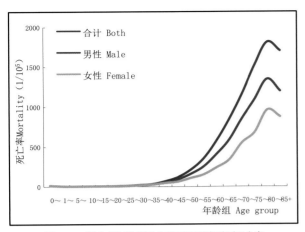

图 3-2a　福建省肿瘤登记地区恶性肿瘤年龄别死亡率
Figure 3-2a　Age-specific mortality of all cancer sites in Fujian cancer registration areas

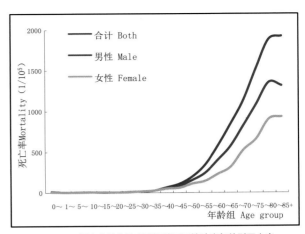

图 3-2b　福建省城市肿瘤登记地区恶性肿瘤年龄别死亡率
Figure 3-2b　Age-specific mortality of all cancer sites in urban areas of Fujian cancer registries

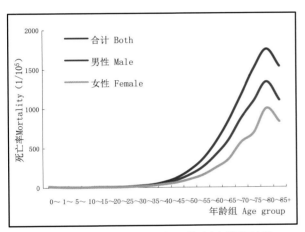

图 3-2c　福建省农村肿瘤登记地区恶性肿瘤年龄别死亡率
Figure 3-2c　Age-specific mortality of all cancer sites in rural areas of Fujian cancer registries

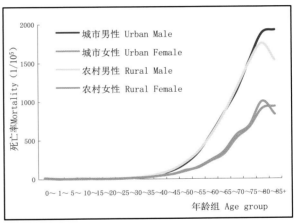

图 3-2d　福建省城市和农村肿瘤登记地区恶性肿瘤年龄别死亡率
Figure 3-2d　Age-specific mortality of all cancer sites in urban and rural areas of Fujian cancer registries

第二节　福建省肿瘤登记地区前 10 位恶性肿瘤

Section 2　The 10 most common cancers in Fujian cancer registration areas

一、前 10 位恶性肿瘤发病情况

福建省肿瘤登记地区 2019 年恶性肿瘤发病第 1 位是肺癌，其次是乳腺癌、结直肠癌、甲状腺癌和胃癌，发病前 10 位恶性肿瘤占全部恶性肿瘤的 77.23%。居男性恶性肿瘤发病第 1 位的是肺癌，其次是结直肠癌、胃癌、肝癌和食管癌，男性发病前 10 位恶性肿瘤占全部恶性肿瘤的 82.46%。居女性恶性肿瘤发病第 1 位的是甲状腺癌，其次是乳腺癌、肺癌、结直肠癌和子宫颈癌，女性发病前 10 位恶性肿瘤占全部恶性肿瘤的 83.00%（表 3-5，图 3-3a~ 图 3-3f）。

1. Incidence of the 10 most common cancers

Lung cancer was the most common cancer followed by cancers of female breast, colorectum, thyroid and stomach in Fujian cancer registration areas in 2019. The top 10 most common cancers accounted for 77.23% of all new cancers. For males, Lung cancer was the most common cancer followed by cancers of colorectum, stomach, liver and esophagus. The top 10 most common cancers accounted for 82.46% of all new cancers for males. While for females, thyroid cancer was most common cancer followed by cancers of the breast, lung, colorectum and cervix. The top 10 most common cancers accounted for 83.00% of all new cancers for females (Table 3-5, Figure 3-3a~3-3f).

表 3-5　2019 年福建省肿瘤登记地区前 10 位恶性肿瘤发病主要指标
Table 3-5　Incidence of the 10 most common cancers in Fujian cancer registration areas, 2019

顺位 Rank	合计 All				男性 Male				女性 Female			
	部位 Site	发病率 Incidence (1/10⁵)	构成 Freq. (%)	中标率 ASR China (1/10⁵)	部位 Site	发病率 Incidence (1/10⁵)	构成 Freq. (%)	中标率 ASR China (1/10⁵)	部位 Site	发病率 Incidence (1/10⁵)	构成 Freq. (%)	中标率 ASR China (1/10⁵)
1	肺 Lung	54.69	17.96	37.54	肺 Lung	67.85	21.28	47.88	甲状腺 Thyroid	51.83	17.91	44.54
2	乳腺 Breast	41.37	6.66	31.56	结直肠 Colon-rectum	41.40	12.99	29.35	乳腺 Breast	41.37	14.30	31.56
3	结直肠 Colon-rectum	35.70	11.73	24.42	胃 Stomach	39.51	12.39	27.76	肺 Lung	40.80	14.10	27.54
4	甲状腺 Thyroid	33.40	10.97	29.26	肝 Liver	39.09	12.26	28.79	结直肠 Colon-rectum	29.69	10.26	19.64
5	胃 Stomach	28.31	9.30	19.28	食管 Esophagus	24.48	7.68	16.69	子宫颈 Cervix	20.11	6.95	14.66
6	肝 Liver	24.97	8.20	17.72	甲状腺 Thyroid	15.94	5.00	14.36	胃 Stomach	16.49	5.70	11.04
7	子宫颈 Cervix	20.11	3.21	14.66	前列腺 Prostate	11.18	3.51	7.52	子宫体 Uterus	10.13	3.50	6.98
8	食管 Esophagus	17.36	5.70	11.34	淋巴瘤 Lymphoma	8.32	2.61	6.41	肝 Liver	10.06	3.48	6.74
9	前列腺 Prostate	11.18	1.89	7.52	脑 Brain	7.55	2.37	6.28	脑 Brain	9.89	3.42	7.46
10	子宫体 Uterus	10.13	1.62	6.98	鼻咽 Nasopharynx	7.55	2.37	6.12	食管 Esophagus	9.85	3.40	6.09

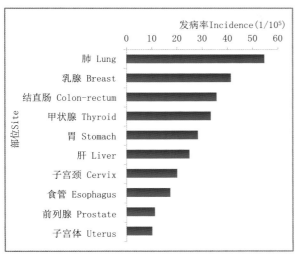

图 3-3a　福建省肿瘤登记地区前 10 位恶性肿瘤发病率
Figure 3-3a　Incidence of the 10 most common cancers in Fujian cancer registration areas

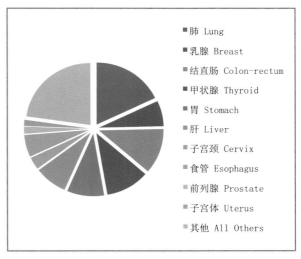

图 3-3b　福建省肿瘤登记地区发病前 10 位恶性肿瘤构成（%）
Figure 3-3b　Proportion of the 10 most common cancers in Fujian cancer registration areas (%)

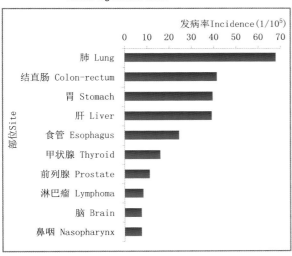

图 3-3c　福建省肿瘤登记地区男性前 10 位恶性肿瘤发病率
Figure 3-3c　Incidence of the 10 most common cancers for males in Fujian cancer registration areas

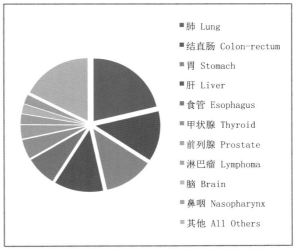

图 3-3b　福建省肿瘤登记地区发病前 10 位恶性肿瘤构成（%）
Figure 3-3d　Proportion of the 10 most common cancers for males in Fujian cancer registration areas (%)

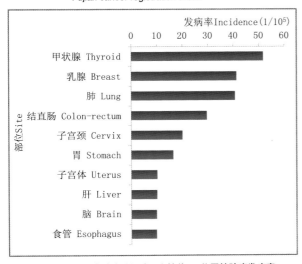

图 3-3e　福建省肿瘤登记地区女性前 10 位恶性肿瘤发病率
Figure 3-3e　Incidence of the 10 most common cancers for females in Fujian cancer registration areas

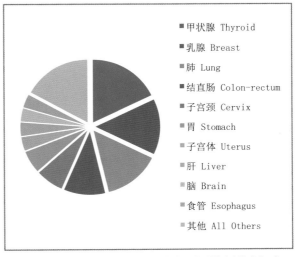

图 3-3f　福建省肿瘤登记地区女性发病前 10 位恶性肿瘤构成（%）
Figure 3-3f　Proportion of the 10 most common cancers for females in Fujian cancer registration areas (%)

31

二、前 10 位恶性肿瘤死亡情况

福建省肿瘤登记地区 2019 年恶性肿瘤死亡第 1 位是肺癌，其次是肝癌、胃癌、食管癌和结直肠癌，死亡前 10 位恶性肿瘤占全部恶性肿瘤的 80.42%。居男性恶性肿瘤死亡第 1 位的是肺癌，其次是肝癌、胃癌、食管癌和结直肠癌，男性死亡前 10 位恶性肿瘤占全部恶性肿瘤的 86.59%。居女性恶性肿瘤死亡第 1 位的是肺癌，其次是结直肠癌、胃癌、肝癌和食管癌，女性死亡前 10 位恶性肿瘤占全部恶性肿瘤的 78.29%（表 3-6，图 3-4a~ 图 3-4f）。

2. Top 10 leading causes of cancer deaths

Lung cancer was the leading cause of cancer deaths followed by cancers of liver, stomach, esophagus and colorectum in Fujian cancer registration areas in 2019. The top 10 leading causes of cancer deaths accounted for 80.42% of all cancer deaths. For males, lung cancer was the leading cause of cancer deaths followed by cancers of liver, stomach, esophagus and colorectum. The top 10 leading causes of cancer deaths accounted for 86.59% of cancer deaths for males. While for females, lung cancer was the leading cause of cancer deaths followed by cancers of colorectum, stomach, liver and esophagus. The top 10 leading causes of cancer deaths accounted for 78.29% of cancer deaths for females (Table 3-6, Figure 3-4a~3-4f).

表 3-6　2019 年福建省肿瘤登记地区前 10 位恶性肿瘤死亡主要指标
Table 3-6　Mortality of the top 10 leading cancer sites in Fujian cancer registration areas, 2019

顺位 Rank	合计 All				男性 Male				女性 Female			
	部位 Site	死亡率 Mortality（1/10^5）	构成 Freq.（%）	中标率 ASR China（1/10^5）	部位 Site	死亡率 Mortality（1/10^5）	构成 Freq.（%）	中标率 ASR China（1/10^5）	部位 Site	死亡率 Mortality（1/10^5）	构成 Freq.（%）	中标率 ASR China（1/10^5）
1	肺 Lung	39.17	24.22	25.59	肺 Lung	57.11	27.29	39.31	肺 Lung	20.24	18.13	12.34
2	肝 Liver	23.08	14.27	15.98	肝 Liver	35.42	16.93	25.78	结直肠 Colon-rectum	12.98	11.63	7.80
3	胃 Stomach	20.88	12.91	13.49	胃 Stomach	28.82	13.77	19.73	胃 Stomach	12.50	11.20	7.53
4	食管 Esophagus	15.56	9.62	9.70	食管 Esophagus	21.11	10.09	14.07	肝 Liver	10.06	9.01	6.27
5	结直肠 Colon-rectum	15.42	9.53	9.88	结直肠 Colon-rectum	17.74	8.48	12.06	食管 Esophagus	9.70	8.69	5.46
6	乳腺 Breast	7.23	2.20	5.02	胰腺 Pancreas	4.52	2.16	3.10	乳腺 Breast	7.23	6.48	5.02
7	子宫颈 Cervix	5.53	1.66	3.75	前列腺 Prostate	4.38	2.09	2.65	子宫颈 Cervix	5.53	4.95	3.75
8	前列腺 Prostate	4.38	1.39	2.65	脑 Brain	4.28	2.05	3.32	脑 Brain	3.21	2.88	2.29
9	脑 Brain	3.76	2.32	2.80	淋巴瘤 Lymphoma	4.04	1.93	2.93	白血病 Leukemia	3.09	2.77	2.42
10	胰腺 Pancreas	3.71	2.29	2.41	白血病 Leukemia	3.76	1.80	3.03	胰腺 Pancreas	2.85	2.55	1.75

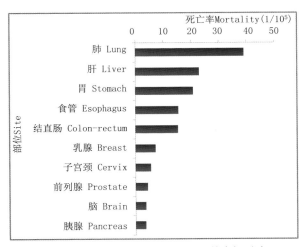

图 3-4a 福建省肿瘤登记地区前 10 位恶性肿瘤死亡率
Figure 3-4a Mortality of the top 10 leading cancer sites in Fujian cancer registration areas

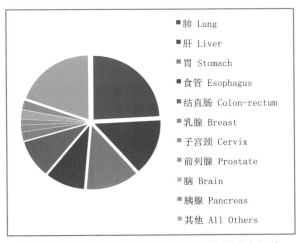

图 3-4b 福建省肿瘤登记地区死亡前 10 位恶性肿瘤构成（%）
Figure 3-4b Proportion of the top 10 leading causes of cancer deaths in Fujian cancer registration areas (%)

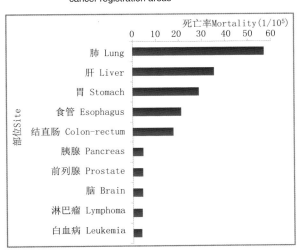

图 3-4c 福建省肿瘤登记地区男性前 10 位恶性肿瘤死亡率
Figure 3-4c Mortality of the top 10 leading cancer sites for males in Fujian cancer registration areas

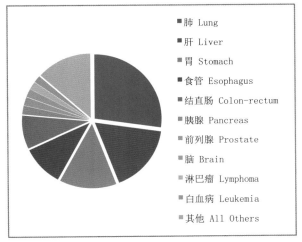

图 3-4d 福建省肿瘤登记地区男性死亡前 10 位恶性肿瘤构〔%〕
Figure 3-4d Proportion of the top 10 leading causes of cancer deaths for males in Fujian cancer registration areas (%)

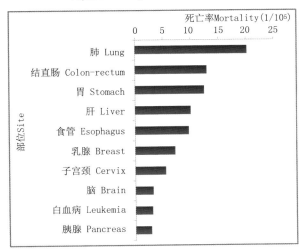

图 3-4e 福建省肿瘤登记地区女性前 10 位恶性肿瘤死亡率
Figure 3-4e Mortality of the top 10 leading cancer sites for females in Fujian cancer registration areas

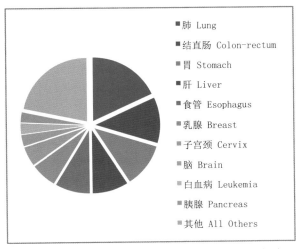

图 3-4f 福建省肿瘤登记地区女性死亡前 10 位恶性肿瘤构成（%）
Figure 3-4f Proportion of the top 10 leading causes of cancer deaths for females in Fujian cancer registration areas (%)

三、城市肿瘤登记地区前 10 位恶性肿瘤发病情况

城市肿瘤登记地区 2019 年恶性肿瘤发病第 1 位是肺癌，其次是乳腺癌、甲状腺癌、结直肠癌和胃癌，发病前 10 位恶性肿瘤占全部恶性肿瘤的 77.97%。居男性恶性肿瘤发病第 1 位的是肺癌，其次是结直肠癌、肝癌、胃癌和食管癌，男性发病前 10 位恶性肿瘤占全部恶性肿瘤的 83.01%。居女性恶性肿瘤发病第 1 位的是甲状腺癌，其次是肺癌、乳腺癌、结直肠癌和子宫颈癌，女性发病前 10 位恶性肿瘤占全部恶性肿瘤的 84.16%（表 3-7，图 3-5a~ 图 3-5f）。

3. Incidence of the 10 most common cancers in urban areas

Lung cancer was the most common cancer followed by cancers of female breast, thyroid, colorectum and stomach in urban areas of Fujian cancer registries in 2019. The top 10 most common cancers accounted for 77.97% of all new cancers. For males, Lung cancer was the most common cancer followed by cancers of colorectum, liver, stomach and esophagus. The top 10 most common cancers accounted for 83.01% of all new cancers for males. While for females, thyroid cancer was the most common cancer followed by cancers of lung, breast, colorectum and cervix. The top 10 most common cancers accounted for 84.16% of all new cancers for females (Table 3-7, Figure 3-5a~3-5f).

表 3-7　2019 年福建省城市肿瘤登记地区前 10 位恶性肿瘤发病主要指标
Table 3-7　Incidence of the 10 most common cancers in urban areas of Fujian cancer registries, 2019

顺位 Rank	合计 All				男性 Male				女性 Female			
	部位 Site	发病率 Incidence（1/10^5）	构成 Freq.（%）	中标率 ASR China（1/10^5）	部位 Site	发病率 Incidence（1/10^5）	构成 Freq.（%）	中标率 ASR China（1/10^5）	部位 Site	发病率 Incidence（1/10^5）	构成 Freq.（%）	中标率 ASR China（1/10^5）
1	肺 Lung	61.73	18.19	41.80	肺 Lung	73.21	20.77	50.26	甲状腺 Thyroid	65.35	20.04	55.86
2	乳腺 Breast	49.67	7.31	37.39	结直肠 Colon-rectum	47.71	13.53	32.85	肺 Lung	50.08	15.36	33.81
3	甲状腺 Thyroid	43.61	12.85	37.91	肝 Liver	42.09	11.94	30.16	乳腺 Breast	49.67	15.23	37.39
4	结直肠 Colon-rectum	40.16	11.83	26.88	胃 Stomach	40.43	11.47	27.39	结直肠 Colon-rectum	32.50	9.97	21.22
5	胃 Stomach	28.67	8.45	19.01	食管 Esophagus	26.73	7.58	17.92	子宫颈 Cervix	18.17	5.57	13.48
6	肝 Liver	26.70	7.87	18.54	甲状腺 Thyroid	22.18	6.29	19.70	胃 Stomach	16.73	5.13	11.06
7	子宫颈 Cervix	18.17	2.66	13.48	前列腺 Prostate	13.67	3.88	8.89	脑 Brain	11.53	3.54	8.89
8	食管 Esophagus	17.65	5.20	11.42	淋巴瘤 Lymphoma	10.02	2.84	7.56	肝 Liver	11.09	3.40	7.30
9	前列腺 Prostate	13.67	2.03	8.89	脑 Brain	8.29	2.35	6.61	子宫体 Uterus	10.88	3.33	7.55
10	子宫体 Uterus	10.88	1.59	7.55	膀胱 Bladder	8.26	2.34	5.67	食管 Esophagus	8.44	2.59	5.13

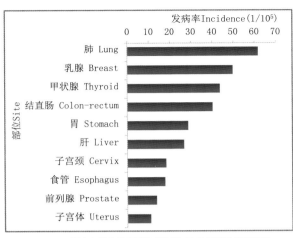

图 3-5a　福建省城市肿瘤登记地区前 10 位恶性肿瘤发病率
Figure 3-5a　Incidence of the 10 most common cancers in urban areas of Fujian cancer registries

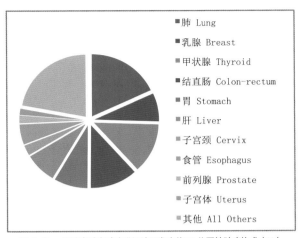

图 3-5b　福建省城市肿瘤登记地区发病前 10 位恶性肿瘤构成（%）
Figure 3-5b　Proportion of the 10 most common cancers in urban areas of Fujian cancer registries(%)

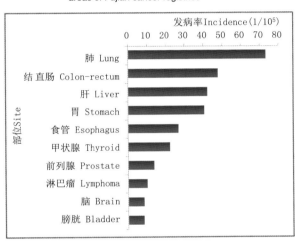

图 3-5c　福建省城市肿瘤登记地区男性前 10 位恶性肿瘤发病率
Figure 3-5c　Incidence of the 10 most common cancers for males in urban areas of Fujian cancer registries

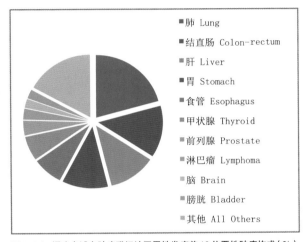

图 3-5d　福建省城市肿瘤登记地区男性发病前 10 位恶性肿瘤构成（%）
Figure 3-5d　Proportion of the 10 most common cancers for males in urban areas of Fujian cancer registries(%)

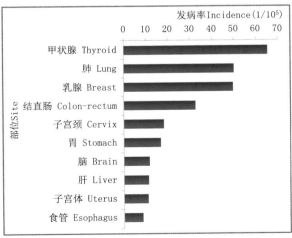

图 3-5e　福建省城市肿瘤登记地区女性前 10 位恶性肿瘤发病率
Figure 3-5e　Incidence of the 10 most common cancers for females in urban areas of Fujian cancer registries

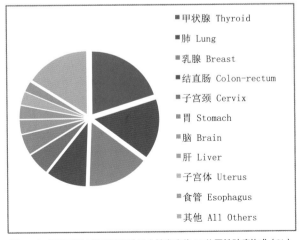

图 3-5f　福建省城市肿瘤登记地区女性发病前 10 位恶性肿瘤构成（%）
Figure 3-5f　Proportion of the 10 most common cancers for females in urban areas of Fujian cancer registries(%)

四、城市肿瘤登记地区前 10 位恶性肿瘤死亡情况

城市肿瘤登记地区 2019 年恶性肿瘤死亡第 1 位是肺癌，其次是肝癌、胃癌、结直肠癌和食管癌，死亡前 10 位恶性肿瘤占全部恶性肿瘤的 79.13%。居男性恶性肿瘤死亡第 1 位的是肺癌，其次是肝癌、胃癌、食管癌和结直肠癌，男性死亡前 10 位恶性肿瘤占全部恶性肿瘤的 85.84%。居女性恶性肿瘤死亡第 1 位的是肺癌，其次是结直肠癌、胃癌、肝癌和乳腺癌，女性死亡前 10 位恶性肿瘤占全部恶性肿瘤的 76.26%（表 3-8，图 3-6a~ 图 3-6f）。

4. Top 10 leading causes of cancer deaths in urban areas

Lung cancer was the leading cause of cancer deaths followed by cancers of liver, stomach, colorectum and esophagus in urban areas of Fujian cancer registries in 2019. The top 10 leading causes of cancer deaths accounted for 79.13% of all cancer death. For males, lung cancer was the leading cause of cancer deaths followed by cancers of liver, stomach, esophagus and colorectum. The top 10 leading causes of cancer deaths accounted for 85.84% of cancer deaths for males. While for females, lung cancer was the leading cause of cancer deaths followed by cancers of colorectum, stomach, liver and breast. The top 10 leading causes of cancer deaths accounted for 76.26% of cancer deaths for females (Table 3-8, Figure 3-6a~3-6f).

表 3-8　2019 年福建省城市肿瘤登记地区前 10 位恶性肿瘤死亡主要指标

Table 3-8　Mortality of the top 10 leading cancer sites in urban areas of Fujian cancer registries, 2019

顺位 Rank	合计 All				男性 Male				女性 Female			
	部位 Site	死亡率 Mortality (1/10^5)	构成 Freq. (%)	中标率 ASR China (1/10^5)	部位 Site	死亡率 Mortality (1/10^5)	构成 Freq. (%)	中标率 ASR China (1/10^5)	部位 Site	死亡率 Mortality (1/10^5)	构成 Freq. (%)	中标率 ASR China (1/10^5)
1	肺 Lung	39.11	24.02	25.01	肺 Lung	57.36	26.76	38.37	肺 Lung	20.60	18.64	12.37
2	肝 Liver	22.35	13.73	15.15	肝 Liver	34.90	16.28	24.59	结直肠 Colon-rectum	13.18	11.93	7.73
3	胃 Stomach	20.03	12.31	12.73	胃 Stomach	28.69	13.39	19.02	胃 Stomach	11.25	10.18	6.85
4	结直肠 Colon-rectum	16.43	10.09	10.17	食管 Esophagus	21.29	9.93	13.83	肝 Liver	9.63	8.71	6.05
5	食管 Esophagus	13.89	8.53	8.56	结直肠 Colon-rectum	19.63	9.16	12.79	乳腺 Breast	8.63	7.81	5.90
6	乳腺 Breast	8.63	2.66	5.90	前列腺 Prostate	5.04	2.35	2.83	食管 Esophagus	6.39	5.78	3.55
6	前列腺 Prostate	5.04	1.56	2.83	胰腺 Pancreas	4.70	2.19	3.16	子宫颈 Cervix	4.43	4.00	3.10
8	子宫颈 Cervix	4.43	1.35	3.10	淋巴瘤 Lymphoma	4.39	2.05	3.04	淋巴瘤 Lymphoma	3.68	3.33	2.29
9	淋巴瘤 Lymphoma	4.04	2.48	2.66	脑 Brain	4.09	1.91	3.09	白血病 Leukemia	3.40	3.07	2.78
10	胰腺 Pancreas	3.91	2.40	2.51	白血病 Leukemia	3.90	1.82	2.91	胰腺 Pancreas	3.12	2.82	1.90

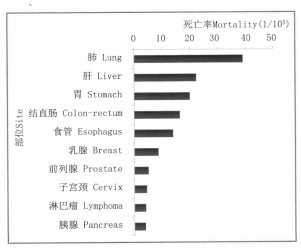

图 3-6a 福建省城市肿瘤登记地区前 10 位恶性肿瘤死亡率
Figure 3-6a Mortality of the top 10 leading cancer sites in urban areas of Fujian cancer registries

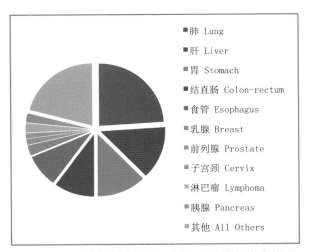

图 3-6b 福建省城市肿瘤登记地区死亡前 10 位恶性肿瘤构成（%）
Figure 3-6b Proportion of the top 10 leading causes of cancer deaths in urban areas of Fujian cancer registries(%)

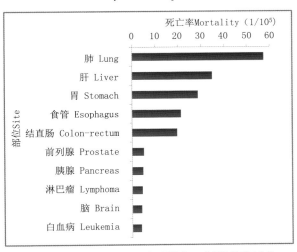

图 3-6c 福建省城市肿瘤登记地区男性前 10 位恶性肿瘤死亡率
Figure 3-6c Mortality of the top 10 leading cancer sites for males in urban areas of Fujian cancer registries

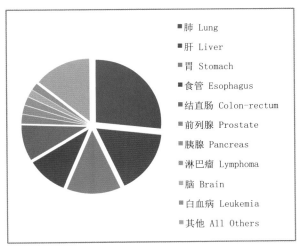

图 3-6d 福建省城市肿瘤登记地区男性死亡前 10 位恶性肿瘤构成（%）
Figure 3-6d Proportion of the top 10 leading causes of cancer deaths for males in urban areas of Fujian cancer registries(%)

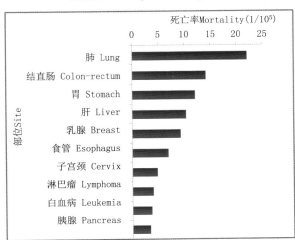

图 3-6e 福建省城市肿瘤登记地区女性前 10 位恶性肿瘤死亡率
Figure 3-6e Mortality of the top 10 leading cancer sites for females in urban areas of Fujian cancer registries

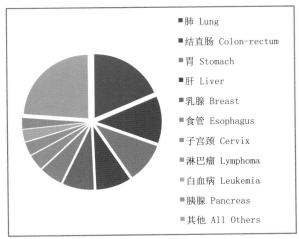

图 3-6f 福建省城市肿瘤登记地区女性死亡前 10 位恶性肿瘤构成（%）
Figure 3-6f Proportion of the top 10 leading causes of cancer deaths for females in urban areas of Fujian cancer registries(%)

五、农村肿瘤登记地区前 10 位恶性肿瘤发病情况

农村肿瘤登记地区 2019 年恶性肿瘤发病第 1 位是肺癌，其次是乳腺癌、结直肠癌、胃癌和甲状腺癌，发病前 10 位恶性肿瘤占全部恶性肿瘤的 76.58%。居男性恶性肿瘤发病第 1 位的是肺癌，其次是胃癌、肝癌、结直肠癌和食管癌，男性发病前 10 位恶性肿瘤占全部恶性肿瘤的 82.36%。居女性恶性肿瘤发病第 1 位的是甲状腺癌，其次是乳腺癌、肺癌、结直肠癌和子宫颈癌，女性发病前 10 位恶性肿瘤占全部恶性肿瘤的 81.93%（表 3-9，图 3-7a~ 图 3-7f）。

5. Incidence of the 10 most common cancers in rural areas

Lung cancer was the most common cancer followed by cancers of female breast, colorectum, stomach and thyroid in rural areas of Fujian cancer registries in 2019. The top 10 most common cancers accounted for 76.58% of all new cancers. For males, Lung cancer was the most common cancer followed by cancers of stomach, liver, colorectum, and esophagus. The top 10 most common cancers accounted for 82.36% of all new cancers for males. While for females, thyroid cancer was the most common cancer followed by cancers of breast, lung, colorectum and cervix. The top 10 most common cancers accounted for 81.93% of all new cancers for females (Table 3-9, Figure 3-7a~3-7f).

表 3-9 2019 年福建省农村肿瘤登记地区前 10 位恶性肿瘤发病主要指标

Table 3-9 Incidence of the 10 most common cancers in rural areas of Fujian cancer registries, 2019

顺位 Rank	合计 All				男性 Male				女性 Female			
	部位 Site	发病率 Incidence（1/10^5）	构成 Freq.（%）	中标率 ASR China（1/10^5）	部位 Site	发病率 Incidence（1/10^5）	构成 Freq.（%）	中标率 ASR China（1/10^5）	部位 Site	发病率 Incidence（1/10^5）	构成 Freq.（%）	中标率 ASR China（1/10^5）
1	肺 Lung	49.61	17.76	34.36	肺 Lung	64.11	21.71	46.10	甲状腺 Thyroid	41.73	15.93	36.00
2	乳腺 Breast	35.17	6.09	27.14	胃 Stomach	38.87	13.16	28.01	乳腺 Breast	35.17	13.43	27.14
3	结直肠 Colon-rectum	32.49	11.63	22.59	肝 Liver	37.01	12.53	27.79	肺 Lung	33.87	12.93	22.76
4	胃 Stomach	28.06	10.05	19.48	结直肠 Colon-rectum	37.01	12.53	26.77	结直肠 Colon-rectum	27.58	10.53	18.44
5	甲状腺 Thyroid	26.04	9.32	22.96	食管 Esophagus	22.91	7.76	15.83	子宫颈 Cervix	21.55	8.23	15.49
6	肝 Liver	23.72	8.49	17.13	甲状腺 Thyroid	11.59	3.93	10.61	胃 Stomach	16.32	6.23	11.03
7	子宫颈 Cervix	21.55	3.70	15.49	前列腺 Prostate	9.45	3.20	6.51	食管 Esophagus	10.89	4.16	6.81
8	食管 Esophagus	17.15	6.14	11.29	鼻咽 Nasopharynx	8.10	2.74	6.67	子宫体 Uterus	9.57	3.65	6.54
9	子宫体 Uterus	9.57	1.64	6.54	淋巴瘤 Lymphoma	7.14	2.42	5.61	肝 Liver	9.29	3.55	6.32
10	前列腺 Prostate	9.45	1.76	6.51	脑 Brain	7.03	2.38	6.04	脑 Brain	8.66	3.31	6.43

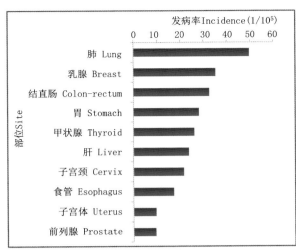

图 3-7a　福建省农村肿瘤登记地区前 10 位恶性肿瘤发病率
Figure 3-7a　Incidence of the 10 most common cancers in rural areas of Fujian cancer registries

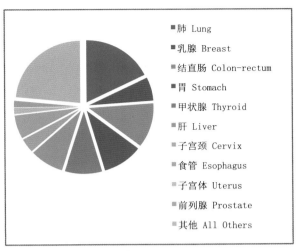

图 3-7b　福建省农村肿瘤登记地区发病前 10 位恶性肿瘤构成（%）
Figure 3-7b　Proportion of the 10 most common cancers in rural areas of Fujian cancer registries(%)

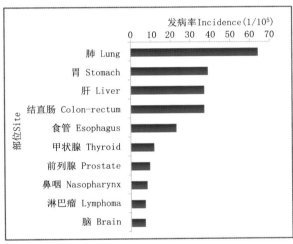

图 3-7c　福建省农村肿瘤登记地区男性前 10 位恶性肿瘤发病率
Figure 3-7c　Incidence of the 10 most common cancers for males in rural areas of Fujian cancer registries

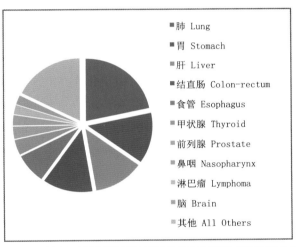

图 3-7d　福建省农村肿瘤登记地区男性发病前 10 位恶性肿瘤构成（%）
Figure 3-7d　Proportion of the 10 most common cancers for males in rural areas of Fujian cancer registries(%)

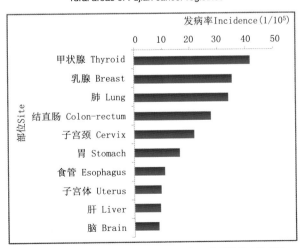

图 3-7e　福建省农村肿瘤登记地区女性前 10 位恶性肿瘤发病率
Figure 3-7e　Incidence of the 10 most common cancers for females in rural areas of Fujian cancer registries

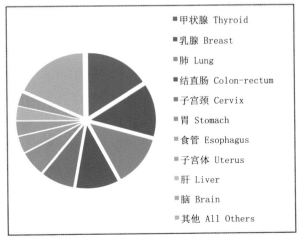

图 3-7f　福建省农村肿瘤登记地区女性发病前 10 位恶性肿瘤构成（%）
Figure 3-7f　Proportion of the 10 most common cancers for females in rural areas of Fujian cancer registries(%)

六、农村肿瘤登记地区前10位恶性肿瘤死亡情况

农村肿瘤登记地区2019年恶性肿瘤死亡第1位是肺癌，其次是肝癌、胃癌、食管癌和结直肠癌，死亡前10位恶性肿瘤占全部恶性肿瘤的81.59%。居男性恶性肿瘤死亡第1位的是肺癌，其次是肝癌、胃癌、食管癌和结直肠癌，男性死亡前10位恶性肿瘤占全部恶性肿瘤的87.20%。居女性恶性肿瘤死亡第1位的是肺癌，其次是胃癌、结直肠癌、食管癌和肝癌，女性死亡前10位恶性肿瘤占全部恶性肿瘤的80.27%（表3–10，图3–8a~图3–8f）。

6. Top 10 leading causes of cancer deaths in rural areas

Lung cancer was the leading cause of cancer deaths followed by cancers of liver, stomach, esophagus and colorectum in rural areas of Fujian cancer registries in 2019. The top 10 leading causes of cancer deaths accounted for 81.59% of all cancer death. For males, lung cancer was the leading cause of cancer deaths followed by cancers of liver, stomach, esophagus and colorectum. The top 10 leading causes of cancer deaths accounted for 87.20% of cancer deaths for males. While for females, lung cancer was the leading cause of cancer deaths followed by cancers of stomach, colorectum, esophagus and liver. The top 10 leading causes of cancer deaths accounted for 80.27% of cancer deaths for females (Table 3–10, Figure 3–8a~3–8f).

表 3–10　2019 年福建省农村肿瘤登记地区前 10 位恶性肿瘤死亡主要指标
Table 3–10　Mortality of the top 10 leading cancer sites in rural areas of Fujian cancer registries, 2019

顺位 Rank	合计 All				男性 Male				女性 Female			
	部位 Site	死亡率 Mortality (1/10⁵)	构成 Freq. (%)	中标率 ASR China (1/10⁵)	部位 Site	死亡率 Mortality (1/10⁵)	构成 Freq. (%)	中标率 ASR China (1/10⁵)	部位 Site	死亡率 Mortality (1/10⁵)	构成 Freq. (%)	中标率 ASR China (1/10⁵)
1	肺 Lung	39.22	24.36	26.00	肺 Lung	56.93	27.68	39.99	肺 Lung	19.97	17.76	12.30
2	肝 Liver	23.61	14.66	16.60	肝 Liver	35.79	17.40	26.62	胃 Stomach	13.43	11.94	8.04
3	胃 Stomach	21.49	13.35	14.06	胃 Stomach	28.91	14.06	20.24	结直肠 Colon-rectum	12.82	11.41	7.85
4	食管 Esophagus	16.76	10.41	10.55	食管 Esophagus	20.98	10.20	14.27	食管 Esophagus	12.17	10.83	6.90
5	结直肠 Colon-rectum	14.69	9.13	9.66	结直肠 Colon-rectum	16.41	7.98	11.53	肝 Liver	10.38	9.23	6.44
6	子宫颈 Cervix	6.35	1.89	4.22	脑 Brain	4.41	2.15	3.50	子宫颈 Cervix	6.35	5.65	4.22
7	乳腺 Breast	6.19	1.86	4.37	胰腺 Pancreas	4.39	2.14	3.05	乳腺 Breast	6.19	5.51	4.37
8	脑 Brain	3.94	2.45	2.99	前列腺 Prostate	3.92	1.91	2.51	脑 Brain	3.42	3.04	2.49
9	前列腺 Prostate	3.92	1.27	2.51	淋巴瘤 Lymphoma	3.79	1.84	2.85	白血病 Leukemia	2.86	2.55	2.17
10	胰腺 Pancreas	3.56	2.21	2.34	鼻咽 Nasopharynx	3.79	1.84	2.79	胰腺 Pancreas	2.65	2.36	1.65

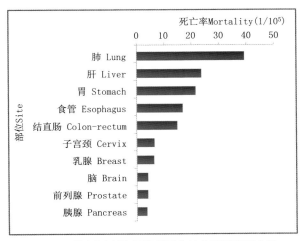

图 3-8a 福建省农村肿瘤登记地区前 10 位恶性肿瘤死亡率
Figure 3-8a Mortality of the top 10 leading cancer sites in rural areas of Fujian cancer registries

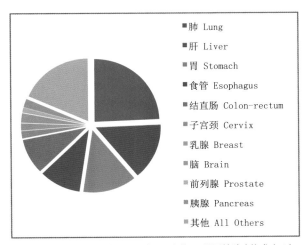

图 3-8b 福建省农村肿瘤登记地区死亡前 10 位恶性肿瘤构成（%）
Figure 3-8b Proportion of the top 10 leading causes of cancer deaths in rural areas of Fujian cancer registries(%)

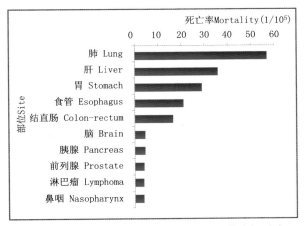

图 3-8c 福建省农村肿瘤登记地区男性前 10 位恶性肿瘤死亡率
Figure 3-8c Mortality of the top 10 leading cancer sites for males in rural areas of Fujian cancer registries

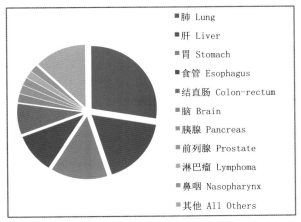

图 3-8d 福建省农村肿瘤登记地区男性死亡前 10 位恶性肿瘤构成（%）
Figure 3-8d Proportion of the top 10 leading causes of cancer deaths for males in rural areas of Fujian cancer registries(%)

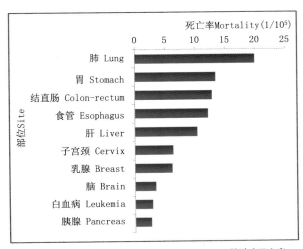

图 3-8e 福建省农村肿瘤登记地区女性前 10 位恶性肿瘤死亡率
Figure 3-8e Mortality of the top 10 leading cancer sites for females in rural areas of Fujian cancer registries

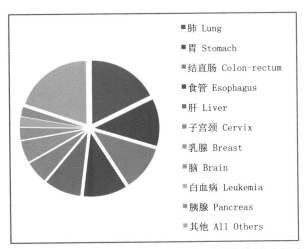

图 3-8f 福建省农村肿瘤登记地区女性死亡前 10 位恶性肿瘤构成（%）
Figure 3-8f Proportion of the top 10 leading causes of cancer deaths for females in rural areas of Fujian cancer registries(%)

第四章 各部位恶性肿瘤的发病与死亡
Chapter 4 Cancer Incidence and Mortality by Site

第一节 气管、支气管、肺

Section 1 Trachea, Bronchus & Lung

2019 年福建省肿瘤登记地区肺癌发病率为 54.69/10 万，中标率为 37.54/10 万，世标率为 37.32/10 万，占全部恶性肿瘤发病的 17.96%，居发病第 1 位。其中男性发病率为 67.85/10 万，女性发病率为 40.80/10 万，男性为女性的 1.66 倍。城市地区发病率为 61.73/10 万，农村地区发病率为 49.61/10 万，城市地区比农村地区高 24.43%，年龄标化后高 21.65%。2019 年全省估计新发肺癌病例 21246 例，其中男性 13672 例，女性 7574 例。

同期肿瘤登记地区肺癌死亡率为 39.17/10 万，中标率为 25.59/10 万，世标率为 25.42/10 万，占全部恶性肿瘤死亡的 24.22%，居死亡第 1 位。其中男性死亡率为 57.11/10 万，女性死亡率为 20.24/10 万，男性为女性的 2.82 倍。城市地区死亡率为 39.11/10 万，农村地区死亡率为 39.22/10 万，年龄标化后农村地区比城市地区高 3.96%。2019 年全省估计肺癌死亡 15669 例，其中男性 11731 例，女性 3938 例（表 4-1）。

Lung cancer was the 1st most common cancer in the registration areas of Fujian Province in 2019. The crude incidence rate was 54.69 per 100,000 (37.54 per 100,000 for ASR China and 37.32 per 100,000 for ASR World), accounting for 17.96% of all new cancer cases. The crude incidence rate was 67.85 per 100,000 for males and 40.80 per 100,000 for females, 1.66 times higher for males than females.The crude incidence rate was 61.73 per 100,000 in urban areas and 49.61 per 100,000 in rural areas, 24.43% higher in urban areas than in rural areas and 21.65% higher after age standardization. There were an estimated 21,246 new cases diagnosed as lung cancer in Fujian Province in 2019 (13,672 males and 7,574 females).

Lung cancer was the first most common cause of cancer deaths in the registration areas of Fujian Province in 2019. The crude mortality rate was 39.17 per 100,000 (25.59 per 100,000 for ASR China and 25.42 per 100,000 for ASR World), accounting for 24.22% of all cancer deaths. The crude mortality rate was 57.11 per 100,000 for males and 20.24 per 100,000 for females, 2.82 times higher for males than females. The crude mortality rate was 39.11 per 100,000 in urban areas and 39.22 per 100,000 in rural areas, 3.96% higher in rural areas than in urban areas after age standardization. There were an estimated 15,669 cases died of lung cancer in 2019 (11,731 males and 3,938 females)(Table 4−1).

表 4-1　2019 年福建省肿瘤登记地区肺癌发病与死亡

Table 4-1　Incidence and mortality of lung cancer in Fujian cancer registration areas, 2019

地区 Areas	性别 Sex	全省估计病例数 Estimated cases in Fujian Province	肿瘤登记 地区病例数 Cases	粗率 Crude rate (1/10⁵)	构成 Freq. (%)	中标率 ASR China (1/10⁵)	世标率 ASR world (1/10⁵)	累积率 Cum. rate (0~74, %)
发病 Incidence								
全省 All	合计 Both	21246	8437	54.69	17.96	37.54	37.32	4.77
	男性 Male	13672	5375	67.85	21.28	47.88	47.97	6.26
	女性 Female	7574	3062	40.80	14.10	27.54	26.99	3.29
城市 Urban areas	合计 Both	8078	3990	61.73	18.19	41.80	41.45	5.26
	男性 Male	4808	2383	73.21	20.77	50.26	50.35	6.53
	女性 Female	3270	1607	50.08	15.36	33.81	33.05	4.03
农村 Rural areas	合计 Both	13168	4447	49.61	17.76	34.36	34.24	4.41
	男性 Male	8864	2992	64.11	21.71	46.10	46.20	6.06
	女性 Female	4304	1455	33.87	12.93	22.76	22.40	2.73
死亡 Mortality								
全省 All	合计 Both	15669	6043	39.17	24.22	25.59	25.42	3.14
	男性 Male	11731	4524	57.11	27.29	39.31	39.21	4.88
	女性 Female	3938	1519	20.24	18.13	12.34	12.14	1.41
城市 Urban areas	合计 Both	5185	2528	39.11	24.02	25.01	24.86	3.04
	男性 Male	3806	1867	57.36	26.76	38.37	38.33	4.79
	女性 Female	1379	661	20.60	18.64	12.37	12.17	1.35
农村 Rural areas	合计 Both	10484	3515	39.22	24.36	26.00	25.82	3.22
	男性 Male	7925	2657	56.93	27.68	39.99	39.84	4.94
	女性 Female	2559	858	19.97	17.76	12.30	12.12	1.47

　　肺癌年龄别发病率在 50 岁以前处于较低水平，50 岁以后快速上升，在 70~ 岁组达到高峰。肺癌年龄别死亡率在 55 岁以前处于较低水平，55 岁以后迅速上升，在 75~ 岁组达到高峰。城市地区、农村地区年龄别发病率均在 70~ 岁年龄组达到高峰，年龄别死亡率分别在 80+ 岁和 75~ 岁组达到高峰（图 4-1a~图 4-1f）。

　　The age-specific incidence rate was relatively low before 50 years old, but dramatically increased after 50 years old, and reached the peak at the age group of 70-years. The age-specific mortality rate was relatively low before 55 years old, while sharply increased after 55 years old, and reached the peak at the age group of 75-years. The age-specific incidence rate reached the peak at the age group of 70-years in both urban and rural areas, while the age-specific mortality rate reached the peak at the age group of 80+ years and 75- years in urban and rural areas, respectively(Figure 4-1a~4-1f).

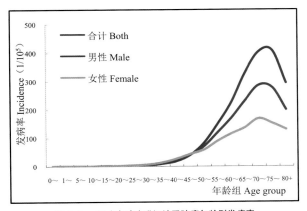

图 4-1a　福建省肿瘤登记地区肺癌年龄别发病率
Figure 4-1a　Age-specific incidence of lung cancer in Fujian cancer registration areas

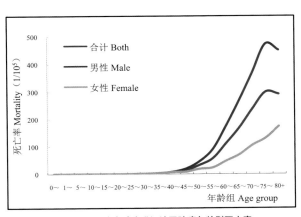

图 4-1b　福建省肿瘤登记地区肺癌年龄别死亡率
Figure 4-1b　Age-specific mortality of lung cancer in Fujian cancer registration areas

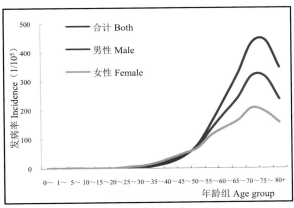

图 4-1c　福建省城市地区肺癌年龄别发病率
Figure 4-1c　Age-specific incidence of lung cancer in urban areas of Fujian cancer registries

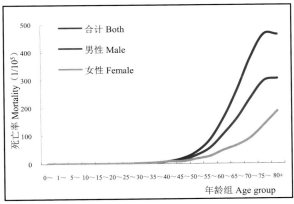

图 4-1d　福建省城市地区肺癌年龄别死亡率
Figure 4-1d　Age-specific mortality of lung cancer in urban areas of Fujian cancer registries

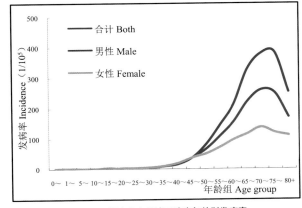

图 4-1e　福建省农村地区肺癌年龄别发病率
Figure 4-1e　Age-specific incidence of lung cancer in rural areas of Fujian cancer registries

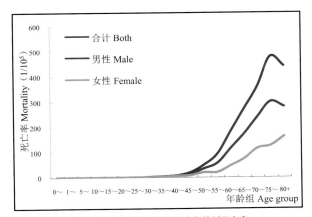

图 4-1f　福建省农村地区肺癌年龄别死亡率
Figure 4-1f　Age-specific mortality of lung cancer in rural areas of Fujian cancer registries

肺癌病例中，有明确亚部位的病例占48.76%。其中肺上叶病例最多，占55.44%，其次下叶占33.96%，中叶占5.88%（图4-1g）。

About 48.76% cases were assigned to specified categories of lung cancer sites. Among those, the upper lobe was the most common subsite, accounting for 55.44% of all cases, followed by the lower lobe(33.96%) and the middle lobe (5.88%) (Figure 4-1g).

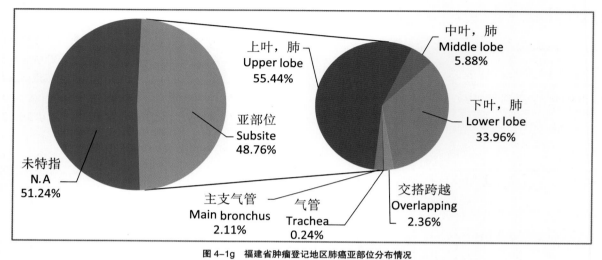

图4-1g　福建省肿瘤登记地区肺癌亚部位分布情况

Figure 4-1g　Distribution of subsites of lung cancer in Fujian cancer registration areas

肺癌病例中，有明确组织学类型的病例占72.75%。其中腺癌病例最多，占68.33%，其次鳞癌占17.79%，小细胞癌占6.94%，其他类型病例占5.67%（图4-1h）。

About 72.75% of cases of lung cancer had morphological verification. Among those, adenocarcinoma was the most common histological type, accounting for 68.33% of all cases, followed by squamous cell carcinoma (17.79%), small cell carcinoma (6.94%) and others (5.67%) (Figure 4-1h).

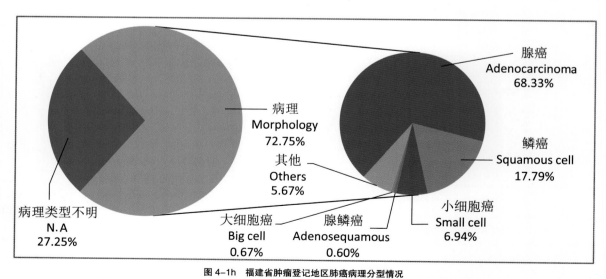

图4-1h　福建省肿瘤登记地区肺癌病理分型情况

Figure 4-1h　Distribution of histological subtypes of lung cancer in Fujian cancer registration areas

第二节　乳房

2019 年福建省肿瘤登记地区女性乳腺癌发病率为 41.37/10 万，中标率为 31.56/10 万，世标率为 28.78/10 万，占女性恶性肿瘤发病的 14.30%，居女性发病第 2 位。其中城市地区发病率为 49.67/10 万，农村地区发病率为 35.17/10 万，城市地区比农村地区高 41.23%，年龄标化后高 37.77%。2019 年全省估计新发女性乳腺癌病例 7634 例。

同期肿瘤登记地区乳腺癌死亡率为 7.23/10 万，中标率为 5.02/10 万，世标率为 4.78/10 万，占女性恶性肿瘤死亡的 6.48%，居女性死亡第 6 位。其中城市地区死亡率为 8.63/10 万，农村地区死亡率为 6.19/10 万，城市地区比农村地区高 39.42%，年龄标化后高 35.01%。2019 年全省估计女性乳腺癌死亡病例 1356 例（表 4-2）。

Section 2　Breast

Female breast cancer was the 2nd most common cancer among females in the registration areas of Fujian Province in 2019. The crude incidence rate was 41.37 per 100,000 (31.56 per 100,000 for ASR China and 28.78 per 100,000 for ASR World), accounting for 14.30% of all new female cancer cases. The crude incidence rate was 49.67 per 100,000 in urban areas and 35.17 per 100,000 in rural areas, 41.23% higher in urban areas than in rural areas and 37.77% higher after age standardization. There were an estimated 7,634 new cases diagnosed as female breast cancer in Fujian Province in 2019.

Female breast cancer was the 6th most common cause of cancer deaths among females in the registration areas of Fujian Province in 2019. The crude mortality rate was 7.23 per 100,000 (5.02 per 100,000 for ASR China and 4.78 per 100,000 for ASR World), accounting for 6.48% of all female cancer deaths. The crude mortality rate was 8.63 per 100,000 in urban areas and 6.19 per 100,000 in rural areas, 39.42% higher in urban areas than in rural areas and 35.01% higher after age standardization. There were an estimated 1,356 females died of breast cancer in 2019(Table 4-2).

表 4-2　2019 年福建省肿瘤登记地区女性乳腺癌发病与死亡
Table 4-2　Incidence and mortality of female breast cancer in Fujian cancer registration areas, 2019

地区 Areas	全省估计病例数 Estimated cases in Fujian Province	肿瘤登记 地区病例数 Cases	粗率 Crude rate （1/10⁵）	构成 Freq. （%）	中标率 ASR China （1/10⁵）	世标率 ASR world （1/10⁵）	累积率 Cum.rate （0~74，%）
发病 Incidence							
全省 All	7634	3105	41.37	14.30	31.56	28.78	2.93
城市 Urban areas	3205	1594	49.67	15.23	37.39	34.32	3.53
农村 Rural areas	4429	1511	35.17	13.43	27.14	24.61	2.48
死亡 Mortality							
全省 All	1356	543	7.23	6.48	5.02	4.78	0.52
城市 Urban areas	576	277	8.63	7.81	5.90	5.64	0.60
农村 Rural areas	780	266	6.19	5.51	4.37	4.15	0.46

女性乳腺癌年龄别发病率在 30 岁以前处于较低水平，30 岁以后逐渐上升，45~ 岁组达到高峰，后缓慢下降。女性乳腺癌年龄别死亡率在 45 岁以前处于较低水平，45 岁以后上升，在 80+ 岁组达到高峰。城市地区、农村地区年龄别发病率均在 45~ 岁组达到高峰，年龄别死亡率分别在 80+ 岁和 60~ 岁组达到高峰（图 4-2a~ 图 4-2b）。

The age-specific incidence rate was relatively low before 30 years old, and gradually increased after 30 years old, reached the peak at the age group of 45– years, and then slowly decreased. The age-specific mortality rate was relatively low before 45 years old, while increased after 45 years old, and reached the peak at the age group of 80+ years. The age-specific incidence rate reached the peak at the age group of 45– years in both urban and rural areas, while the age-specific mortality rate reached the peak at the age group of 80+ years and 60– years in urban and rural areas, respectively(Figure 4-2a~4-2b).

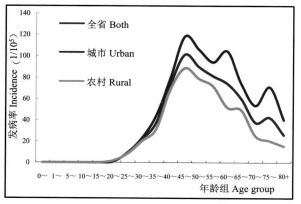
图 4-2a　福建省城市和农村地区女性乳腺癌年龄别发病率
Figure 4-2a　Age-specific incidence of female breast cancer in urban and rural areas of Fujian cancer registries

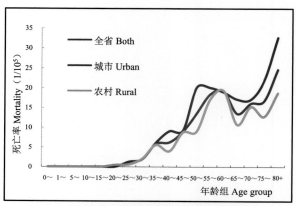
图 4-2b　福建省城市和农村地区女性乳腺癌年龄别死亡率
Figure 4-2b　Age-specific mortality of female breast cancer in urban and rural areas of Fujian cancer registries

乳腺癌病例中，有明确组织学类型的病例占 79.45%。其中导管癌病例最多，占 85.08%，小叶癌、佩吉特病和髓样癌分别占 3.97%、0.97% 和 0.65%（图 4-2c）。

About 79.45% cases of female breast cancer had morphological verification. Among those, ductal cancer was the most common histological type, accounting for 85.08% of all cases, followed by lobular carcinoma (3.97%), Paget's disease (0.97%) and medullary carcinoma (0.65%) (Figure 4-2c).

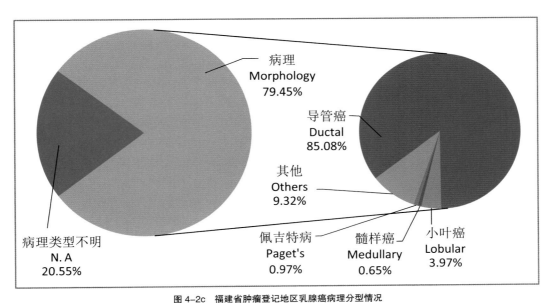

图 4-2c　福建省肿瘤登记地区乳腺癌病理分型情况

Figure 4-2c　Distribution of histological subtypes of female breast cancer in Fujian cancer registration areas

第三节　结直肠肛门

2019 年福建省肿瘤登记地区结直肠癌发病率为 35.70/10 万，中标率为 24.42/10 万，世标率为 23.97/10 万，占全部恶性肿瘤发病的 11.73%，居发病第 3 位。其中男性发病率为 41.40/10 万，女性发病率为 29.69/10 万，男性为女性的 1.39 倍。城市地区发病率为 40.16/10 万，农村地区发病率为 32.49/10 万，城市地区比农村地区高 23.61%，年龄标化后高 18.99%。2019 年全省估计新发结直肠癌病例 13764 例，其中男性 8196 例，女性 5568 例。

同期肿瘤登记地区结直肠癌死亡率为 15.42/10 万，中标率为 9.88/10 万，世标率为 9.69/10 万，占全部恶性肿瘤死亡的 9.53%，居死亡第 5 位。其中男性死亡率为 17.74/10 万，女性死亡率为 12.98/10 万，男性为女性的 1.37 倍。城市地区死亡率为 16.43/10 万，农村地区死亡率为 14.69/10 万，城市地区比农村地区高 11.84%，年龄标化后高 5.28%。2019 年全省估计结直肠癌死亡 6024 例，其中男性 3531 例，女性 2493 例（表 4-3）。

Section 3 Colon, Rectum & Anus

Colorectal cancer was the 3rd most common cancer in the registration areas of Fujian Province in 2019. The crude incidence rate was 35.70 per 100,000 (24.42 per 100,000 for ASR China and 23.97 per 100,000 for ASR World), accounting for 11.73% of all new cancer cases. The crude incidence rate was 41.40 per 100,000 for males and 29.69 per 100,000 for females, 1.39 times higher for males than females. The crude incidence rate was 40.16 per 100,000 in urban areas and 32.49 per 100,000 in rural areas,23.61% higher in urban areas than in rural areas and 18.99% higher after age standardization. There were an estimated 13,764 new cases diagnosed as colorectal cancer in Fujian Province in 2019 (8,196 males and 5,568 females).

Colorectal cancer was the 5th most common cause of cancer deaths in the registration areas of Fujian Province in 2019. The crude mortality rate was 15.42 per 100,000 (9.88 per 100,000 for ASR China and 9.69 per 100,000 for ASR World), accounting for 9.53% of all cancer deaths. The crude mortality rate was 17.74 per 100,000 for males and 12.98 per 100,000 for females, 1.37 times higher for males than females. The crude mortality rate was 16.43 per 100,000 in urban areas and 14.69 per 100,000 in rural areas,11.84% higher in urban areas than in rural areas and 5.28% higher after age standardization. There were an estimated 6,024 cases died of colorectal cancer in 2019 (3,531 males and 2,493 females) (Table 4-3).

表4-3　2019年福建省肿瘤登记地区结直肠癌发病与死亡

Table 4-3　Incidence and mortality of colorectal cancer in Fujian cancer registration areas, 2019

地区 Areas	性别 Sex	全省估计病例数 Estimated cases in Fujian Province	肿瘤登记 地区病例数 Cases	粗率 Crude rate （1/10⁵）	构成 Freq. （%）	中标率 ASR China （1/10⁵）	世标率 ASR world （1/10⁵）	累积率 Cum.rate （0~74,%）
发病 Incidence								
全省 All	合计 Both	13764	5508	35.70	11.73	24.42	23.97	2.94
	男性 Male	8196	3280	41.40	12.99	29.35	29.06	3.59
	女性 Female	5568	2228	29.69	10.26	19.64	19.04	2.30
城市 Urban areas	合计 Both	5183	2596	40.16	11.83	26.88	26.44	3.21
	男性 Male	3089	1553	47.71	13.53	32.85	32.54	3.97
	女性 Female	2094	1043	32.50	9.97	21.22	20.68	2.47
农村 Rural areas	合计 Both	8581	2912	32.49	11.63	22.59	22.14	2.75
	男性 Male	5107	1727	37.01	12.53	26.77	26.51	3.32
	女性 Female	3474	1185	27.58	10.53	18.44	17.80	2.17
死亡 Mortality								
全省 All	合计 Both	6024	2379	15.42	9.53	9.88	9.69	1.08
	男性 Male	3531	1405	17.74	8.48	12.06	11.93	1.31
	女性 Female	2493	974	12.98	11.63	7.80	7.57	0.85
城市 Urban areas	合计 Both	2142	1062	16.43	10.09	10.17	10.05	1.11
	男性 Male	1275	639	19.63	9.16	12.79	12.77	1.40
	女性 Female	867	423	13.18	11.93	7.73	7.53	0.84
农村 Rural areas	合计 Both	3882	1317	14.69	9.13	9.66	9.43	1.06
	男性 Male	2256	766	16.41	7.98	11.53	11.32	1.25
	女性 Female	1626	551	12.82	11.41	7.85	7.61	0.86

结直肠癌年龄别发病率在60岁以前处于较低水平，60岁以后逐步上升，到75~岁组达到高峰。结直肠癌年龄别死亡率在65岁以前处于较低水平，65岁以后逐步上升，在80+岁组达到高峰。城市地区、农村地区年龄别发病率分别在80+岁组和75~岁组达到高峰，年龄别死亡率均在80+岁组达到高峰（图4-3a~图4-3f）。

The age-specific incidence rate was relatively low before 60 years old, but gradually increased after 60 years old, and reached the peak at the age group of 75- years. The age-specific mortality rate was relatively low before 65 years old, while gradually increased after 65 years old, and reached the peak at the age group of 80+ years. The age-specific incidence rate reached the peak at the age group of 80+ years and 75- years in urban and rural areas, respectively, and the age-specific mortality rate reached the peak at the age group of 80+ years in both urban and rural areas(Figure 4-3a~4-3f).

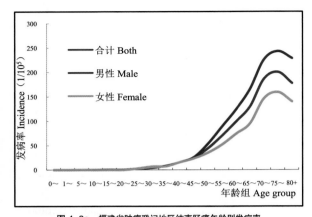

图 4-3a　福建省肿瘤登记地区结直肠癌年龄别发病率
Figure 4-3a　Age-specific incidence of colorectal cancer in Fujian cancer registration areas

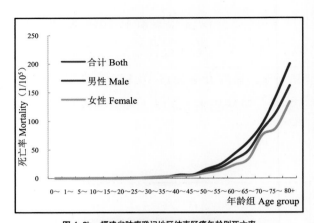

图 4-3b　福建省肿瘤登记地区结直肠癌年龄别死亡率
Figure 4-3b　Age-specific mortality of colorectal cancer in Fujian cancer registration areas

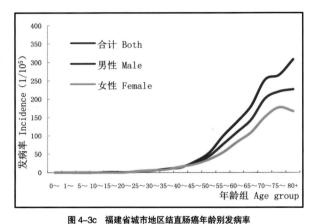

图 4-3c　福建省城市地区结直肠癌年龄别发病率
Figure 4-3c　Age-specific incidence of colorectal cancer in urban areas of Fujian cancer registries

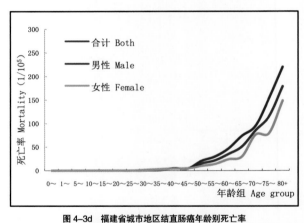

图 4-3d　福建省城市地区结直肠癌年龄别死亡率
Figure 4-3d　Age-specific mortality of colorectal cancer in urban areas of Fujian cancer registries

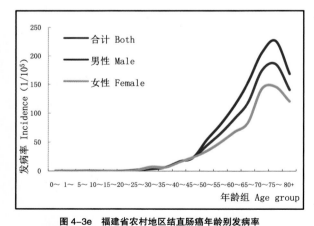

图 4-3e　福建省农村地区结直肠癌年龄别发病率
Figure 4-3e　Age-specific incidence of colorectal cancer in rural areas of Fujian cancer registries

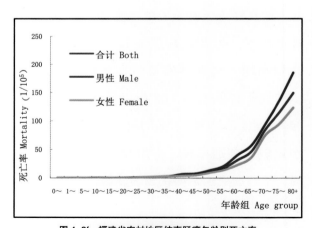

图 4-3f　福建省农村地区结直肠癌年龄别死亡率
Figure 4-3f　Age-specific mortality of colorectal cancer in rural areas of Fujian cancer registries

结直肠癌病例中，有明确亚部位的病例占 43.77%。其中乙状结肠病例最多，占 39.49%，其次升结肠占 16.47%，交搭跨越占 9.79%，降结肠占 8.30%，横结肠 7.92%（图 4-3g）。

About 43.77% cases were assigned to specified categories of colorectal cancer site. Among those, the sigmoid colon was the most common site, accounting for 39.49% of all cases, followed by the ascending colon (16.47%), the overlapping (9.79%), the descending colon (8.30%) and the transverse colon (7.92%)(Figure 4-3g).

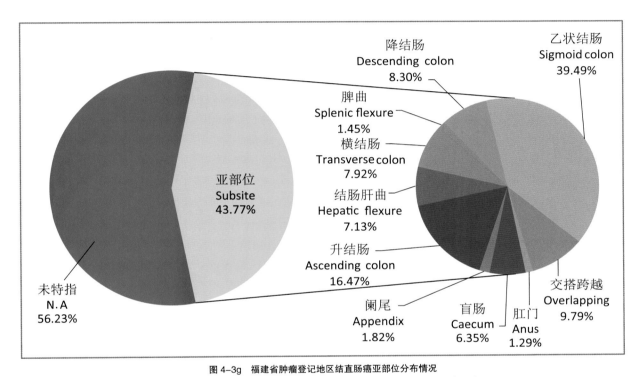

图 4-3g　福建省肿瘤登记地区结直肠癌亚部位分布情况
Figure 4-3g　Distribution of subsites of colorectal cancer in Fujian cancer registration areas

第四节　甲状腺

Section 4　Thyroid

2019 年福建省肿瘤登记地区甲状腺癌发病率为 33.40/10 万，中标率为 29.26/10 万，世标率为 25.43/10 万，占全部恶性肿瘤发病的 10.97%，居发病第 4 位。其中男性发病率为 15.94/10 万，女性发病率为 51.83/10 万，女性为男性的 3.25 倍。城市地区发病率为 43.61/10 万，农村地区发病率为 26.04/10 万，城市地区比农村地区高 67.47%，年龄标化后高 65.11%。2019 年全省估计新发甲状腺癌病例 12491 例，其中男性 3043 例，女性 9448 例。同期肿瘤登记地区甲状腺癌死亡率为 0.70/10 万，仅占全部恶性肿瘤死亡的 0.43%（表 4-4）。

Thyroid cancer was the 4th most common cancer in the registration areas of Fujian Province in 2019. The crude incidence rate was 33.40 per 100,000 (29.26 per 100,000 for ASR China and 25.43 per 100,000 for ASR World), accounting for 10.97% of all new cancer cases. The crude incidence rate was 15.94 per 100,000 for males and 51.83 per 100,000 for females, 3.25 times higher for females than males. The crude incidence rate was 43.61 per 100,000 in urban areas and 26.04 per 100,000 in rural areas, 67.47% higher in urban areas than in rural areas and 65.11% higher after age standardization. There were an estimated 12,491 new cases diagnosed as thyroid cancer in Fujian Province in 2019 (3,043 males and 9,448 females). The crude mortality rate was 0.70 per 100,000 in 2019, accounting for 0.43% of all cancer deaths (Table 4-4).

表 4-4　2019 年福建省肿瘤登记地区甲状腺癌发病与死亡
Table 4-4　Incidence and mortality of thyroid cancer in Fujian cancer registration areas, 2019

地区 Areas	性别 Sex	全省估计病例数 Estimated cases in Fujian Province	肿瘤登记 地区病例数 Cases	粗率 Crude rate （1/10⁵）	构成 Freq. （%）	中标率 ASR China （1/10⁵）	世标率 ASR world （1/10⁵）	累积率 Cum.rate （0~74，%）
发病 Incidence								
全省 All	合计 Both	12491	5153	33.40	10.97	29.26	25.43	2.39
	男性 Male	3043	1263	15.94	5.00	14.36	12.47	1.18
	女性 Female	9448	3890	51.83	17.91	44.54	38.72	3.61
城市 Urban areas	合计 Both	5557	2819	43.61	12.85	37.91	33.06	3.10
	男性 Male	1420	722	22.18	6.29	19.70	17.25	1.64
	女性 Female	4137	2097	65.35	20.04	55.86	48.70	4.54
农村 Rural areas	合计 Both	6934	2334	26.04	9.32	22.96	19.92	1.87
	男性 Male	1623	541	11.59	3.93	10.61	9.13	0.86
	女性 Female	5311	1793	41.73	15.93	36.00	31.29	2.92
死亡 Mortality								
全省 All	合计 Both	280	108	0.70	0.43	0.46	0.46	0.05
	男性 Male	132	50	0.63	0.30	0.45	0.45	0.05
	女性 Female	148	58	0.77	0.69	0.47	0.47	0.05
城市 Urban areas	合计 Both	118	55	0.85	0.52	0.54	0.55	0.07
	男性 Male	47	22	0.68	0.32	0.46	0.48	0.06
	女性 Female	71	33	1.03	0.93	0.60	0.61	0.08
农村 Rural areas	合计 Both	162	53	0.59	0.37	0.41	0.40	0.04
	男性 Male	85	28	0.60	0.29	0.44	0.43	0.05
	女性 Female	77	25	0.58	0.52	0.36	0.36	0.03

甲状腺癌年龄别发病率在35岁以前处于较低水平，35岁以后上升，尤其女性上升速度较快，发病率在50~岁组达到高峰。城市地区、农村地区年龄别发病率分别在45~岁组和40~岁组达到高峰。甲状腺癌预后较好，不同年龄组死亡率均较低（图4-4a～图4-4c）。

The age-specific incidence rate was relatively low before 35 years old, but gradually increased after 35 years old, especially for females, and reached the peak at the age group of 50– years. The age-specific incidence rate reached the peak at the age group of 45– years and 40– years in urban and rural areas, respectively. Thyroid cancer had a better prognosis with low mortality in different age groups (Figure 4-4a~4-4c).

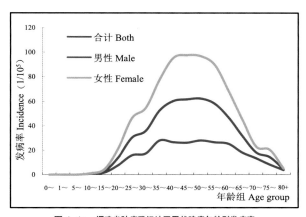

图 4-4a 福建省肿瘤登记地区甲状腺癌年龄别发病率
Figure 4-4a Age-specific incidence of thyroid cancer in Fujian cancer registration areas

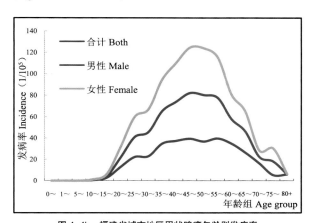

图 4-4b 福建省城市地区甲状腺癌年龄别发病率
Figure 4-4b Age-specific incidence of thyroid cancer in urban areas of Fujian cancer registries

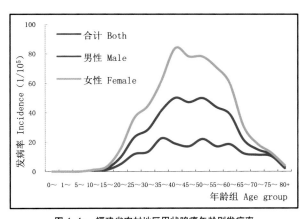

图 4-4c 福建省农村地区甲状腺癌年龄别发病率
Figure 4-4c Age-specific incidence of thyroid cancer in rural areas of Fujian cancer registries

甲状腺癌病例中，有明确组织学类型的病例占90.26%。其中乳头状腺癌是最主要的病理类型，占96.95%，滤泡性腺癌占1.38%（图4-4d）。

About 90.26% cases of thyroid cancer had morphological verification. Among those, papillary thyroid cancer was the most common histological type, accounting for 96.95% of all cases, followed by follicular adenoma (1.38%) (Figure 4-4d).

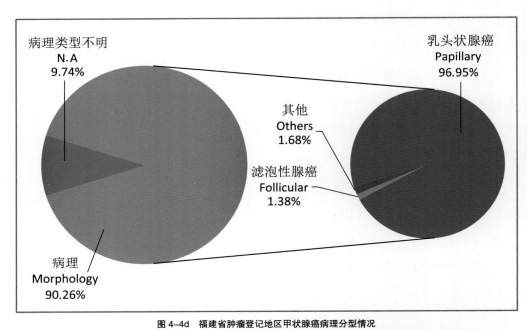

图 4–4d   福建省肿瘤登记地区甲状腺癌病理分型情况

Figure 4–4d   Distribution of histological subtypes of thyroid cancer in Fujian cancer registration areas

第五节　胃

2019 年福建省肿瘤登记地区胃癌发病率为 28.31/10 万，中标率为 19.28/10 万，世标率为 19.13/10 万，占全部恶性肿瘤发病的 9.30%，居发病第 5 位。其中男性发病率为 39.51/10 万，女性发病率为 16.49/10 万，男性为女性的 2.40 倍。城市地区发病率为 28.67/10 万，农村地区发病率为 28.06/10 万，城市地区比农村地区高 2.17%，年龄标化后低 2.41%。2019 年全省估计新发胃癌病例 11403 例，其中男性 8183 例，女性 3220 例。

同期肿瘤登记地区胃癌死亡率为 20.88/10 万，中标率为 13.49/10 万，世标率为 13.22/10 万，占全部恶性肿瘤死亡的 12.91%，居死亡第 3 位。其中男性死亡率为 28.82/10 万，女性死亡率为 12.50/10 万，男性为女性的 2.31 倍。城市地区死亡率为 20.03/10 万，农村地区死亡率为 21.49/10 万，城市地区比农村地区低 6.79%，年龄标化后低 9.46%。2019 年全省估计胃癌死亡 8529 例，其中男性 6036 例，女性 2493 例（表 4-5）。

Section 5 Stomach

Stomach cancer was the 5th most common cancer in the registration areas of Fujian Province in 2019. The crude incidence rate was 28.31 per 100,000 (19.28 per 100,000 for ASR China and 19.13 per 100,000 for ASR World), accounting for 9.30% of all new cancer cases. The crude incidence rate was 39.51 per 100,000 for males and 16.49 per 100,000 for females, 2.40 times higher for males than females. The crude incidence rate was 28.67 per 100,000 in urban areas and 28.06 per 100,000 in rural areas, 2.17% higher in urban areas than in rural areas and 2.41% lower after age standardization. There were an estimated 11,403 new cases diagnosed as stomach cancer in Fujian Province in 2019 (8,183 males and 3,220 females).

Stomach cancer was the 3rd most common cause of cancer deaths in the registration areas of Fujian Province in 2019. The crude mortality rate was 20.88 per 100,000 (13.49 per 100,000 for ASR China and 13.22 per 100,000 for ASR World), accounting for 12.91% of all cancer deaths. The crude mortality rate was 28.82 per 100,000 for males and 12.50 per 100,000 for females, 2.31 times higher for males than females. The crude mortality rate was 20.03 per 100,000 in urban areas and 21.49 per 100,000 in rural areas,6.79% lower in urban areas than in rural areas and 9.46% lower after age standardization. There were an estimated 8,529 cases died of stomach cancer in 2019 (6,036 males and 2,493 females) (Table 4-5).

表 4-5　2019 年福建省肿瘤登记地区胃癌发病与死亡

Table 4-5　Incidence and mortality of stomach cancer in Fujian cancer registration areas, 2019

地区 Areas	性别 Sex	全省估计病例数 Estimated cases in Fujian Province	肿瘤登记 地区病例数 Cases	粗率 Crude rate （1/10⁵）	构成 Freq. （%）	中标率 ASR China （1/10⁵）	世标率 ASR world （1/10⁵）	累积率 Cum.rate （0~74，%）
发病 Incidence								
全省 All	合计 Both	11403	4368	28.31	9.30	19.28	19.13	2.46
	男性 Male	8183	3130	39.51	12.39	27.76	27.85	3.62
	女性 Female	3220	1238	16.49	5.70	11.04	10.68	1.30
城市 Urban areas	合计 Both	3859	1853	28.67	8.45	19.01	18.97	2.42
	男性 Male	2733	1316	40.43	11.47	27.39	27.64	3.57
	女性 Female	1126	537	16.73	5.13	11.06	10.76	1.29
农村 Rural areas	合计 Both	7544	2515	28.06	10.05	19.48	19.26	2.49
	男性 Male	5450	1814	38.87	13.16	28.01	27.99	3.65
	女性 Female	2094	701	16.32	6.23	11.03	10.61	1.31
死亡 Mortality								
全省 All	合计 Both	8529	3221	20.88	12.91	13.49	13.22	1.54
	男性 Male	6036	2283	28.82	13.77	19.73	19.44	2.26
	女性 Female	2493	938	12.50	11.20	7.53	7.31	0.82
城市 Urban areas	合计 Both	2723	1295	20.03	12.31	12.73	12.44	1.43
	男性 Male	1967	934	28.69	13.39	19.02	18.67	2.11
	女性 Female	756	361	11.25	10.18	6.85	6.67	0.77
农村 Rural areas	合计 Both	5806	1926	21.49	13.35	14.06	13.81	1.62
	男性 Male	4069	1349	28.91	14.06	20.24	19.99	2.37
	女性 Female	1737	577	13.43	11.94	8.04	7.81	0.86

胃癌年龄别发病率在 50 岁以前处于较低水平，50 岁以后迅速上升，在 75~ 岁组达到高峰。胃癌年龄别死亡率在 60 岁以前处于较低水平，60 岁以后迅速上升，在 80+ 岁组达到高峰。城市地区、农村地区年龄别发病率均在 75~ 岁组达到高峰，年龄别死亡率均在 80+ 岁组达到高峰（图 4-5a~ 图 4-5f）。

The age-specific incidence rate was relatively low before 50 years old, but dramatically increased after 50 years old, and reached the peak at the age group of 75- years. The age-specific mortality rate was relatively low before 60 years old, while sharply increased after 60 years old, and reached the peak at the age group of 80+ years. The age-specific incidence rate reached the peak at the age group of 75- years in both urban and rural areas, and the age-specific mortality rate reached the peak at the age group of 80+ years (Figure 4-5a~4-5f).

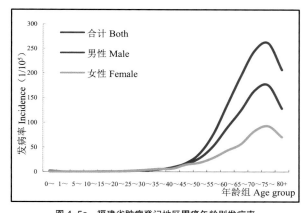

图 4-5a　福建省肿瘤登记地区胃癌年龄别发病率
Figure 4-5a　Age-specific incidence of stomach cancer in Fujian cancer registration areas

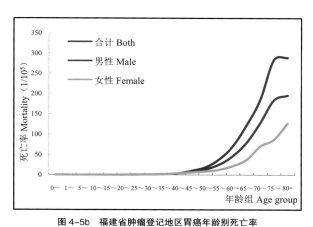

图 4-5b　福建省肿瘤登记地区胃癌年龄别死亡率
Figure 4-5b　Age-specific mortality of stomach cancer in Fujian cancer registration areas

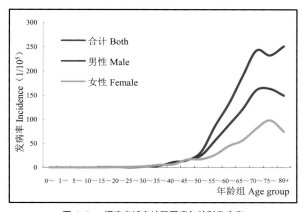

图 4-5c　福建省城市地区胃癌年龄别发病率
Figure 4-5c　Age-specific incidence of stomach cancer in urban areas of Fujian cancer registries

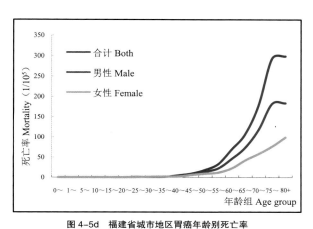

图 4-5d　福建省城市地区胃癌年龄别死亡率
Figure 4-5d　Age-specific mortality of stomach cancer in urban areas of Fujian cancer registries

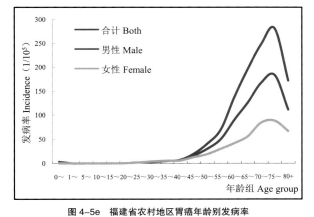

图 4-5e　福建省农村地区胃癌年龄别发病率
Figure 4-5e　Age-specific incidence of stomach cancer in rural areas of Fujian cancer registries

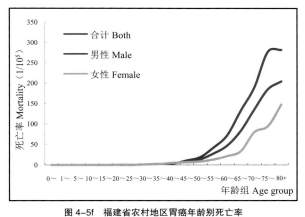

图 4-5f　福建省农村地区胃癌年龄别死亡率
Figure 4-5f　Age-specific mortality of stomach cancer in rural areas of Fujian cancer registries

胃癌病例中，有明确亚部位的病例占 57.17%。其中贲门病例最多，占38.57%，其次幽门窦占22.51%，胃体占18.78%，交搭跨越占11.85%，胃小弯占3.76%，胃底占3.36%（图4-5g）。

About 57.17% of the stomach cancer cases had complete information on subsite. Among those, cardia was the most common subsite and accounted for 38.57% of the total cases, followed by pyloric antrum (22.51%), body (18.78%), overlapping (11.85%), lesser curvature (3.76%) and fundus (3.36%) (Figure 4-5g).

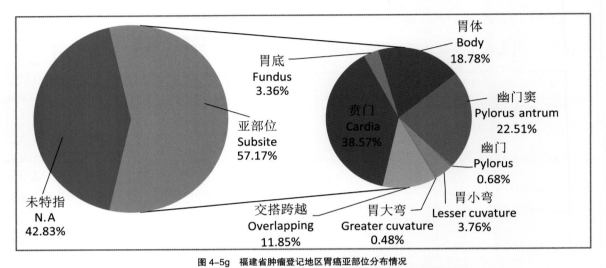

图4-5g 福建省肿瘤登记地区胃癌亚部位分布情况
Figure 4-5g Distribution of subsites of stomach cancer in Fujian cancer registration areas

胃癌病例中，有明确组织学类型的病例占72.78%。其中腺癌病例最多，占92.07%，其次胃肠道间质瘤占2.45%，神经内分泌肿瘤占1.70%，鳞癌占1.16%（图4-5h）。

About 72.78% of the stomach cancer cases had morphological verification. Among those, adenocarcinoma was the most common histological type, accounting for 92.07% of all cases, followed by gastrointestinal stromal tumors (2.45%), neuroendocrine tumors (1.70%) and squamous cell carcinoma (1.16%) (Figure 4-5h).

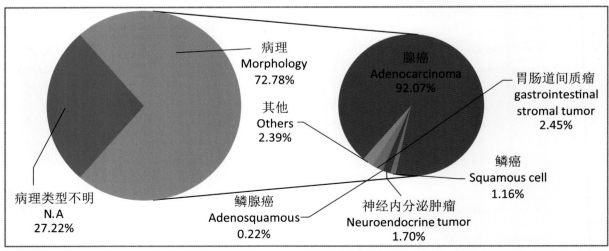

图4-5h 福建省肿瘤登记地区胃癌病理分型情况
Figure 4-5h Distribution of histological subtypes of stomach cancer in Fujian cancer registration areas

第六节　肝脏

2019 年福建省肿瘤登记地区肝癌发病率为 24.97/10 万，中标率为 17.72/10 万，世标率为 17.22/10 万，占全部恶性肿瘤发病的 8.20%，居发病第 6 位。其中男性发病率为 39.09/10 万，女性发病率为 10.06/10 万，男性为女性的 3.89 倍。城市地区发病率为 26.70/10 万，农村地区发病率为 23.72/10 万，城市地区比农村地区发病率高 12.56%，年龄标化后高 8.23%。2019 年全省估计新发肝癌病例 9803 例，其中男性 7879 例，女性 1924 例。

同期肿瘤登记地区肝癌死亡率为 23.08/10 万，中标率为 15.98/10 万，世标率为 15.53/10 万，占全部恶性肿瘤死亡的 14.27%，居死亡第 2 位。其中男性死亡率为 35.42/10 万，女性死亡率为 10.06/10 万，男性为女性的 3.52 倍。城市地区死亡率为 22.35/10 万，农村地区死亡率为 23.61/10 万，城市地区比农村地区死亡率低 5.34%，年龄标化后低 8.73%。2019 年全省估计肝癌死亡 9257 例，其中男性 7286 例，女性 1971 例（表 4-6）。

Section 6 Liver

Liver cancer was the 6th most common cancer in the registration areas of Fujian Province in 2019. The crude incidence rate was 24.97 per 100,000 (17.72 per 100,000 for ASR China and 17.22 per 100,000 for ASR World), accounting for 8.20% of all new cancer cases. The crude incidence rate was 39.09 per 100,000 for males and 10.06 per 100,000 for females, 3.89 times higher for males than females.The crude incidence rate was 26.70 per 100,000 in urban areas and 23.72 per 100,000 in rural areas,12.56% higher in urban areas than in rural areas and 8.23% higher after age standardization. There were an estimated 9,803 new cases diagnosed as liver cancer in Fujian Province in 2019 (7,879 males and 1,924 females).

Liver cancer was the 2nd most common cause of cancer deaths in the registration areas of Fujian Province in 2019. The crude mortality rate was 23.08 per 100,000 (15.98 per 100,000 for ASR China and 15.53 per 100,000 for ASR World), accounting for 14.27% of all cancer deaths. The crude mortality rate was 35.42 per 100,000 for males and 10.06 per 100,000 for females, 3.52 times higher for males than females. The crude mortality rate was 22.35 per 100,000 in urban areas and 23.61 per 100,000 in rural areas,5.34% lower in urban areas than in rural areas and 8.73% lower after age standardization. There were an estimated 9,257 cases died of liver cancer in 2019 (7,286 males and 1,971 females) (Table 4–6).

表 4-6　2019 年福建省肿瘤登记地区肝癌发病与死亡

Table 4-6　Incidence and mortality of liver cancer in Fujian cancer registration areas, 2019

地区 Areas	性别 Sex	全省估计病例数 Estimated cases in Fujian Province	肿瘤登记 地区病例数 Cases	粗率 Crude rate （1/10⁵）	构成 Freq. （%）	中标率 ASR China （1/10⁵）	世标率 ASR world （1/10⁵）	累积率 Cum.rate （0~74，%）
发病 Incidence								
	合计 Both	9803	3852	24.97	8.20	17.72	17.22	2.00
全省 All	男性 Male	7879	3097	39.09	12.26	28.79	28.00	3.25
	女性 Female	1924	755	10.06	3.48	6.74	6.53	0.75
	合计 Both	3495	1726	26.70	7.87	18.54	18.11	2.08
城市 Urban areas	男性 Male	2751	1370	42.09	11.94	30.16	29.49	3.40
	女性 Female	744	356	11.09	3.40	7.30	7.12	0.80
	合计 Both	6308	2126	23.72	8.49	17.13	16.55	1.94
农村 Rural areas	男性 Male	5128	1727	37.01	12.53	27.79	26.91	3.14
	女性 Female	1180	399	9.29	3.55	6.32	6.09	0.71
死亡 Mortality								
	合计 Both	9257	3561	23.08	14.27	15.98	15.53	1.82
全省 All	男性 Male	7286	2806	35.42	16.93	25.78	25.06	2.94
	女性 Female	1971	755	10.06	9.01	6.27	6.11	0.70
	合计 Both	2940	1445	22.35	13.73	15.15	14.80	1.72
城市 Urban areas	男性 Male	2294	1136	34.90	16.28	24.59	24.06	2.78
	女性 Female	646	309	9.63	8.71	6.05	5.90	0.69
	合计 Both	6317	2116	23.61	14.66	16.60	16.07	1.89
农村 Rural areas	男性 Male	4992	1670	35.79	17.40	26.62	25.77	3.05
	女性 Female	1325	446	10.38	9.23	6.44	6.27	0.71

肝癌年龄别发病率在 50 岁以前处于较低水平，50 岁以后迅速上升，在 75~ 岁组达到高峰。肝癌年龄别死亡率在 55 岁以前处于较低水平，55 岁以后迅速上升，在 80+ 岁组达到高峰。城市地区、农村地区年龄别发病率均在 75~ 岁组达到高峰，年龄别死亡率均在 80+ 岁组达到高峰（图 4-6a~ 图 4-6f）。

The age-specific incidence rate was relatively low before 50 years old, but dramatically increased after 50 years old, and reached the peak at the age group of 75- years. The age-specific mortality rate was relatively low before 55 years old, while sharply increased after 55 years old, and reached the peak at the age group of 80+ years. The age-specific incidence rate reached the peak at the age group of 75- years in both urban and rural areas, and the age-specific mortality rate reached the peak at the age group of 80+ years (Figure 4-6a~4-6f).

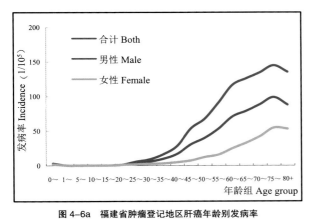

图 4-6a　福建省肿瘤登记地区肝癌年龄别发病率
Figure 4-6a　Age-specific incidence of liver cancer in Fujian cancer registration areas

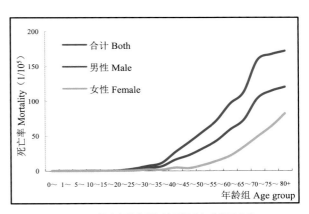

图 4-6b　福建省肿瘤登记地区肝癌年龄别死亡率
Figure 4-6b　Age-specific mortality of liver cancer in Fujian cancer registration areas

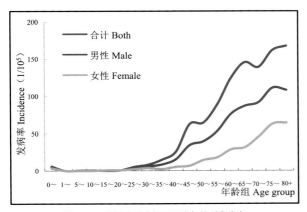

图 4-6c　福建省城市地区肝癌年龄别发病率
Figure 4-6c　Age-specific incidence of liver cancer in urban areas of Fujian cancer registries

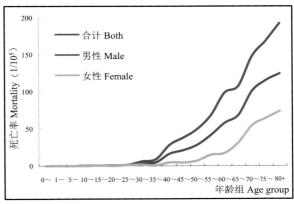

图 4-6d　福建省城市地区肝癌年龄别死亡率
Figure 4-6d　Age-specific mortality of liver cancer in urban areas of Fujian cancer registries

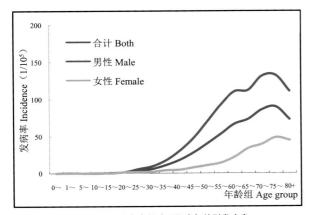

图 4-6e　福建省农村地区肝癌年龄别发病率
Figure 4-6e　Age-specific incidence of liver cancer in rural areas of Fujian cancer registries

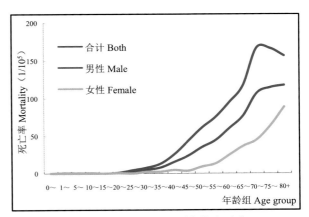

图 4-6f　福建省农村地区肝癌年龄别死亡率
Figure 4-6f　Age-specific mortality of liver cancer in rural areas of Fujian cancer registries

第七节　子宫颈

2019 年福建省肿瘤登记地区子官颈癌发病率为 20.11/10 万，中标率为 14.66/10 万，世标率为 13.79/10 万，占女性恶性肿瘤发病的 6.95%，居女性发病第 5 位。其中城市地区发病率为 18.17/10 万，农村地区发病率为 21.55/10 万，城市地区比农村地区低 15.68%，年龄标化后低 12.98%。2019 年全省估计新发子宫颈癌病例 3878 例。

同期肿瘤登记地区子宫颈癌死亡率为 5.53/10 万，中标率为 3.75/10 万，世标率为 3.64/10 万，占女性恶性肿瘤死亡的 4.95%，居女性死亡第 7 位。其中城市地区死亡率为 4.43/10 万，农村地区死亡率为 6.35/10 万，城市地区比农村地区低 30.24%，年龄标化后低 26.54%。2019 年全省估计子宫颈癌死亡病例 1085 例（表 4−7）。

Section 7　Cervix

Cervix cancer was the 5th most common cancer of females in the registration areas of Fujian Province in 2019. The crude incidence rate was 20.11 per 100,000 (14.66 per 100,000 for ASR China and 13.79 per 100,000 for ASR World), accounting for 6.95% of all new female cancer cases. The crude incidence rate was 18.17 per 100,000 in urban areas and 21.55 per 100,000 in rural areas, 15.68% lower in urban areas than in rural areas and 12.98% lower after age standardization. There were an estimated 3,878 new cases diagnosed as cervix cancer in Fujian Province in 2019.

Cervix cancer was the 7th most common cause of cancer deaths among females in the registration areas of Fujian Province in 2019. The crude mortality rate was 5.53 per 100,000 (3.75 per 100,000 for ASR China and 3.64 per 100,000 for ASR World), accounting for 4.95% of all female cancer deaths. The crude mortality rate was 4.43 per 100,000 in urban areas and 6.35 per 100,000 in rural areas, 30.24% lower in urban areas than in rural areas and 26.54% lower after age standardization. There were an estimated 1,085 females died of cervix cancer in 2019 (Table 4−7).

表 4−7　2019 年福建省肿瘤登记地区子宫颈癌发病与死亡
Table 4−7　Incidence and mortality of cervix cancer in Fujian cancer registration areas, 2019

地区 Areas	全省估计病例数 Estimated cases in Fujian Province	肿瘤登记 地区病例数 Cases	粗率 Crude rate （1/10⁵）	构成 Freq. （%）	中标率 ASR China （1/10⁵）	世标率 ASR world （1/10⁵）	累积率 Cum.rate （0~74，%）
发病 Incidence							
全省 All	3878	1509	20.11	6.95	14.66	13.79	1.50
城市 Urban areas	1155	583	18.17	5.57	13.48	12.48	1.34
农村 Rural areas	2723	926	21.55	8.23	15.49	14.73	1.62
死亡 Mortality							
全省 All	1085	415	5.53	4.95	3.75	3.64	0.44
城市 Urban areas	286	142	4.43	4.00	3.10	2.95	0.35
农村 Rural areas	799	273	6.35	5.65	4.22	4.16	0.51

子宫颈癌年龄别发病率在 45 岁以前处于较低水平，45 岁以后快速上升，55~ 岁组达到高峰后缓慢下降。子宫颈癌年龄别死亡率在 45 岁以前处于较低水平，45 岁以后开始上升，在 70~ 岁组达到高峰。城市地区、农村地区年龄别发病率分别在 55~ 岁组和 50~ 岁组达到高峰，年龄别死亡率均在 70~ 岁组达到高峰（图 4-7a~ 图 4-7b）。

The age-specific incidence rate was relatively low before 45 years old, dramatically increased after 45 years old, reached the peak at the age group of 55– years, and then slowly decreased. The age-specific mortality rate was relatively low before 45 years old, while increased after 45 years old, and reached the peak at the age group of 70– years. The age-specific incidence rate reached the peak at the age group of 55– years and 50– years in urban and rural areas, respectively, and the age-specific mortality rate reached the peak at the age group of 70– years in both urban and rural areas(Figure 4-7a~4-7b).

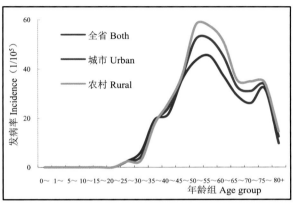

图 4-7a 福建省城市和农村地区子宫颈癌年龄别发病率
Figure 4-7a Age-specific incidence of cervix cancer in urban and rural areas of Fujian cancer registries

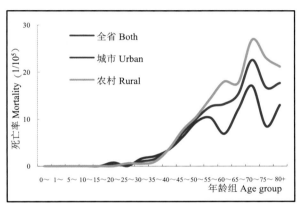

图 4-7b 福建省城市和农村地区子宫颈癌年龄别死亡率
Figure 4-7b Age-specific mortality of cervix cancer in urban and rural areas of Fujian cancer registries

第八节　食管

2019 年福建省肿瘤登记地区食管癌发病率为 17.36/10 万，中标率为 11.34/10 万，世标率为 11.60/10 万，占全部恶性肿瘤发病的 5.70%，居发病第 8 位。其中男性发病率为 24.48/10 万，女性发病率为 9.85/10 万，男性为女性的 2.49 倍。城市地区发病率为 17.65/10 万，农村地区发病率为 17.15/10 万，城市地区比农村地区高 2.92%，年龄标化城市地区比农村地区高 1.15%。2019 年全省估计新发食管癌病例 7129 例，其中男性 5105 例，女性 2024 例。

同期肿瘤登记地区食管癌死亡率为 15.56/10 万，中标率为 9.70/10 万，世标率为 9.79/10 万，占全部恶性肿瘤死亡的 9.62%，居死亡第 4 位。其中男性死亡率为 21.11/10 万，女性死亡率为 9.70/10 万，男性为女性的 2.18 倍。城市地区死亡率为 13.89/10 万，农村地区死亡率为 16.76/10 万，城市地区比农村地区低 17.12%，年龄标化后低 18.86%。2019 年全省估计食管癌死亡病例 6552 例，其中男性 4480 例，女性 2072 例（表 4-8）。

Section 8　Esophagus

Esophageal cancer was the 8th most common cancer in the registration areas of Fujian Province in 2019. The crude incidence rate was 17.36 per 100,000 (11.34 per 100,000 for ASR China and 11.60 per 100,000 for ASR World), accounting for 5.70% of all new cancer cases. The crude incidence rate was 24.48 per 100,000 for males and 9.85 per 100,000 for females, 2.49 times higher for males than females. The crude incidence rate was 17.65 per 100,000 in urban areas and 17.15 per 100,000 in rural areas, 2.92% higher in urban areas than in rural areas and 1.15% higher after age standardization. There were an estimated 7,129 new cases diagnosed as esophageal cancer in Fujian Province in 2019 (5,105 males and 2,024 females).

Esophageal cancer was the 4th most common cause of cancer deaths in the registration areas of Fujian Province in 2019. The crude mortality rate was 15.56 per 100,000 (9.70 per 100,000 for ASR China and 9.79 per 100,000 for ASR World), accounting for 9.62% of all cancer deaths. The crude mortality rate was 21.11 per 100,000 for males and 9.70 per 100,000 for females, 2.18 times higher for males than females. The crude mortality rate was 13.89 per 100,000 in urban areas and 16.76 per 100,000 in rural areas,17.12% lower in urban areas than in rural areas and 18.86% lower after age standardization. There were an estimated 6,552 cases died of esophageal cancer in 2019 (4,480 males and 2,072 females) (Table 4-8).

表 4-8　2019 年福建省肿瘤登记地区食管癌发病与死亡

Table 4-8　Incidence and mortality of esophageal cancer in Fujian cancer registration areas, 2019

地区 Areas	性别 Sex	全省估计病例数 Estimated cases in Fujian Province	肿瘤登记 地区病例数 Cases	粗率 Crude rate （1/10^5）	构成 Freq. （%）	中标率 ASR China （1/10^5）	世标率 ASR world （1/10^5）	累积率 Cum.rate （0~74，%）
发病 Incidence								
全省 All	合计 Both	7129	2678	17.36	5.70	11.34	11.60	1.49
	男性 Male	5105	1939	24.48	7.68	16.69	17.20	2.16
	女性 Female	2024	739	9.85	3.40	6.09	6.12	0.81
城市 Urban areas	合计 Both	2446	1141	17.65	5.20	11.42	11.61	1.45
	男性 Male	1850	870	26.73	7.58	17.92	18.35	2.26
	女性 Female	596	271	8.44	2.59	5.13	5.10	0.66
农村 Rural areas	合计 Both	4683	1537	17.15	6.14	11.29	11.61	1.51
	男性 Male	3255	1069	22.91	7.76	15.83	16.38	2.09
	女性 Female	1428	468	10.89	4.16	6.81	6.90	0.92
死亡 Mortality								
全省 All	合计 Both	6552	2400	15.56	9.62	9.70	9.79	1.15
	男性 Male	4480	1672	21.11	10.09	14.07	14.36	1.69
	女性 Female	2072	728	9.70	8.69	5.46	5.39	0.61
城市 Urban areas	合计 Both	1939	898	13.89	8.53	8.56	8.71	1.04
	男性 Male	1478	693	21.29	9.93	13.83	14.24	1.70
	女性 Female	461	205	6.39	5.78	3.55	3.48	0.40
农村 Rural areas	合计 Both	4613	1502	16.76	10.41	10.55	10.60	1.22
	男性 Male	3002	979	20.98	10.20	14.27	14.46	1.68
	女性 Female	1611	523	12.17	10.83	6.90	6.83	0.76

食管癌年龄别发病率在 55 岁以前处于较低水平，55 岁以后快速上升，在 75~ 岁组达到高峰。食管癌年龄别死亡率在 60 岁以前处于较低水平，60 岁以后快速上升，在 80+ 岁组达到高峰。城市地区、农村地区年龄别发病率均在 75~ 岁组达到高峰，年龄别死亡率均在 80+ 岁组达到高峰（图 4-8a~ 图 4-8f）。

The age-specific incidence rate was relatively low before 55 years old, but dramatically increased after 55 years old, and reached the peak at the age group of 75- years. The age-specific mortality rate was relatively low before 60 years old, while sharply increased after 60 years old, and reached the peak at the age group of 80+ years. The age-specific incidence rate reached the peak at the age group of 75- years in both urban and rural areas, and the age-specific mortality rate reached the peak at the age group of 80+ years (Figure 4-8a~4-8f).

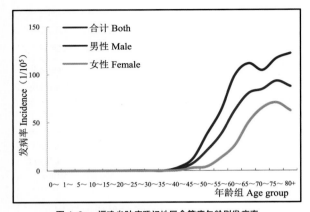

图 4-8a　福建省肿瘤登记地区食管癌年龄别发病率
Figure 4-8a　Age-specific incidence of esophageal cancer in Fujian cancer registration areas

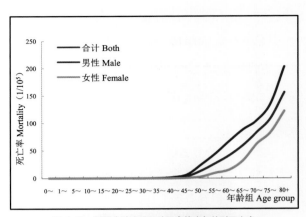

图 4-8b　福建省肿瘤登记地区食管癌年龄别死亡率
Figure 4-8b　Age-specific mortality of esophageal cancer in Fujian cancer registration areas

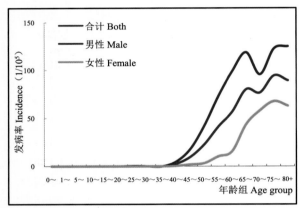

图 4-8c　福建省城市地区食管癌年龄别发病率
Figure 4-8c　Age-specific incidence of esophageal cancer in urban areas of Fujian cancer registries

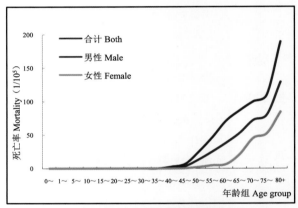

图 4-8d　福建省城市地区食管癌年龄别死亡率
Figure 4-8d　Age-specific mortality of esophageal cancer in urban areas of Fujian cancer registries

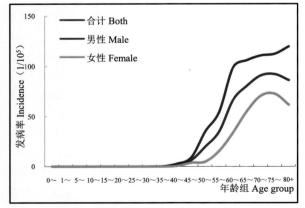

图 4-8e　福建省农村地区食管癌年龄别发病率
Figure 4-8e　Age-specific incidence of esophageal cancer in rural areas of Fujian cancer registries

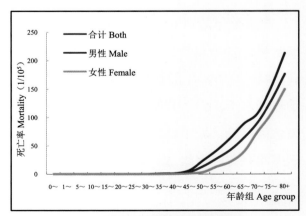

图 4-8f　福建省农村地区食管癌年龄别死亡率
Figure 4-8f　Age-specific mortality of esophageal cancer in rural areas of Fujian cancer registries

食管癌病例中，有明确亚部位的病例占 32.45%。其中胸中段病例最多，占 36.02%，其次交搭跨越占 24.63%，胸下段占 22.44%，胸上段占 11.97%（图 4-8g）。

There were 32.45% of esophageal cancer cases having specific subsite information. Esophageal cancer occurred most frequently in the middle third (36.02%), followed by overlapping (24.63%), lower third (22.44%), and upper third (11.97%)(Figure 4-8g).

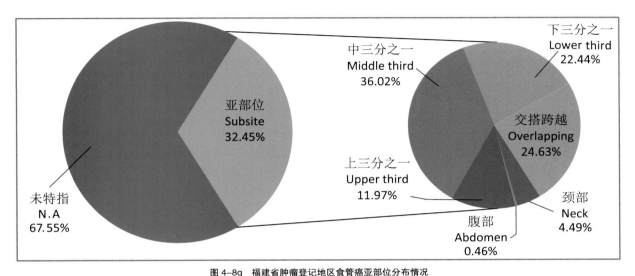

图 4-8g　福建省肿瘤登记地区食管癌亚部位分布情况
Figure 4-8g　Distribution of subsites of esophageal cancer in Fujian cancer registration areas

食管癌病例中，有明确组织学类型的病例占 71.06%。其中鳞癌病例最多，占 91.70%，其次腺癌占 5.20%，腺鳞癌占 0.89%（图 4-8h）。

About 71.06% of the esophageal cancer cases had morphological verification. Among those, esophageal squamous cell carcinoma was the most common type, accounting for 91.70% of all cases, followed by adenocarcinoma (5.20%) and adenosquamous carcinoma (0.89%) (Figure 4-8h).

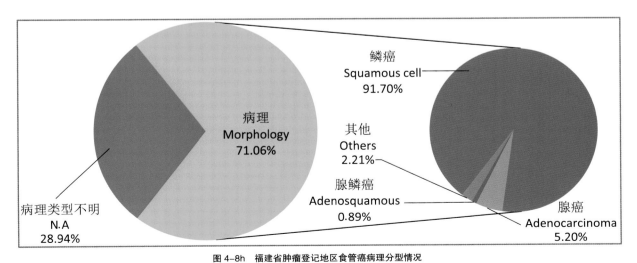

图 4-8h　福建省肿瘤登记地区食管癌病理分型情况
Figure 4-8h　Distribution of histological subtypes of esophageal cancer in Fujian cancer registration areas

第九节　前列腺

2019 年福建省肿瘤登记地区前列腺癌发病率为 11.18/10 万，中标率为 7.52/10 万，世标率为 7.39/10 万，占男性恶性肿瘤发病的 3.51%，居男性发病第 7 位。其中城市地区发病率为 13.67/10 万，农村地区发病率为 9.45/10 万，城市地区比农村地区高 44.66%，年龄标化后高 36.56%。2019 年全省估计新发前列腺癌病例 2182 例。

同期肿瘤登记地区前列腺癌死亡率为 4.38/10 万，中标率为 2.65/10 万，世标率为 2.68/10 万，占男性恶性肿瘤死亡的 2.09%，居男性死亡第 7 位。其中城市地区死亡率为 5.04/10 万，农村地区死亡率为 3.92/10 万，城市地区比农村地区高 28.57%，年龄标化后高 12.75%。2019 年全省估计前列腺癌死亡 885 例（表 4-9）。

Section 9　Prostate

Prostate cancer was the 7th of the male cancer cases in the registration areas of Fujian Province in 2019. The crude incidence rate was 11.18 per 100,000 (7.52 per 100,000 for ASR China and 7.39 per 100,000 for ASR World), accounting for 3.51% of all male cancer cases. The crude incidence rate was 13.67 per 100,000 in urban areas and 9.45 per 100,000 in rural areas,44.66% higher in urban areas than in rural areas and 36.56% higher after age standardization. There were an estimated 2,182 new cases diagnosed as prostate cancer in Fujian Province in 2019.

Prostate cancer was the 7th most common cause of cancer deaths among males in the registration areas of Fujian Province in 2019. The crude mortality rate was 4.38 per 100,000 (2.65 per 100,000 for ASR China and 2.68 per 100,000 for ASR World), accounting for 2.09% of all male cancer deaths. The crude mortality rate was 5.04 per 100,000 in urban areas and 3.92 per 100,000 in rural areas,28.57% higher in urban areas than in rural areas and 12.75% higher after age standardization. There were an estimated 885 males died of prostate cancer in 2019 (Table 4-9).

表 4-9　2019 年福建省肿瘤登记地区前列腺癌发病与死亡
Table 4-9　Incidence and mortality of prostate cancer in Fujian cancer registration areas, 2019

地区 Areas	全省估计病例数 Estimated cases in Fujian Province	肿瘤登记 地区病例数 Cases	粗率 Crude rate （1/10^5）	构成 Freq. （%）	中标率 ASR China （1/10^5）	世标率 ASR world （1/10^5）	累积率 Cum.rate （0~74，%）
发病 Incidence							
全省 All	2182	886	11.18	3.51	7.52	7.39	0.83
城市 Urban areas	875	445	13.67	3.88	8.89	8.70	0.96
农村 Rural areas	1307	441	9.45	3.20	6.51	6.42	0.74
死亡 Mortality							
全省 All	885	347	4.38	2.09	2.65	2.68	0.21
城市 Urban areas	340	164	5.04	2.35	2.83	2.92	0.21
农村 Rural areas	545	183	3.92	1.91	2.51	2.50	0.21

前列腺癌年龄别发病率在 60 岁以前处于较低水平，60 岁以后迅速上升，在 80+ 岁组达到高峰。前列腺癌年龄别死亡率在 65 岁以前处于较低水平，65 岁以后迅速上升，在 80+ 岁组达到高峰。城市地区、农村地区年龄别发病率均在 80+ 组达到高峰，年龄别死亡率均在80+ 岁组达到高峰（图 4-9a~ 图 4-9b ）。

The age-specific incidence rate was relatively low before 60 years old, and dramatically increased after 60 years old, reached the peak at the age group of 80+ years. The age-specific mortality rate was relatively low before 65 years old, while increased after 65 years old, and reached the peak at the age group of 80+ years. In both urban and rural areas, the age-specific incidence and age-specific mortality peaked in the age group of 80+ years (Figure 4-9a~4-9b).

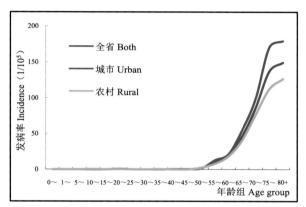

图 4-9a　福建省城市和农村地区前列腺癌年龄别发病率
Figure 4-9a　Age-specific incidence of prostate cancer in urban and rural areas of Fujian cancer registries

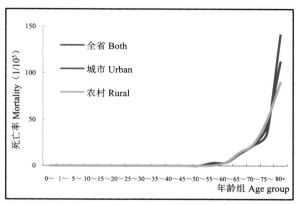

图 4-9b　福建省城市和农村地区前列腺癌年龄别死亡率
Figure 4-9b　Age-specific mortality of prostate cancer in urban and rural areas of Fujian cancer registries

第十节　子宫体

2019 年福建省肿瘤登记地区子宫体癌发病率为 10.13/10 万，中标率为 6.98/10 万，世标率为 6.83/10 万，占女性恶性肿瘤发病的 3.50%，居女性发病第 7 位。其中城市地区发病率为 10.88/10 万，农村地区发病率为 9.57/10 万，城市地区比农村地区高 13.69%，年龄标化后高 15.44%。2019 年全省估计新发子宫体癌病例 1904 例。

同期肿瘤登记地区子宫体癌死亡率为 2.28/10 万，中标率为 1.48/10 万，世标率为 1.44/10 万，占女性恶性肿瘤死亡的 2.04%，居女性死亡第 13 位。其中城市地区死亡率为 2.03/10 万，农村地区死亡率为 2.47/10 万，城市地区比农村地区低 17.81%，年龄标化后低 20.37%。2019 年全省估计子宫体癌死亡病例 439 例（表 4-10）。

Section 10　Corpus Uterus

Corpus uterus cancer was the 7th common cancer of females in the registration areas of Fujian Province in 2019. The crude incidence rate was 10.13 per 100,000 (6.98 per 100,000 for ASR China and 6.83 per 100,000 for ASR World), accounting for 3.50% of all female cancer cases. The crude incidence rate was 10.88 per 100,000 in urban areas and 9.57 per 100,000 in rural areas, 13.69% higher in urban areas than in rural areas and 15.44% higher after age standardization. There were an estimated 1,904 new cases diagnosed as corpus uterus cancer in Fujian Province in 2019.

Corpus uterus cancer was the 13th most common cause of cancer deaths among females in the registration areas of Fujian Province in 2019. The crude mortality rate was 2.28 per 100,000 (1.48 per 100,000 for ASR China and 1.44 per 100,000 for ASR World), accounting for 2.04% of all female cancer deaths. The crude mortality rate was 2.03 per 100,000 in urban areas and 2.47 per 100,000 in rural areas, 17.81% lower in urban areas than in rural areas and 20.37% lower after age standardization. There were an estimated 439 females died of corpus uterus cancer in 2019 (Table 4-10).

表 4-10　2019 年福建省肿瘤登记地区子宫体癌发病与死亡

Table 4-10　Incidence and mortality of corpus uterus cancer in Fujian cancer registration areas, 2019

地区 Areas	全省估计病例数 Estimated cases in Fujian Province	肿瘤登记地区病例数 Cases	粗率 Crude rate （1/10^5）	构成 Freq. （%）	中标率 ASR China （1/10^5）	世标率 ASR world （1/10^5）	累积率 Cum.rate （0~74，%）
发病 Incidence							
全省 All	1904	760	10.13	3.50	6.98	6.83	0.77
城市 Urban areas	709	349	10.88	3.33	7.55	7.43	0.87
农村 Rural areas	1195	411	9.57	3.65	6.54	6.37	0.69
死亡 Mortality							
全省 All	439	171	2.28	2.04	1.48	1.44	0.17
城市 Urban areas	129	65	2.03	1.83	1.29	1.29	0.16
农村 Rural areas	310	106	2.47	2.19	1.62	1.55	0.18

子宫体癌年龄别发病率在 40 岁以前处于较低水平，40 岁以后迅速上升，在 55~ 岁组达到高峰。年龄别死亡率在 45 岁以前处于较低水平，45 岁以后迅速上升，在 75~ 岁组达到高峰。城市地区、农村地区年龄别发病率分别在 50~ 岁和 55~ 岁组达到高峰，年龄别死亡率分别在 80+ 岁和 75~ 岁组达到高峰（图4-10a~ 图 4-10b ）。

The age-specific incidence rate was relatively low before 40 years old, and dramatically increased after 40 years old, reached the peak at the age group of 55- years. The age-specific mortality rate was relatively low before 45 years old, while sharply increased after 45 years old, and reached the peak at the age group of 75- years. The age-specific incidence rate in urban and rural areas reached the peak at the age group of 50- years and 55- years, and the age-specific mortality rate reached the peak at the age group of 80+ years and 75- years, respectively (Figure 4-10a~4-10b).

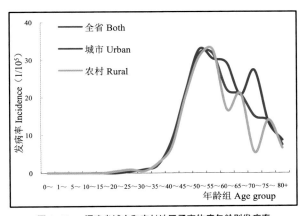

图 4-10a 福建省城市和农村地区子宫体癌年龄别发病率
Figure 4-10a Age-specific incidence of corpus uterus cancer in urban and rural areas of Fujian cancer registries

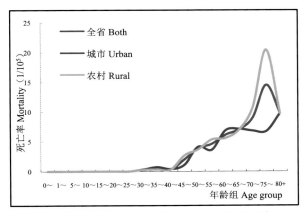

图 4-10b 福建省城市和农村地区子宫体癌年龄别死亡率
Figure 4-10b Age-specific mortality of corpus uterus cancer in urban and rural areas of Fujian cancer registries

第十一节　脑及中枢神经系统

2019 年福建省肿瘤登记地区脑及中枢神经系统肿瘤（简称脑瘤）发病率为 8.69/10 万，中标率为 6.88/10 万，世标率为 6.65/10 万，占全部恶性肿瘤发病的 2.85%，居发病第 11 位。其中男性发病率为 7.55/10 万，女性发病率为 9.89/10 万，女性比男性高 30.99%。城市地区发病率为 9.90/10 万，农村地区发病率为 7.81/10 万，城市地区比农村地区高 26.76%，年龄标化后高 23.76%。2019 年全省估计脑瘤新发病例 3326 例，其中男性 1493 例，女性 1833 例。

同期肿瘤登记地区脑瘤死亡率为 3.76/10 万，中标率为 2.80/10 万，世标率为 2.78/10 万，占全部恶性肿瘤死亡的 2.32%，居死亡第 9 位。其中男性死亡率为 4.28/10 万，女性死亡率为 3.21/10 万，男性比女性高 33.3%。城市地区死亡率为 3.51/10 万，农村地区死亡率为 3.94/10 万，城市地区比农村地区低 10.91%，年龄标化后低 14.72%。2019 年全省估计脑瘤死亡例数 1500 例，其中男性 871 例，女性 629 例（表 4-11）。

Section 11　Brain & Central Nervous System

Brain and central nervous system tumor (below named as brain tumor) was the 11th most common cancer in the registration areas of Fujian Province in 2019. The crude incidence rate was 8.69 per 100,000 (6.88 per 100,000 for ASR China and 6.65 per 100,000 for ASR World), accounting for 2.85% of all new cancer cases. The crude incidence rate was 7.55 per 100,000 for males and 9.89 per 100,000 for females, 30.99% higher for females than males. The crude incidence rate was 9.90 per 100,000 in urban areas and 7.81 per 100,000 in rural areas, 26.76% higher in urban areas than in rural areas and 23.76% higher after age standardization. There were an estimated 3,326 new cases diagnosed as brain tumor in Fujian Province in 2019 (1,493 males and 1,833 females).

Brain tumor was the 9th most common cause of cancer deaths in the registration areas of Fujian Province in 2019. The crude mortality rate was 3.76 per 100,000 (2.80 per 100,000 for ASR China and 2.78 per 100,000 for ASR World), accounting for 2.32% of all cancer deaths. The crude mortality rate was 4.28 per 100,000 for males and 3.21 per 100,000 for females, 33.3% higher for males than females. The crude mortality rate was 3.51 per 100,000 in urban areas and 3.94 per 100,000 in rural areas, 10.91% lower in urban areas than in rural areas and 14.72% lower after age standardization. There were an estimated 1,500 cases died of brain tumor in 2019 (871 males and 629 females) (Table 4-11).

表 4-11 2019 年福建省肿瘤登记地区脑瘤发病与死亡

Table 4-11 Incidence and mortality of brain tumor in Fujian cancer registration areas, 2019

地区 Areas	性别 Sex	全省估计病例数 Estimated cases in Fujian Province	肿瘤登记 地区病例数 Cases	粗率 Crude rate （1/10^5）	构成 Freq. （%）	中标率 ASR China （1/10^5）	世标率 ASR world （1/10^5）	累积率 Cum.rate （0~74，%）
发病 Incidence								
全省 All	合计 Both	3326	1340	8.69	2.85	6.88	6.65	0.69
	男性 Male	1493	598	7.55	2.37	6.28	6.11	0.61
	女性 Female	1833	742	9.89	3.42	7.46	7.16	0.77
城市 Urban areas	合计 Both	1273	640	9.90	2.92.	7.76	7.49	0.79
	男性 Male	532	270	8.29	2.35	6.61	6.44	0.67
	女性 Female	741	370	11.53	3.54	8.89	8.55	0.90
农村 Rural areas	合计 Both	2053	700	7.81	2.80	6.27	6.05	0.62
	男性 Male	961	328	7.03	2.38	6.04	5.87	0.56
	女性 Female	1092	372	8.66	3.31	6.43	6.17	0.67
死亡 Mortality								
全省 All	合计 Both	1500	580	3.76	2.32	2.80	2.78	0.30
	男性 Male	871	339	4.28	2.05	3.32	3.30	0.36
	女性 Female	629	241	3.21	2.88	2.29	2.26	0.24
城市 Urban areas	合计 Both	455	227	3.51	2.16	2.55	2.49	0.26
	男性 Male	260	133	4.09	1.91	3.09	3.04	0.33
	女性 Female	195	94	2.93	2.65	2.02	1.95	0.19
农村 Rural areas	合计 Both	1045	353	3.94	2.45	2.99	3.00	0.33
	男性 Male	611	206	4.41	2.15	3.50	3.50	0.39
	女性 Female	434	147	3.42	3.04	2.49	2.49	0.27

全省、城市、农村地区脑瘤发病病例中，45~64 岁年龄组所占比例均最大，分别为 47.09%、44.53% 和 49.43%。在脑瘤死亡病例中，全省、城市、农村地区 65+ 岁年龄组所占比例均最大，分别为 46.38%、50.22% 和 43.91%（图 4-11a~ 图 4-11f）。

The largest proportions of brain tumor new cases in Fujian Province, urban and rural areas were at the age group of 45-64 years, with 47.09%, 44.53% and 49.43%, respectively. Among the cases of brain tumor deaths, the largest proportions were at the age group of 65+ years in Fujian Province, urban, and rural areas, with 46.38%, 50.22% and 43.91%, respectively (Figure 4-11a~4-11f).

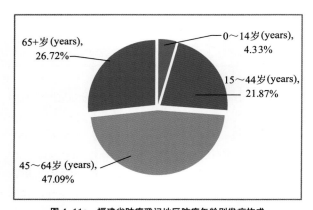

图 4-11a　福建省肿瘤登记地区脑瘤年龄别发病构成
Figure 4-11a　Distribution of age-specific incidence of brain tumor in Fujian cancer registration areas

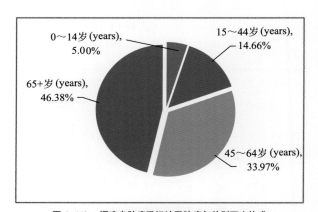

图 4-11b　福建省肿瘤登记地区脑瘤年龄别死亡构成
Figure 4-11b　Distribution of age-specific mortality of brain tumor in Fujian cancer registration areas

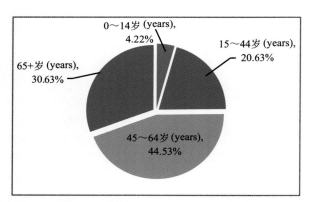

图 4-11c　福建省城市地区脑瘤年龄别发病构成
Figure 4-11c　Distribution of age-specific incidence of brain tumor in urban areas of Fujian cancer registries

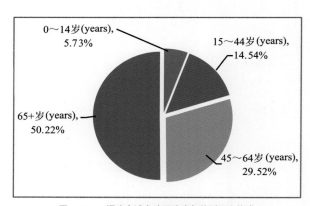

图 4-11d　福建省城市地区脑瘤年龄别死亡构成
Figure 4-11d　Distribution of age-specific mortality of brain tumor in urban areas of Fujian cancer registries

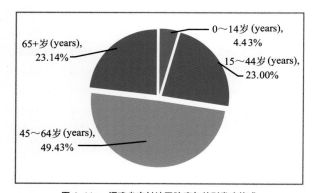

图 4-11e　福建省农村地区脑瘤年龄别发病构成
Figure 4-11e　Distribution of age-specific incidence of brain tumor in rural areas of Fujian cancer registries

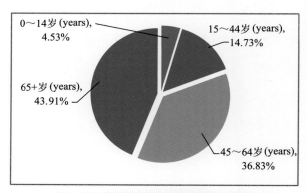

图 4-11f　福建省农村地区脑瘤年龄别死亡构成
Figure 4-11f　Distribution of age-specific mortality of brain tumor in rural areas of Fujian cancer registries

第十二节　淋巴瘤

2019 年福建省肿瘤登记地区淋巴瘤发病率为 7.23/10 万，中标率为 5.40/10 万，世标率为 5.22/10 万，占全部恶性肿瘤发病的 2.38%，居发病第 12 位。其中男性发病率为 8.32/10 万，女性发病率为 6.09/10 万，男性比女性高 36.62%。城市地区发病率为 8.54/10 万，农村地区发病率为 6.29/10 万，城市地区比农村地区高 35.77%，年龄标化后高 30.48%。2019 年全省估计新发淋巴瘤病例 2792 例，其中男性 1655 例，女性 1137 例。

同期肿瘤登记地区淋巴瘤死亡率为 3.42/10 万，中标率为 2.36/10 万，世标率为 2.31/10 万，占全部恶性肿瘤死亡的 2.11%，居死亡第 12 位。其中男性死亡率为 4.04/10 万，女性死亡率为 2.76/10 万，男性为女性的 1.46 倍。城市地区死亡率为 4.04/10 万，农村地区死亡率为 2.97/10 万，城市地区比农村地区高 36.03%，年龄标化后高 24.88%。2019 年全省估计淋巴瘤死亡例数 1327 例，其中男性 820 例，女性 507 例（表 4-12）。

Section12　Lymphoma

Lymphoma was the 12th most common cancer in the registration areas of Fujian Province in 2019. The crude incidence rate was 7.23 per 100,000 (5.40 per 100,000 for ASR China and 5.22 per 100,000 for ASR World), accounting for 2.38% of all new cancer cases. The crude incidence rate was 8.32 per 100,000 for males and 6.09 per 100,000 for females, 36.62% higher for males than females. The crude incidence rate was 8.54 per 100,000 in urban areas and 6.29 per 100,000 in rural areas, 35.77% higher in urban areas than in rural areas and 30.48% higher after age standardization. There were an estimated 2,792 new cases diagnosed as lymphoma in Fujian Province in 2019 (1,655 males and 1,137 females).

Lymphoma was the12th most common cause of cancer deaths in the registration areas of Fujian Province in 2019. The crude mortality rate was 3.42 per 100,000 (2.36 per 100,000 for ASR China and 2.31 per 100,000 for ASR World), accounting for 2.11% of all cancer deaths. The crude mortality rate was 4.04 per 100,000 for males and 2.76 per 100,000 for females, 1.46 times higher for males than females. The crude mortality rate was 4.04 per 100,000 in urban areas and 2.97 per 100,000 in rural areas,36.03% higher in urban areas than in rural areas and 24.88% higher after age standardization. There were an estimated 1,327 cases died of lymphoma in 2019 (820 males and 507 females) (Table 4-12).

表 4-12　2019 年福建省肿瘤登记地区淋巴瘤发病与死亡

Table 4-12　Incidence and mortality of lymphoma in Fujian cancer registration areas, 2019

地区 Areas	性别 Sex	全省估计病例数 Estimated cases in Fujian Province	肿瘤登记 地区病例数 Cases	粗率 Crude rate （1/10⁵）	构成 Freq. （%）	中标率 ASR China （1/10⁵）	世标率 ASR world （1/10⁵）	累积率 Cum.rate （0~74,%）
发病 Incidence								
全省 All	合计 Both	2792	1116	7.23	2.38	5.40	5.22	0.60
	男性 Male	1655	659	8.32	2.61	6.41	6.23	0.71
	女性 Female	1137	457	6.09	2.10	4.40	4.22	0.49
城市 Urban areas	合计 Both	1122	552	8.54	2.52	6.25	6.07	0.70
	男性 Male	663	326	10.02	2.84	7.56	7.40	0.84
	女性 Female	459	226	7.04	2.16	4.98	4.79	0.55
农村 Rural areas	合计 Both	1670	564	6.29	2.25	4.79	4.61	0.53
	男性 Male	992	333	7.14	2.42	5.61	5.41	0.63
	女性 Female	678	231	5.38	2.05	3.96	3.80	0.44
死亡 Mortality								
全省 All	合计 Both	1327	527	3.42	2.11	2.36	2.31	0.27
	男性 Male	820	320	4.04	1.93	2.93	2.87	0.35
	女性 Female	507	207	2.76	2.47	1.79	1.75	0.19
城市 Urban areas	合计 Both	536	261	4.04	2.48	2.66	2.59	0.27
	男性 Male	292	143	4.39	2.05	3.04	2.94	0.32
	女性 Female	244	118	3.68	3.33	2.29	2.25	0.22
农村 Rural areas	合计 Both	791	266	2.97	1.84	2.13	2.10	0.27
	男性 Male	528	177	3.79	1.84	2.85	2.81	0.37
	女性 Female	263	89	2.07	1.84	1.40	1.37	0.16

全省、城市、农村地区淋巴瘤发病病例中，45~64 岁年龄组所占比例均最大，分别为 45.07%、44.38% 和 45.74%。在淋巴瘤死亡病例中，全省、城市、农村地区 65+ 岁年龄组所占比例均最大，分别为 54.84%、61.30% 和 48.50%（图 4-12a~ 图 4-12f）。

The largest proportions of lymphoma new cases in Fujian Province, urban and rural areas were in the age group of 45-64 years, with 45.07%, 44.38% and 45.74%, respectively. Among the cases of lymphoma deaths, the largest proportions were at the age group of 65+ years in Fujian Province, urban, and rural areas, with 54.84%, 61.30% and 48.50%, respectively (Figure 4-12a~4-12f).

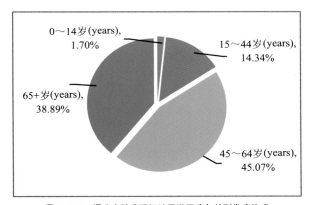

图 4-12a　福建省肿瘤登记地区淋巴瘤年龄别发病构成
Figure 4-12a　Distribution of age-specific incidence of lymphoma in Fujian cancer registration areas

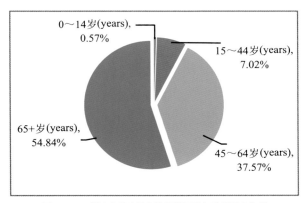

图 4-12b　福建省肿瘤登记地区淋巴瘤年龄别死亡构成
Figure 4-12b　Distribution of age-specific mortality of lymphoma in Fujian cancer registration areas

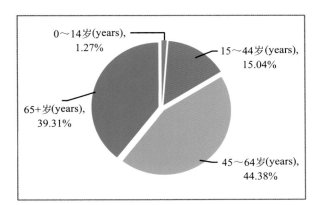

图 4-12c　福建省城市地区淋巴瘤年龄别发病构成
Figure 4-12c　Distribution of age-specific incidence of lymphoma in urban areas of Fujian cancer registries

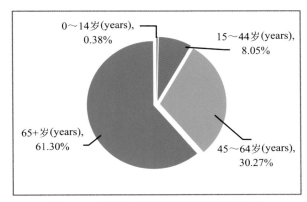

图 4-12d　福建省城市地区淋巴瘤年龄别死亡构成
Figure 4-12d　Distribution of age-specific mortality of lymphoma in urban areas of Fujian cancer registries

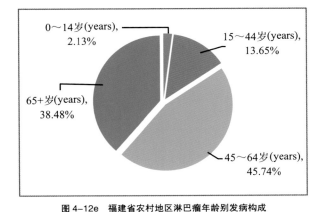

图 4-12e　福建省农村地区淋巴瘤年龄别发病构成
Figure 4-12e　Distribution of age-specific incidence of lymphoma in rural areas of Fujian cancer registries

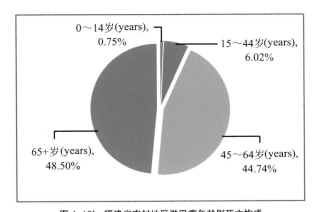

图 4-12f　福建省农村地区淋巴瘤年龄别死亡构成
Figure 4-12f　Distribution of age-specific mortality of lymphoma in rural areas of Fujian cancer registries

淋巴瘤病例中，有明确组织学类型的病例占 76.52%。其中非霍奇金 B 细胞淋巴瘤病例最多，占 46.96%，多发性骨髓瘤和恶性浆细胞瘤占 27.40%，非霍奇金淋巴瘤的其他和未特指类型占 11.83%，非霍奇金 T 细胞淋巴瘤占 8.20%，霍奇金淋巴瘤占 3.86%（图 4-12g）。

About 76.52% of the lymphoma cases had morphological verification. Among them, the non-Hodgkin's B-cell lymphoma was the most common histological type, accounting for 46.96% of all cases, followed by the multiple myeloma and malignant plasma cell neoplasms (27.40%), other and unspecified types of non-Hodgkin's lymphoma (11.83%), the non-Hodgkin's T-cell lymphoma (8.20%) and the Hodgkin's lymphoma (3.86%) (Figure 4-12g).

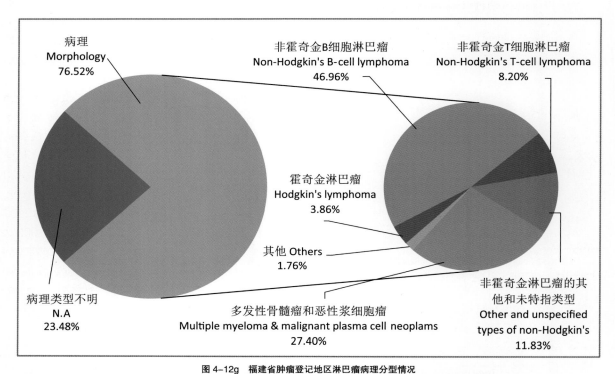

图 4-12g　福建省肿瘤登记地区淋巴瘤病理分型情况

Figure 4-12g　Distribution of histological subtypes of lymphoma in Fujian cancer registration areas

第十三节　卵巢

2019 年福建省肿瘤登记地区卵巢癌发病率为 6.04/10 万，中标率为 4.65/10 万，世标率为 4.46/10 万，占女性恶性肿瘤发病的 2.09%，居女性发病第 12 位。其中城市地区发病率为 6.42/10 万，农村地区发病率为 5.75/10 万，城市地区比农村地区高 11.65%，年龄标化后高 11.76%。2019 年全省估计新发卵巢癌病例 1132 例。

同期肿瘤登记地区卵巢癌死亡率为 2.73/10 万，中标率为 1.84/10 万，世标率为 1.82/10 万，占女性恶性肿瘤死亡的 2.45%，居女性死亡第 12 位。其中城市地区死亡率为 2.90/10 万，农村地区死亡率为 2.61/10 万，城市地区比农村地区高 11.11%，年龄标化后高 9.66%。2019 年全省估计卵巢癌死亡病例 515 例（表 4–13）。

Section 13　Ovary

Ovarian cancer was the 12th of female cancer cases in the registration areas of Fujian Province in 2019. The crude incidence rate was 6.04 per 100,000 (4.65 per 100,000 for ASR China and 4.46 per 100,000 for ASR World), accounting for 2.09% of all female cancer cases. The crude incidence rate was 6.42 per 100,000 in urban areas and 5.75 per 100,000 in rural areas, 11.65% higher in urban areas than in rural areas and 11.76% higher after age standardization. There were an estimated 1,132 new cases diagnosed as ovarian cancer in Fujian Province in 2019.

Ovarian cancer was the 12th most common cause of cancer deaths among females in the registration areas of Fujian Province in 2019. The crude mortality rate was 2.73 per 100,000 (1.84 per 100,000 for ASR China and 1.82 per 100,000 for ASR World), accounting for 2.45% of all female cancer deaths. The crude mortality rate was 2.90 per 100,000 in urban areas and 2.61 per 100,000 in rural areas, 11.11% higher in urban areas than in rural areas and 9.66% higher after age standardization. There were an estimated 515 females died of ovarian cancer in 2019 (Table 4–13).

表 4–13　2019 年福建省肿瘤登记地区卵巢癌发病与死亡

Table 4–13　Incidence and mortality of ovarian cancer in Fujian cancer registration areas, 2019

地区 Areas	全省估计病例数 Estimated cases in Fujian Province	肿瘤登记 地区病例数 Cases	粗率 Crude rate （1/10⁵）	构成 Freq. （%）	中标率 ASR China （1/10⁵）	世标率 ASR world （1/10⁵）	累积率 Cum.rate （0~74，%）
发病 Incidence							
全省 All	1132	453	6.04	2.09	4.65	4.46	0.48
城市 Urban areas	411	206	6.42	1.97	4.94	4.73	0.49
农村 Rural areas	721	247	5.75	2.19	4.42	4.25	0.47
死亡 Mortality							
全省 All	515	205	2.73	2.45	1.84	1.82	0.22
城市 Urban areas	188	93	2.90	2.62	1.93	1.89	0.23
农村 Rural areas	327	112	2.61	2.32	1.76	1.75	0.21

全省、城市、农村地区卵巢癌发病病例中，45~64 岁年龄组所占比例均最大，分别为 52.10%、50.49% 和 53.44%。全省、城市、农村地区卵巢癌死亡病例中，45~64 岁年龄组所占比例最大，分别为 52.68%、48.39% 和 56.25%（图 4-13a~ 图 4-13f）。

The largest proportions of ovarian cancer new cases in Fujian Province, urban and rural areas were at the age group of 45–64 years, with 52.10%, 50.49% and 53.44%, respectively. Among the cases of ovarian cancer deaths, the largest proportions were at the age group of 45–64 years in Fujian Province, urban, and rural areas, with 52.68%, 48.39% and 56.25%, respectively (Figure 4–13a~4–13f).

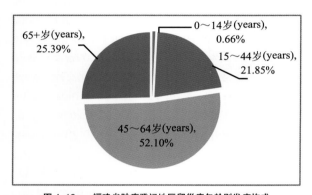

图 4-13a 福建省肿瘤登记地区卵巢癌年龄别发病构成
Figure 4-13a Distribution of age-specific incidence of ovarian cancer in Fujian cancer registration areas

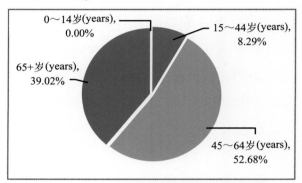

图 4-13b 福建省肿瘤登记地区卵巢癌年龄别死亡构成
Figure 4-13b Distribution of age-specific mortality of ovarian cancer in Fujian cancer registration areas

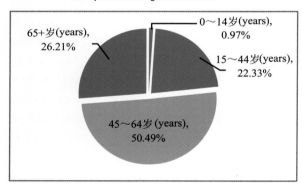

图 4-13c 福建省城市地区卵巢癌年龄别发病构成
Figure 4-13c Distribution of age-specific incidence of ovarian cancer in urban areas of Fujian cancer registries

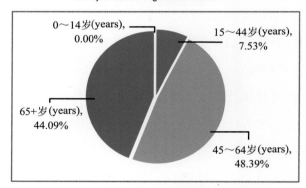

图 4-13d 福建省城市地区卵巢癌年龄别死亡构成
Figure 4-13d Distribution of age-specific mortality of ovarian cancer in urban areas of Fujian cancer registrie

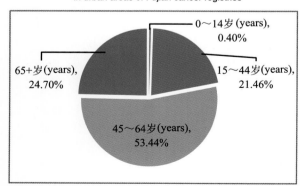

图 4-13e 福建省农村地区卵巢癌年龄别发病构成
Figure 4-13e Distribution of age-specific incidence of ovarian cancer in rural areas of Fujian cancer registries

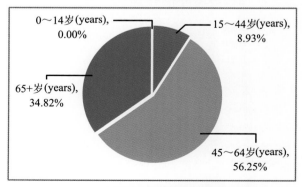

图 4-13f 福建省农村地区卵巢癌年龄别死亡构成
Figure 4-13f Distribution of age-specific mortality of ovarian cancer in rural areas of Fujian cancer registries

第十四节 白血病

2019 年福建省肿瘤登记地区白血病发病率为 5.09/10 万,中标率为 4.40/10 万,世标率为 4.67/10 万,占全部恶性肿瘤发病的 1.67%,居发病第 14 位。其中男性发病率为 5.68/10 万,女性发病率为 4.46/10 万,男性比女性高 27.35%。城市地区发病率为 5.45/10 万,农村地区发病率为 4.83/10 万,城市地区比农村地区高 12.84%,年龄标化后高 7.26%。2019 年全省估计新发白血病 1972 例,其中男性 1139 例,女性 833 例。

同期肿瘤登记地区白血病死亡率为 3.44/10 万,中标率为 2.72/10 万,世标率为 2.77/10 万,占全部恶性肿瘤死亡的 2.12%,居死亡第 11 位。其中男性死亡率为 3.76/10 万,女性死亡率为 3.09/10 万,男性比女性高 21.68%。城市地区死亡率为 3.65/10 万,农村地区死亡率为 3.28/10 万,城市地区比农村地区高 11.28%,年龄标化后高 6.04%。2019 年全省估计白血病死亡 1352 例,其中男性 765 例,女性 587 例(表 4-14)。

Section 14   Leukaemia

Leukaemia was the 14th most common cancer in the registration areas of Fujian Province in 2019. The crude incidence rate was 5.09 per 100,000 (4.40 per 100,000 for ASR China and 4.67 per 100,000 for ASR World), accounting for 1.67% of all new cancer cases. The crude incidence rate was 5.68 per 100,000 for males and 4.46 per 100,000 for females, 27.35% higher for males than females. The crude incidence rate was 5.45 per 100,000 in urban areas and 4.83 per 100,000 in rural areas,12.84% higher in urban areas than in rural areas and 7.26% higher after age standardization. There were an estimated 1,972 new cases diagnosed as leukaemia in Fujian Province in 2019 (1,139 males and 833 females).

Leukaemia was the 11th most common cause of cancer deaths in the registration areas of Fujian Province in 2019. The crude mortality rate was 3.44 per 100,000 (2.72 per 100,000 for ASR China and 2.77 per 100,000 for ASR World), accounting for 2.12% of all cancer deaths. The crude mortality rate was 3.76 per 100,000 for males and 3.09 per 100,000 for females, 21.68% higher for males than females. The crude mortality rate was 3.65 per 100,000 in urban areas and 3.28 per 100,000 in rural areas,11.28% higher in urban areas than in rural areas and 6.04% higher after age standardization. There were an estimated 1,352 cases died of leukaemia in 2019 (765 males and 587 females) (Table 4-14).

表 4-14　2019 年福建省肿瘤登记地区白血病发病与死亡

Table 4-14　Incidence and mortality of leukemia in Fujian cancer registration areas, 2019

地区 Areas	性别 Sex	全省估计病例数 Estimated cases in Fujian Province	肿瘤登记 地区病例数 Cases	粗率 Crude rate （1/10^5）	构成 Freq. （%）	中标率 ASR China （1/10^5）	世标率 ASR world （1/10^5）	累积率 Cum.rate （0~74，%）
发病 Incidence								
全省 All	合计 Both	1972	785	5.09	1.67	4.40	4.67	0.40
	男性 Male	1139	450	5.68	1.78	4.89	5.23	0.46
	女性 Female	833	335	4.46	1.54	3.90	4.11	0.34
城市 Urban areas	合计 Both	703	352	5.45	1.60	4.58	4.86	0.44
	男性 Male	389	195	5.99	1.70	5.12	5.33	0.50
	女性 Female	314	157	4.89	1.50	4.04	4.41	0.39
农村 Rural areas	合计 Both	1269	433	4.83	1.73	4.27	4.54	0.37
	男性 Male	750	255	5.46	1.85	4.74	5.18	0.43
	女性 Female	519	178	4.14	1.58	3.77	3.84	0.30
死亡 Mortality								
全省 All	合计 Both	1352	530	3.44	2.12	2.72	2.77	0.26
	男性 Male	765	298	3.76	1.80	3.03	3.04	0.28
	女性 Female	587	232	3.09	2.77	2.42	2.54	0.23
城市 Urban areas	合计 Both	482	236	3.65	2.24	2.81	2.92	0.28
	男性 Male	259	127	3.90	1.82	2.91	3.02	0.28
	女性 Female	223	109	3.40	3.07	2.78	2.89	0.28
农村 Rural areas	合计 Both	870	294	3.28	2.04	2.65	2.68	0.24
	男性 Male	506	171	3.66	1.78	3.11	3.04	0.29
	女性 Female	364	123	2.86	2.55	2.17	2.30	0.19

全省、城市、农村地区白血病发病病例中，45~64 岁年龄组所占比例均最大，分别为 33.76%、36.65%、31.41%。在白血病死亡病例中，全省、城市、农村地区 65+ 岁年龄组所占比例均最大，分别为 43.02%、44.92% 和 41.50%（图 4-14a~ 图 4-14f ）。

The largest proportions of leukaemia new cases in Fujian Province, urban and rural areas were at the age group of 45–64 years, with 33.76%, 36.65% and 31.41%, respectively. Among the cases of leukaemia deaths, the largest proportions were at the age group of 65+ years in Fujian Province, urban, and rural areas, with 43.02%, 44.92% and 41.50%, respectively (Figure 4–14a~4–14f).

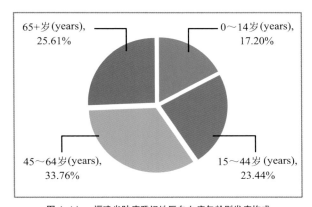

图 4-14a 福建省肿瘤登记地区白血病年龄别发病构成
Figure 4-14a Distribution of age-specific incidence of leukaemia
in Fujian cancer registration areas

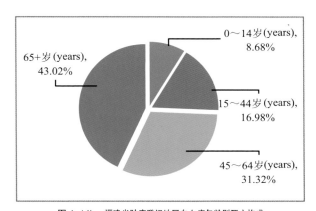

图 4-14b 福建省肿瘤登记地区白血病年龄别死亡构成
Figure 4-14b Distribution of age-specific mortality of leukaemia
in Fujian cancer registration areas

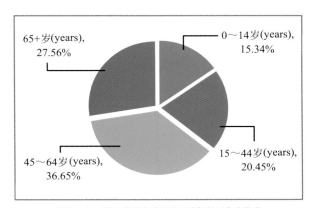

图 4-14c 福建省城市地区白血病年龄别发病构成
Figure 4-14c Distribution of age-specific incidence of leukaemia
in urban areas of Fujian cancer registries

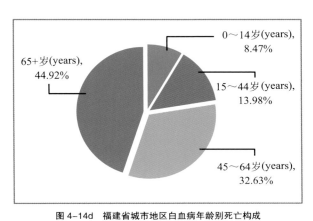

图 4-14d 福建省城市地区白血病年龄别死亡构成
Figure 4-14d Distribution of age-specific mortality of leukaemia
in urban areas of Fujian cancer registries

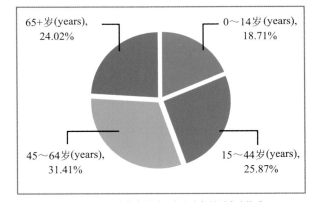

图 4-14e 福建省农村地区白血病年龄别发病构成
Figure 4-14e Distribution of age-specific incidence of leukaemia
in rural areas of Fujian cancer registries

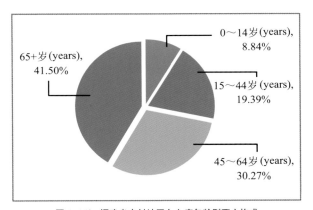

图 4-14f 福建省农村地区白血病年龄别死亡构成
Figure 4-14f Distribution of age-specific mortality of leukaemia in
rural areas of Fujian cancer registries

白血病病例中，髓样白血病占 44.59%，淋巴样白血病占 25.61%，未特指细胞类型白血病占 16.69%，单核细胞白血病占 12.48%（图 4-14g）。

Among the new cases of leukaemia, myeloid leukaemia was the most common histological type, accounting for 44.59%, followed by lymphoid leukaemia (25.61%), unspecified cell type leukaemia (16.69%) and monocytic leukaemia (12.48%)(Figure 4-14g).

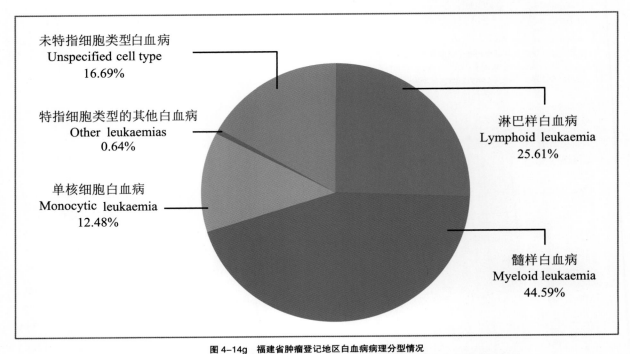

图 4-14g　福建省肿瘤登记地区白血病病理分型情况
Figure 4-14g　Distribution of histological subtypes of leukaemia in Fujian cancer registration areas

第十五节　鼻咽

2019 年福建省肿瘤登记地区鼻咽癌发病率为 5.06/10 万，中标率为 4.06/10 万，世标率为 3.72/10 万，占全部恶性肿瘤发病的 1.66%，居发病第 15 位。其中男性发病率为 7.55/10 万，女性发病率为 2.44/10 万，男性为女性的 3.09 倍。城市地区发病率为 4.41/10 万，农村地区发病率为 5.53/10 万，城市地区比农村地区低 20.25%，年龄标化后低 23.28%。2019 年全省估计新发鼻咽癌病例 2017 例，其中男性 1552 例，女性 465 例。

同期肿瘤登记地区鼻咽癌死亡率为 2.64/10 万，中标率为 1.83/10 万，世标率为 1.80/10 万，占全部恶性肿瘤死亡的 1.64%，居死亡第 14 位。其中男性死亡率为 3.75/10 万，女性死亡率为 1.48/10 万，男性为女性的 2.53 倍。城市地区死亡率为 2.68/10 万，农村地区死亡率为 2.62/10 万。2019 年全省估计鼻咽癌死亡 1033 例，其中男性 759 例，女性 274 例（表 4-15）。

Section 15 Nasopharynx

Nasopharyngeal cancer was the 15th most common cancer in the registration areas of Fujian Province in 2019. The crude incidence rate was 5.06 per 100,000 (4.06 per 100,000 for ASR China and 3.72 per 100,000 for ASR World), accounting for 1.66% of all new cancer cases. The crude incidence rate was 7.55 per 100,000 for males and 2.44 per 100,000 for females, 3.09 times higher for males than females. The crude incidence rate was 4.41 per 100,000 in urban areas and 5.53 per 100,000 in rural areas,20.25% lower in urban areas than in rural areas and 23.28% lower after age standardization. There were an estimated 2,017 new cases diagnosed as nasopharyngeal cancer in Fujian Province in 2019 (1,552 males and 465 females).

Nasopharyngeal cancer was the 14th most common cause of cancer deaths in the registration areas of Fujian Province in 2019. The crude mortality rate was 2.64 per 100,000 (1.83 per 100,000 for ASR China and 1.80 per 100,000 for ASR World), accounting for 1.64% of all cancer deaths. The crude mortality rate was 3.75 per 100,000 for males and 1.48 per 100,000 for females, 2.53 times higher for males than females. The crude mortality rate was 2.68 per 100,000 in urban areas and 2.62 per 100,000 in rural areas. There were an estimated 1,033 cases died of nasopharyngeal cancer in 2019 (759 males and 274 females) (Table 4-15).

表 4-15   2019 年福建省肿瘤登记地区鼻咽癌发病与死亡

Table 4-15   Incidence and mortality of nasopharyngeal cancer in Fujian cancer registration areas, 2019

地区 Areas	性别 Sex	全省估计病例数 Estimated cases in Fujian Province	肿瘤登记 地区病例数 Cases	粗率 Crude rate （1/10^5）	构成 Freq. （%）	中标率 ASR China （1/10^5）	世标率 ASR world （1/10^5）	累积率 Cum.rate （0~74,%）
发病 Incidence								
全省 All	合计 Both	2017	781	5.06	1.66	4.06	3.72	0.39
	男性 Male	1552	598	7.55	2.37	6.12	5.64	0.60
	女性 Female	465	183	2.44	0.84	1.99	1.79	0.19
城市 Urban areas	合计 Both	555	285	4.41	1.30	3.46	3.23	0.36
	男性 Male	432	220	6.76	1.92	5.35	5.02	0.56
	女性 Female	123	65	2.03	0.62	1.61	1.47	0.16
农村 Rural areas	合计 Both	1462	496	5.53	1.98	4.51	4.08	0.42
	男性 Male	1120	378	8.10	2.74	6.67	6.07	0.63
	女性 Female	342	118	2.75	1.05	2.29	2.04	0.21
死亡 Mortality								
全省 All	合计 Both	1033	408	2.64	1.64	1.83	1.80	0.21
	男性 Male	759	297	3.75	1.79	2.69	2.67	0.32
	女性 Female	274	111	1.48	1.32	0.98	0.94	0.11
城市 Urban areas	合计 Both	337	173	2.68	1.64	1.82	1.82	0.22
	男性 Male	234	120	3.69	1.72	2.56	2.60	0.32
	女性 Female	103	53	1.65	1.49	1.11	1.06	0.12
农村 Rural areas	合计 Both	696	235	2.62	1.63	1.84	1.79	0.21
	男性 Male	525	177	3.79	1.84	2.79	2.72	0.32
	女性 Female	171	58	1.35	1.20	0.88	0.85	0.10

全省、城市、农村地区鼻咽癌发病病例中，45~64 岁年龄组所占比例均最大，分别为 54.03%、51.58% 和 55.44%。在鼻咽癌死亡病例中，全省、城市和农村地区 45~64 岁年龄组所占比例均最大，分别为 52.21%、55.49% 和 49.79%（图 4-15a~ 图 4-15f）。

The largest proportions of nasopharyngeal cancer new cases in Fujian Province, urban and rural areas were at the age group of 45–64 years, with 54.03%, 51.58% and 55.44%, respectively. Among the cases of nasopharyngeal cancer deaths, the largest proportions were at the age group of 45–64 years in Fujian Province, urban, and rural areas, with 52.21%, 55.49% and 49.79%, respectively (Figure 4–15a~4–15f).

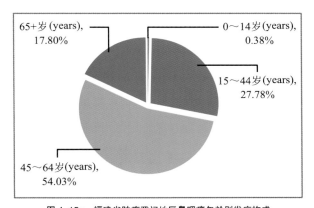

图 4-15a　福建省肿瘤登记地区鼻咽癌年龄别发病构成
Figure 4-15a　Distribution of age-specific incidence of nasopharyngeal cancer in Fujian cancer registration areas

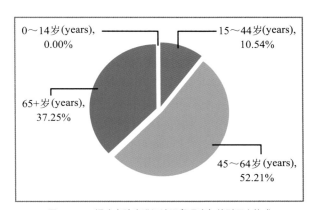

图 4-15b　福建省肿瘤登记地区鼻咽癌年龄别死亡构成
Figure 4-15b　Distribution of age-specific mortality of nasopharyngeal cancer in Fujian cancer registration areas

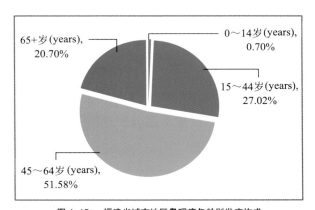

图 4-15c　福建省城市地区鼻咽癌年龄别发病构成
Figure 4-15c　Distribution of age-specific incidence of nasopharyngeal cancer in urban areas of Fujian cancer registries

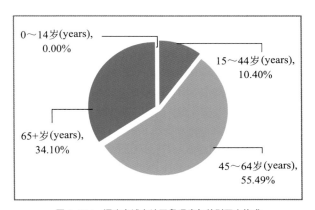

图 4-15d　福建省城市地区鼻咽癌年龄别死亡构成
Figure 4-15d　Distribution of age-specific mortality of nasopharyngeal cancer in urban areas of Fujian cancer registries

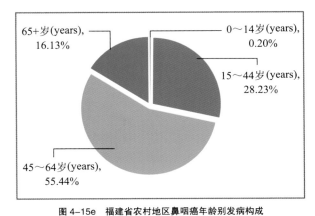

图 4-15e　福建省农村地区鼻咽癌年龄别发病构成
Figure 4-15e　Distribution of age-specific incidence of nasopharyngeal cancer in rural areas of Fujian cancer registries

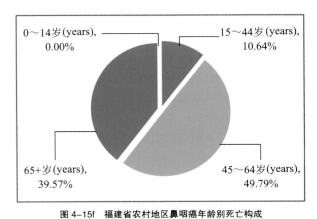

图 4-15f　福建省农村地区鼻咽癌年龄别死亡构成
Figure 4-15f　Distribution of age-specific mortality of nasopharyngeal cancer in rural areas of Fujian cancer registries

第十六节　肾及泌尿系统不明

2019 年福建省肿瘤登记地区肾及泌尿系统不明恶性肿瘤发病率为 5.04/10 万，中标率为 3.66/10 万，世标率为 3.54/10 万，占全部恶性肿瘤发病的 1.65%，居发病第 16 位。其中男性发病率为 6.65/10 万，女性发病率为 3.33/10 万，男性为女性的 2.00 倍。城市地区发病率为 5.94/10 万，农村地区发病率为 4.38/10 万，城市地区比农村地区高 35.62%，年龄标化后高 31.27%。2019 年全省估计新发肾及泌尿系统不明恶性肿瘤 1942 例，其中男性 1312 例，女性 630 例。

同期肿瘤登记地区肾及泌尿系统不明恶性肿瘤死亡率为 1.58/10 万，中标率为 1.01/10 万，世标率为 1.01/10 万，占全部恶性肿瘤死亡的 0.98%，居死亡第 18 位。其中男性死亡率为 2.10/10 万，女性死亡率为 1.04/10 万，男性为女性的 2.02 倍。城市地区死亡率为 2.15/10 万，农村地区死亡率为 1.17/10 万，城市地区比农村地区高 83.76%，年龄标化后高 70.51%。2019 年全省估计肾及泌尿系统不明恶性肿瘤死亡 599 例，其中男性 411 例，女性 188 例（表 4-16）。

Section 16　Kidney & Unspecified Urinary Organs

Cancer of kidney and unspecified urinary organs was the 16th most common cancer in the registration areas of Fujian Province in 2019. The crude incidence rate was 5.04 per 100,000 (3.66 per 100,000 for ASR China and 3.54 per 100,000 for ASR World), accounting for 1.65% of all new cancer cases. The crude incidence rate was 6.65 per 100,000 for males and 3.33 per 100,000 for females, 2.00 times higher for males than females. The crude incidence rate was 5.94 per 100,000 in urban areas and 4.38 per 100,000 in rural areas,35.62% higher in urban areas than in rural areas and 31.27% higher after age standardization. There were an estimated 1,942 new cases diagnosed as cancer of kidney and unspecified urinary organs in Fujian Province in 2019 (1,312 males and 630 females).

Cancer of kidney and unspecified urinary organs was the 18th common cause of cancer deaths in the registration areas of Fujian Province in 2019. The crude mortality rate was 1.58 per 100,000 (1.01 per 100,000 for ASR China and 1.01 per 100,000 for ASR World), accounting for 0.98% of all cancer deaths. The crude mortality rate was 2.10 per 100,000 for males and 1.04 per 100,000 for females, 2.02 times higher for males than females. The crude mortality rate was 2.15 per 100,000 in urban areas and 1.17 per 100,000 in rural areas,83.76% higher in urban areas than in rural areas and 70.51% higher after age standardization. There were an estimated 599 cases died of cancer of the kidney and unspecified urinary organs in 2019 (411 males and 188 females)(Table 4-16).

表4-16 2019年福建省肿瘤登记地区肾及泌尿系统不明恶性肿瘤发病与死亡

Table 4-16 Incidence and mortality of cancer of kidney & unspecified urinary organs in Fujian cancer registration areas, 2019

地区 Areas	性别 Sex	全省估计病例数 Estimated cases in Fujian Province	肿瘤登记 地区病例数 Cases	粗率 Crude rate (1/10⁵)	构成 Freq. (%)	中标率 ASR China (1/10⁵)	世标率 ASR world (1/10⁵)	累积率 Cum.rate (0~74,%)
发病 Incidence								
全省 All	合计 Both	1942	777	5.04	1.65	3.66	3.54	0.42
	男性 Male	1312	527	6.65	2.09	4.97	4.84	0.56
	女性 Female	630	250	3.33	1.15	2.35	2.25	0.27
城市 Urban areas	合计 Both	778	384	5.94	1.75	4.24	4.07	0.44
	男性 Male	538	266	8.17	2.32	6.00	5.79	0.64
	女性 Female	240	118	3.68	1.13	2.53	2.38	0.25
农村 Rural areas	合计 Both	1164	393	4.38	1.57	3.23	3.16	0.40
	男性 Male	774	261	5.59	1.89	4.23	4.16	0.51
	女性 Female	390	132	3.07	1.17	2.22	2.16	0.28
死亡 Mortality								
全省 All	合计 Both	599	244	1.58	0.98	1.01	1.01	0.12
	男性 Male	411	166	2.10	1.00	1.42	1.41	0.16
	女性 Female	188	78	1.04	0.93	0.62	0.64	0.07
城市 Urban areas	合计 Both	286	139	2.15	1.32	1.33	1.31	0.13
	男性 Male	187	91	2.80	1.30	1.83	1.78	0.19
	女性 Female	99	48	1.50	1.35	0.86	0.88	0.08
农村 Rural areas	合计 Both	313	105	1.17	0.73	0.78	0.80	0.11
	男性 Male	224	75	1.61	0.78	1.13	1.15	0.15
	女性 Female	89	30	0.70	0.62	0.45	0.46	0.07

全省、城市、农村地区肾及泌尿系统不明恶性肿瘤发病病例中，45~64岁年龄组所占比例均最大，分别为48.78%、50.00%和47.58%。在全省、城市、农村地区肾及泌尿系统不明恶性肿瘤死亡病例中，65+岁年龄组所占比例均最大，分别为70.90%、73.38%和67.62%（图4-16a~图4-16f）。

The largest proportions of cancer of kidney and unspecified urinary organs new cases in Fujian Province, urban and rural areas were at the age group of 45-64 years, with 48.78%, 50.00% and 47.58%, respectively. Among the cases of cancer of kidney and unspecified urinary organs deaths, the largest proportions were in the age group of 65+ years in Fujian Province, urban, and rural areas, with 70.90%, 73.38% and 67.62%, respectively (Figure 4-16a~4-16f).

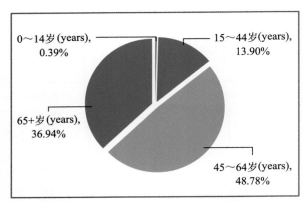

图 4-16a　福建省肿瘤登记地区肾及泌尿系统不明恶性肿瘤年龄别发病构成
Figure 4-16a　Distribution of age-specific incidence of cancer of kidney & unspecified urinary organs in Fujian cancer registration areas

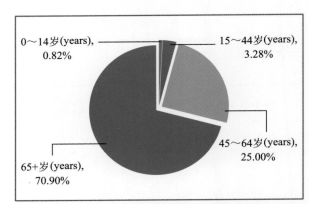

图 4-16b　福建省肿瘤登记地区肾及泌尿系统不明恶性肿瘤年龄别死亡构成
Figure 4-16b　Distribution of age-specific mortality of cancer of kidney & unspecified urinary organs in Fujian cancer registration areas

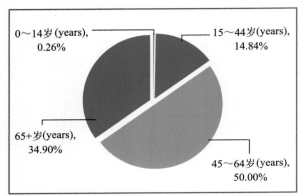

图 4-16c　福建省城市地区肾及泌尿系统不明恶性肿瘤年龄别发病构成
Figure 4-16c　Distribution of age-specific incidence of cancer of kidney & unspecified urinary organs in urban areas of Fujian cancer registries

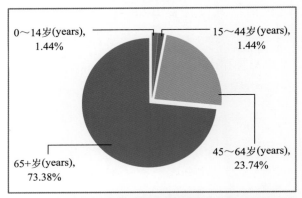

图 4-16d　福建省城市地区肾及泌尿系统不明恶性肿瘤年龄别死亡构成
Figure 4-16d　Distribution of age-specific mortality of cancer of kidney & unspecified urinary organs in urban areas of Fujian cancer registries

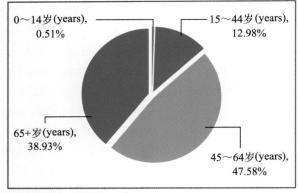

图 4-16e　福建省农村地区肾及泌尿系统不明恶性肿瘤年龄别发病构成
Figure 4-16e　Distribution of age-specific incidence of cancer of kidney & unspecified urinary organs in rural areas of Fujian cancer registries

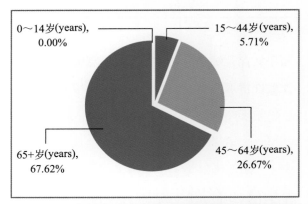

图 4-16f　福建省农村地区肾及泌尿系统不明恶性肿瘤年龄别死亡构成
Figure 4-16f　Distribution of age-specific mortality of cancer of kidney & unspecified urinary organs in rural areas of Fujian cancer registries

第十七节　膀胱

2019年福建省肿瘤登记地区膀胱癌发病率为4.55/10万，中标率为3.05/10万，世标率为3.00/10万，占全部恶性肿瘤发病的1.49%，居发病第17位。其中男性发病率为7.21/10万，女性发病率为1.75/10万，男性为女性的4.12倍。城市地区发病率为5.17/10万，农村地区发病率为4.11/10万，城市地区比农村地区高25.79%，年龄标化后高22.30%。2019年全省估计新发膀胱癌1770例，其中男性1436例，女性334例。

同期肿瘤登记地区膀胱癌死亡率为1.48/10万，中标率为0.85/10万，世标率为0.84/10万，占全部恶性肿瘤死亡的0.91%，居死亡第19位。其中男性死亡率为2.27/10万，女性死亡率为0.64/10万，男性为女性的3.55倍。城市地区死亡率为1.70/10万，农村地区死亡率为1.32/10万，城市地区比农村地区高28.79%，年龄标化后高20.51%。2019年全省估计膀胱癌死亡579例，其中男性462例，女性117例（表4-17）。

Section 17　Bladder

Bladder cancer was the 17th most common cancer in the registration areas of Fujian Province in 2019. The crude incidence rate was 4.55 per 100,000 (3.05 per 100,000 for ASR China and 3.00 per 100,000 for ASR World), accounting for 1.49% of all new cancer cases. The crude incidence rate was 7.21 per 100,000 for males and 1.75 per 100,000 for females, 4.12 times higher for males than females. The crude incidence rate was 5.17 per 100,000 in urban areas and 4.11 per 100,000 in rural areas,25.79% higher in urban areas than in rural areas and 22.30% higher after age standardization. There were an estimated 1,770 new cases diagnosed as bladder cancer in Fujian Province in 2019 (1,436 males and 334 females).

Bladder cancer was the 19th most common cause of cancer deaths in the registration areas of Fujian Province in 2019. The crude mortality rate was 1.48 per 100,000 (0.85 per 100,000 for ASR China and 0.84 per 100,000 for ASR World), accounting for 0.91% of all cancer deaths. The crude mortality rate was 2.27 per 100,000 for males and 0.64 per 100,000 for females, 3.55 times higher for males than females. The crude mortality rate was 1.70 per 100,000 in urban areas and 1.32 per 100,000 in rural areas, 28.79% higher in urban areas than in rural areas and 20.51% higher after age standardization. There were an estimated 579 cases died of bladder cancer in 2019 (462 males and 117 females)(Table 4-17).

表 4-17　2019 年福建省肿瘤登记地区膀胱癌发病与死亡

Table 4-17　Incidence and mortality of bladder cancer in Fujian cancer registration areas, 2019

地区 Areas	性别 Sex	全省估计病例数 Estimated cases in Fujian Province	肿瘤登记 地区病例数 Cases	粗率 Crude rate （1/10⁵）	构成 Freq. （%）	中标率 ASR China （1/10⁵）	世标率 ASR world （1/10⁵）	累积率 Cum.rate （0~74,%）
发病 Incidence								
全省 All	合计 Both	1770	702	4.55	1.49	3.05	3.00	0.35
	男性 Male	1436	571	7.21	2.26	5.07	4.99	0.58
	女性 Female	334	131	1.75	0.60	1.08	1.07	0.13
城市 Urban areas	合计 Both	675	334	5.17	1.52	3.40	3.34	0.39
	男性 Male	538	269	8.26	2.34	5.67	5.59	0.64
	女性 Female	137	65	2.03	0.62	1.23	1.22	0.15
农村 Rural areas	合计 Both	1095	368	4.11	1.47	2.78	2.74	0.32
	男性 Male	898	302	6.47	2.19	4.63	4.55	0.53
	女性 Female	197	66	1.54	0.59	0.95	0.95	0.11
死亡 Mortality								
全省 All	合计 Both	579	228	1.48	0.91	0.85	0.84	0.08
	男性 Male	462	180	2.27	1.09	1.42	1.43	0.14
	女性 Female	117	48	0.64	0.57	0.33	0.32	0.02
城市 Urban areas	合计 Both	228	110	1.70	1.05	0.94	0.95	0.09
	男性 Male	173	83	2.55	1.19	1.55	1.57	0.17
	女性 Female	55	27	0.84	0.76	0.40	0.40	0.02
农村 Rural areas	合计 Both	351	118	1.32	0.82	0.78	0.76	0.07
	男性 Male	289	97	2.08	1.01	1.33	1.33	0.12
	女性 Female	62	21	0.49	0.43	0.28	0.26	0.02

全省、城市、农村地区膀胱癌发病病例中，65+ 岁年龄组所占比例均最大，分别为 55.56%、57.19% 和 54.08%。在全省、城市、农村地区膀胱癌死亡病例中，65+ 岁年龄组所占比例均最大，分别为 82.46%、84.55% 和 80.51%（图 4-17a~ 图 4-17f）。

The largest proportions of bladder cancer new cases in Fujian Province, urban and rural areas were in the age group of 65+ years, with 55.56%, 57.19% and 54.08%, respectively. Among the cases of bladder cancer deaths, the largest proportions were at the age group of 65+ years in Fujian Province, urban, and rural areas, with 82.46%, 84.55% and 80.51%, respectively (Figure 4-17a~4-17f).

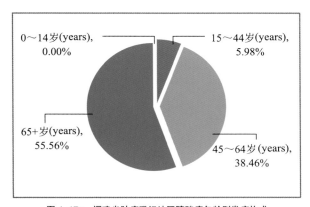

图 4-17a　福建省肿瘤登记地区膀胱癌年龄别发病构成
Figure 4-17a　Distribution of age-specific incidence of bladder cancer
in Fujian cancer registration areas

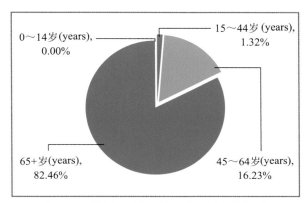

图 4-17b　福建省肿瘤登记地区膀胱癌年龄别死亡构成
Figure 4-17b　Distribution of age-specific mortality of bladder cancer
in Fujian cancer registration areas

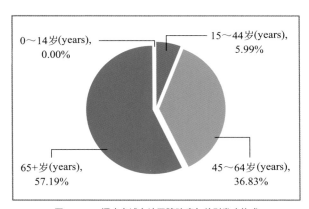

图 4-17c　福建省城市地区膀胱癌年龄别发病构成
Figure 4-17c　Distribution of age-specific incidence of bladder cancer
in urban areas of Fujian cancer registries

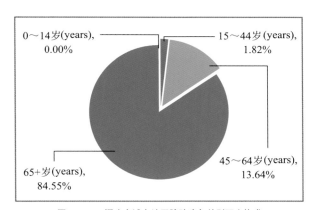

图 4-17d　福建省城市地区膀胱癌年龄别死亡构成
Figure 4-17d　Distribution of age-specific mortality of bladder cancer
in urban areas of Fujian cancer registries

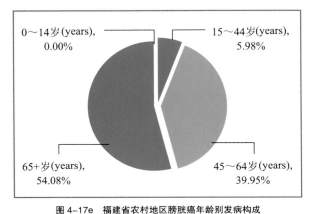

图 4-17e　福建省农村地区膀胱癌年龄别发病构成
Figure 4-17e　Distribution of age-specific incidence of bladder cancer
in rural areas of Fujian cancer registries

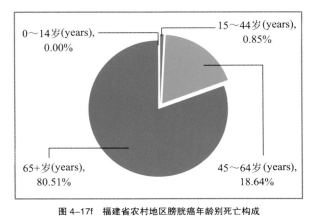

图 4-17f　福建省农村地区膀胱癌年龄别死亡构成
Figure 4-17f　Distribution of age-specific mortality of bladder cancer
in rural areas of Fujian cancer registries

第十八节　口腔和咽（除外鼻咽）

Section 18　Oral Cavity & Pharynx but Nasopharynx

2019 年福建省肿瘤登记地区口腔和咽喉恶性肿瘤发病率为 4.21/10 万，中标率为 2.99/10 万，世标率为 2.94/10 万，占全部恶性肿瘤发病的 1.38%，居发病第 18 位。其中男性发病率为 5.81/10 万，女性发病率为 2.53/10 万，男性是女性的 2.30 倍。城市地区发病率为 4.90/10 万，农村地区发病率为 3.72/10 万，城市地区比农村地区高 31.72%，年龄标化后高 28.95%。2019 年全省估计新发口腔和咽喉恶性肿瘤 1636 例，其中男性 1163 例，女性 473 例。

同期肿瘤登记地区口腔和咽喉恶性肿瘤死亡率为 2.16/10 万，中标率为 1.40/10 万，世标率为 1.42/10 万，占全部恶性肿瘤死亡的 1.33%，居死亡第 16 位。其中男性死亡率为 3.08/10 万，女性死亡率为 1.19/10 万，男性是女性 2.59 倍。城市地区死亡率为 2.65/10 万，农村地区死亡率为 1.81/10 万，城市地区比农村地区高 46.41%，年龄标化后高 42.02%。2019 年全省估计口腔和咽喉恶性肿瘤死亡 840 例，其中男性 610 例，女性 230 例（表 4-18）。

Oral cavity and pharyngeal cancer was the 18th most common cancer in the registration areas of Fujian Province in 2019. The crude incidence rate was 4.21 per 100,000 (2.99 per 100,000 for ASR China and 2.94 per 100,000 for ASR World), accounting for 1.38% of all new cancer cases. The crude incidence rate was 5.81 per 100,000 for males and 2.53 per 100,000 for females, 2.30 times higher for males than females. The crude incidence rate was 4.90 per 100,000 in urban areas and 3.72 per 100,000 in rural areas,31.72% higher in urban areas than in rural areas and 28.95% higher after age standardization. There were an estimated 1,636 new cases diagnosed as oral cavity and pharyngeal cancer in Fujian Province in 2019 (1,163 males and 473 females).

Oral cavity and pharyngeal cancer was the 16th most common cause of cancer deaths in the registration areas of Fujian Province in 2019. The crude mortality rate was 2.16 per 100,000 (1.40 per 100,000 for ASR China and 1.42 per 100,000 for ASR World), accounting for 1.33% of all cancer deaths. The crude mortality rate was 3.08 per 100,000 for males and 1.19 per 100,000 for females, 2.59 times higher for males than females. The crude mortality rate was 2.65 per 100,000 in urban areas and 1.81 per 100,000 in rural areas,46.41% higher in urban areas than in rural areas and 42.02% higher after age standardization. There were an estimated 840 cases died of oral cavity and pharyngeal cancer in 2019 (610 males and 230 females)(Table 4-18).

表 4-18 2019 年福建省肿瘤登记地区口腔和咽喉恶性肿瘤发病与死亡

Table 4-18 Incidence and mortality of oral cavity and pharyngeal cancer in Fujian cancer registration areas, 2019

地区 Areas	性别 Sex	全省估计病例数 Estimated cases in Fujian Province	肿瘤登记 地区病例数 Cases	粗率 Crude rate （1/10⁵）	构成比 Freq. （%）	中标率 ASR China （1/10⁵）	世标率 ASR world （1/10⁵）	累积率 Cum.rate （0~74,%）
发病 Incidence								
全省 All	合计 Both	1636	650	4.21	1.38	2.99	2.94	0.35
	男性 Male	1163	460	5.81	1.82	4.18	4.18	0.51
	女性 Female	473	190	2.53	0.87	1.82	1.72	0.20
城市 Urban areas	合计 Both	647	317	4.90	1.44	3.43	3.37	0.41
	男性 Male	444	219	6.73	1.91	4.78	4.73	0.58
	女性 Female	203	98	3.05	0.94	2.12	2.04	0.24
农村 Rural areas	合计 Both	989	333	3.72	1.33	2.66	2.62	0.31
	男性 Male	719	241	5.16	1.75	3.73	3.77	0.45
	女性 Female	270	92	2.14	0.82	1.58	1.47	0.17
死亡 Mortality								
全省 All	合计 Both	840	333	2.16	1.33	1.40	1.42	0.17
	男性 Male	610	244	3.08	1.47	2.13	2.16	0.26
	女性 Female	230	89	1.19	1.06	0.68	0.67	0.08
城市 Urban areas	合计 Both	354	171	2.65	1.62	1.69	1.72	0.20
	男性 Male	255	125	3.84	1.79	2.57	2.66	0.32
	女性 Female	99	46	1.43	1.30	0.83	0.81	0.08
农村 Rural areas	合计 Both	486	162	1.81	1.12	1.19	1.20	0.14
	男性 Male	355	119	2.55	1.24	1.81	1.81	0.22
	女性 Female	131	43	1.00	0.89	0.57	0.57	0.07

全省、城市、农村地区口腔和咽喉恶性肿瘤发病病例中，45~64 岁年龄组所占比例最大，分别为 51.38%、48.90% 和 53.75%。在全省、城市、农村地区口腔和咽喉恶性肿瘤死亡病例中，65+ 岁年龄组所占比例最大，分别为 53.45%、53.80% 和 53.09%（图 4-18a~图 4-18f）。

The largest proportions of oral cavity and pharyngeal cancer new cases in Fujian Province, urban and rural areas were in the age group of 45-64 years, with 51.38%, 48.90% and 53.75%, respectively. Among the cases of the oral cavity and pharyngeal cancer deaths, the largest proportions were at the age group of 65+ years in Fujian Province, urban, and rural areas, with 53.45%, 53.80% and 53.09%, respectively (Figure 4-18a~4-18f).

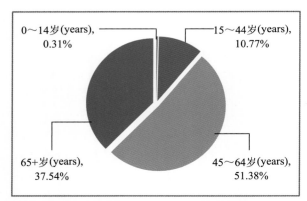

图 4-18a　福建省肿瘤登记地区口腔和咽喉恶性肿瘤年龄别发病构成
Figure 4-18a　Distribution of age-specific incidence of oral cavity and pharyngeal cancer in Fujian cancer registration areas

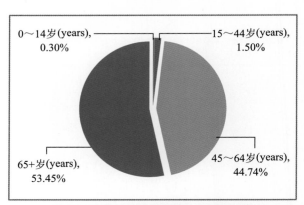

图 4-18b　福建省肿瘤登记地区口腔和咽喉恶性肿瘤年龄别死亡构成
Figure 4-18b　Distribution of age-specific mortality of oral cavity and pharyngeal cancer in Fujian cancer registration areas

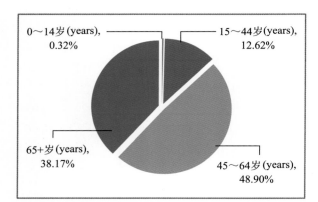

图 4-18c　福建省城市地区口腔和咽喉恶性肿瘤年龄别发病构成
Figure 4-18c　Distribution of age-specific incidence of oral cavity and pharyngeal cancer in urban areas of Fujian cancer registries

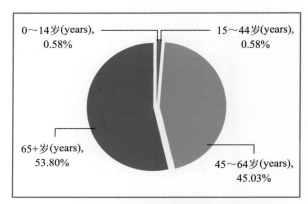

图 4-18d　福建省城市地区口腔和咽喉恶性肿瘤年龄别死亡构成
Figure 4-18d　Distribution of age-specific mortality of oral cavity and pharyngeal cancer in urban areas of Fujian cancer registries

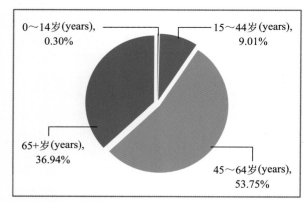

图 4-18e　福建省农村地区口腔和咽喉恶性肿瘤年龄别发病构成
Figure 4-18e　Distribution of age-specific incidence of oral cavity and pharyngeal cancer in rural areas of Fujian cancer registries

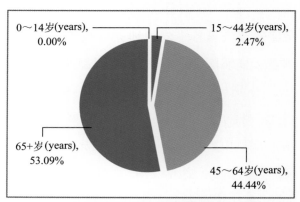

图 4-18f　福建省农村地区口腔和咽喉恶性肿瘤年龄别死亡构成
Figure 4-18f　Distribution of age-specific mortality of oral cavity and pharyngeal cancer in rural areas of Fujian cancer registries

第十九节　胰腺

2019 年福建省肿瘤登记地区胰腺癌发病率为 3.77/10 万，中标率为 2.50/10 万，世标率为 2.47/10 万，占全部恶性肿瘤发病的 1.24%，居发病第 19 位。其中男性发病率为 4.66/10 万，女性发病率为 2.82/10 万，男性比女性高 65.25%。城市地区发病率为 4.21/10 万，农村地区发病率为 3.45/10 万，城市地区比农村地区高 22.03%，年龄标化后高 20.00%。2019 年全省估计新发胰腺癌 1449 例，其中男性 920 例，女性 529 例。

同期肿瘤登记地区胰腺癌死亡率为 3.71/10 万，中标率为 2.41/10 万，世标率为 2.37/10 万，占全部恶性肿瘤死亡的 2.29%，居死亡第 10 位。其中男性死亡率为 4.52/10 万，女性死亡率为 2.85/10 万，男性比女性高 58.60%。城市地区死亡率为 3.91/10 万，农村地区死亡率为 3.56/10 万，城市地区比农村地区高 9.83%，年龄标化后高 7.26%。2019 年全省估计胰腺癌死亡 1460 例，其中男性 913 例，女性 547 例（表 4-19）。

Section 19　Pancreas

Pancreatic cancer was the 19th most common cancer in the registration areas of Fujian Province in 2019. The crude incidence rate was 3.77 per 100,000 (2.50 per 100,000 for ASR China and 2.47 per 100,000 for ASR World), accounting for 1.24% of all new cancer cases. The crude incidence rate was 4.66 per 100,000 for males and 2.82 per 100,000 for females, 65.25% higher for males than females. The crude incidence rate was 4.21 per 100,000 in urban areas and 3.45 per 100,000 in rural areas, 22.03% higher in urban areas than in rural areas and 20.00% higher after age standardization. There were an estimated 1,449 new cases diagnosed as pancreatic cancer in Fujian Province in 2019 (920 males and 529 females).

Pancreatic cancer was the 10th most common cause of cancer deaths in the registration areas of Fujian Province in 2019. The crude mortality rate was 3.71 per 100,000 (2.41 per 100,000 for ASR China and 2.37 per 100,000 for ASR World), accounting for 2.29% of all cancer deaths. The crude mortality rate was 4.52 per 100,000 for males and 2.85 per 100,000 for females, 58.60% higher for males than females. The crude mortality rate was 3.91 per 100,000 in urban areas and 3.56 per 100,000 in rural areas, 9.83% higher in urban areas than in rural areas and 7.26% higher after age standardization. There were an estimated 1,460 cases died of pancreatic cancer in 2019 (913 males and 547 females)(Table 4-19).

表 4-19　2019 年福建省肿瘤登记地区胰腺癌发病与死亡

Table 4-19　Incidence and mortality of pancreatic cancer in Fujian cancer registration areas, 2019

地区 Areas	性别 Sex	全省估计病例数 Estimated cases in Fujian Province	肿瘤登记 地区病例数 Cases	粗率 Crude rate （1/10^5）	构成 Freq. （%）	中标率 ASR China （1/10^5）	世标率 ASR world （1/10^5）	累积率 Cum.rate （0~74，%）
发病 Incidence								
全省 All	合计 Both	1449	581	3.77	1.24	2.50	2.47	0.31
	男性 Male	920	369	4.66	1.46	3.22	3.23	0.40
	女性 Female	529	212	2.82	0.98	1.80	1.75	0.22
城市 Urban areas	合计 Both	545	272	4.21	1.24	2.76	2.71	0.33
	男性 Male	328	167	5.13	1.46	3.45	3.45	0.40
	女性 Female	217	105	3.27	1.00	2.12	2.02	0.25
农村 Rural areas	合计 Both	904	309	3.45	1.23	2.30	2.29	0.29
	男性 Male	592	202	4.33	1.47	3.05	3.06	0.39
	女性 Female	312	107	2.49	0.95	1.56	1.54	0.19
死亡 Mortality								
全省 All	合计 Both	1460	572	3.71	2.29	2.41	2.37	0.28
	男性 Male	913	358	4.52	2.16	3.10	3.08	0.36
	女性 Female	547	214	2.85	2.55	1.75	1.68	0.19
城市 Urban areas	合计 Both	511	253	3.91	2.40	2.51	2.47	0.29
	男性 Male	303	153	4.70	2.19	3.16	3.14	0.37
	女性 Female	208	100	3.12	2.82	1.90	1.84	0.21
农村 Rural areas	合计 Both	949	319	3.56	2.21	2.34	2.29	0.27
	男性 Male	610	205	4.39	2.14	3.05	3.04	0.36
	女性 Female	339	114	2.65	2.36	1.65	1.57	0.18

全省、城市、农村地区胰腺癌发病病例中，65+ 岁年龄组所占比例最大，分别为 60.07%、60.66% 和 59.55%。在全省、城市、农村地区胰腺癌死亡病例中，65+ 岁年龄组所占比例最大，分别为 62.24%、62.45% 和 62.07%（图 4-19a~ 图 4-19f）。

The largest proportions of pancreatic cancer new cases in Fujian Province, urban and rural areas were at the age group of 65+ years, with 60.07%, 60.66% and 59.55%, respectively. Among the cases of pancreatic cancer deaths, the largest proportions were at the age group of 65+ years in Fujian Province, urban, and rural areas, with 62.24%, 62.45% and 62.07%, respectively (Figure 4-19a~4-19f).

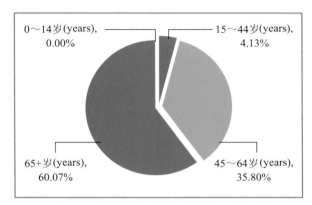

图 4-19a 福建省肿瘤登记地区胰腺癌年龄别发病构成
Figure 4-19a Distribution of age-specific incidence of pancreatic cancer
in Fujian cancer registration areas

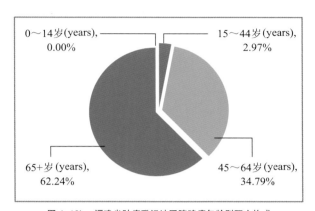

图 4-19b 福建省肿瘤登记地区胰腺癌年龄别死亡构成
Figure 4-19b Distribution of age-specific mortality of pancreatic cancer
in Fujian cancer registration areas

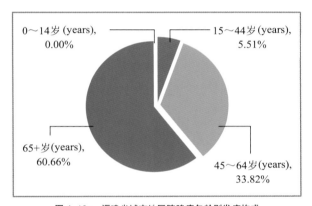

图 4-19c 福建省城市地区胰腺癌年龄别发病构成
Figure 4-19c Distribution of age-specific incidence of pancreatic cancer
in urban areas of Fujian cancer registries

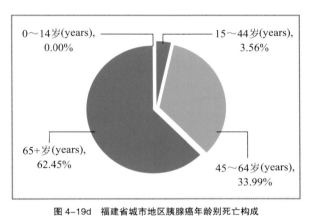

图 4-19d 福建省城市地区胰腺癌年龄别死亡构成
Figure 4-19d Distribution of age-specific mortality of pancreatic cancer
in urban areas of Fujian cancer registries

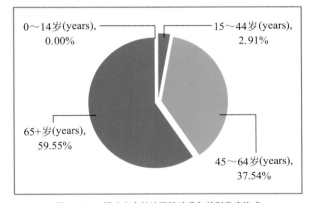

图 4-19e 福建省农村地区胰腺癌年龄别发病构成
Figure 4-19e Distribution of age-specific incidence of pancreatic cancer
in rural areas of Fujian cancer registries

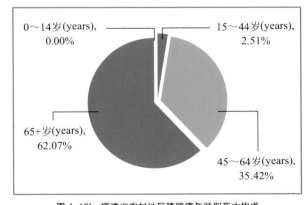

图 4-19f 福建省农村地区胰腺癌年龄别死亡构成
Figure 4-19f Distribution of age-specific mortality of pancreatic cancer
in rural areas of Fujian cancer registries

第二十节　胆囊

2019 年福建省肿瘤登记地区胆囊癌发病率为 2.66/10 万，中标率为 1.77/10 万，世标率为 1.75/10 万，占全部恶性肿瘤发病的 0.87%，居发病第 20 位。其中男性发病率为 2.59/10 万，女性发病率为 2.73/10 万，男性比女性低 5.41%。城市地区发病率为 2.68/10 万，农村地区发病率为 2.64/10 万，城市地区比农村地区高 1.52%，年龄标化后低 2.25%。2019 年全省估计新发胆囊癌 1030 例，其中男性 518 例，女性 512 例。

同期肿瘤登记地区胆囊癌死亡率为 2.01/10 万，中标率为 1.27/10 万，世标率为 1.28/10 万，占全部恶性肿瘤死亡的 1.24%，居死亡第 17 位。其中男性死亡率为 1.99/10 万，女性死亡率为 2.03/10 万，男性比女性低 2.01%。城市地区死亡率为 2.13/10 万，农村地区死亡率为 1.92/10 万，城市地区比农村地区高 10.94%，年龄标化后高 9.84%。2019 年全省估计胆囊癌死亡 782 例，其中男性 395 例，女性 387 例（表 4-20）。

Section 20　Gallbladder

Gallbladder cancer was the 20th most common cancer in the registration areas of Fujian Province in 2019. The crude incidence rate was 2.66 per 100,000 (1.77 per 100,000 for ASR China and 1.75 per 100,000 for ASR World), accounting for 0.87% of all new cancer cases. The crude incidence rate was 2.59 per 100,000 for males and 2.73 per 100,000 for females, 5.41% higher for females than males. The crude incidence rate was 2.68 per 100,000 in urban areas and 2.64 per 100,000 in rural areas,1.52% higher in urban areas than in rural areas and 2.25% lower after age standardization. There were an estimated 1,030 new cases diagnosed as gallbladder cancer in Fujian Province in 2019 (518 males and 512 females).

Gallbladder cancer was the 17th most common cause of cancer deaths in the registration areas of Fujian Province in 2019. The crude mortality rate was 2.01 per 100,000 (1.27 per 100,000 for ASR China and 1.28 per 100,000 for ASR World), accounting for 1.24% of all cancer deaths. The crude mortality rate was 1.99 per 100,000 for males and 2.03 per 100,000 for females, 2.01% higher for females than males. The crude mortality rate was 2.13 per 100,000 in urban areas and 1.92 per 100,000 in rural areas,10.94% higher in urban areas than in rural areas and 9.84% higher after age standardization. There were an estimated 782 cases died of gallbladder cancer in 2019 (395 males and 387 females)(Table 4-20).

表 4-20　2019 年福建省肿瘤登记地区胆囊癌发病与死亡

Table 4-20　Incidence and mortality of gallbladder cancer in Fujian cancer registration areas, 2019

地区 Areas	性别 Sex	全省估计病例数 Estimated cases in Fujian Province	肿瘤登记 地区病例数 Cases	粗率 Crude rate （1/10^5）	构成 Freq. （%）	中标率 ASR China （1/10^5）	世标率 ASR world （1/10^5）	累积率 Cum.rate （0~74,%）
发病 Incidence								
全省 All	合计 Both	1030	410	2.66	0.87	1.77	1.75	0.21
	男性 Male	518	205	2.59	0.81	1.81	1.78	0.21
	女性 Female	512	205	2.73	0.94	1.73	1.73	0.21
城市 Urban areas	合计 Both	344	173	2.68	0.79	1.74	1.73	0.22
	男性 Male	171	86	2.64	0.75	1.81	1.79	0.23
	女性 Female	173	87	2.71	0.83	1.68	1.69	0.21
农村 Rural areas	合计 Both	686	237	2.64	0.95	1.78	1.76	0.21
	男性 Male	347	119	2.55	0.86	1.81	1.78	0.20
	女性 Female	339	118	2.75	1.05	1.77	1.76	0.22
死亡 Mortality								
全省 All	合计 Both	782	310	2.01	1.24	1.27	1.28	0.16
	男性 Male	395	158	1.99	0.95	1.36	1.37	0.17
	女性 Female	387	152	2.03	1.81	1.18	1.21	0.15
城市 Urban areas	合计 Both	280	138	2.13	1.31	1.34	1.36	0.17
	男性 Male	147	73	2.24	1.05	1.51	1.51	0.19
	女性 Female	133	65	2.03	1.83	1.19	1.24	0.16
农村 Rural areas	合计 Both	502	172	1.92	1.19	1.22	1.22	0.15
	男性 Male	248	85	1.82	0.89	1.26	1.27	0.15
	女性 Female	254	87	2.02	1.80	1.17	1.18	0.15

　　全省、城市、农村地区胆囊癌发病病例中，65+ 岁年龄组所占比例最大，分别为 59.02%、59.54% 和 58.65%。在全省、城市、农村地区胆囊癌死亡病例中，65+ 岁年龄组所占比例最大，分别为 69.68%、68.12% 和 70.93%（图 4-20a~ 图 4-20f）。

The largest proportions of gallbladder cancer new cases in Fujian Province, urban and rural areas were at the age group of 65+ years, with 59.02%, 59.54% and 58.65%, respectively. Among the cases of gallbladder cancer deaths, the largest proportions were at the age group of 65+ years in Fujian Province, urban, and rural areas, with 69.68%, 68.12% and 70.93%, respectively (Figure 4-20a~4-20f).

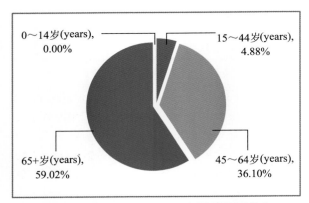

图 4-20a 福建省肿瘤登记地区胆囊癌年龄别发病构成
Figure 4-20a Distribution of age-specific incidence of gallbladder cancer in Fujian cancer registration areas

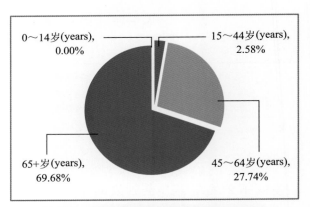

图 4-20b 福建省肿瘤登记地区胆囊癌年龄别死亡构成
Figure 4-20b Distribution of age-specific mortality of gallbladder cancer in Fujian cancer registration areas

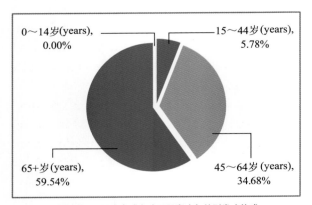

图 4-20c 福建省城市地区胆囊癌年龄别发病构成
Figure 4-20c Distribution of age-specific incidence of gallbladder cancer in urban areas of Fujian cancer registries

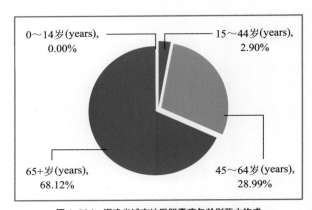

图 4-20d 福建省城市地区胆囊癌年龄别死亡构成
Figure 4-20d Distribution of age-specific mortality of gallbladder cancer in urban areas of Fujian cancer registries

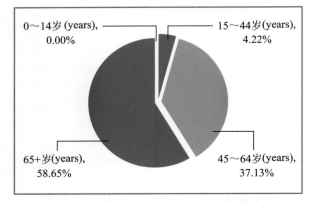

图 4-20e 福建省农村地区胆囊癌年龄别发病构成
Figure 4-20e Distribution of age-specific incidence of gallbladder cancer in rural areas of Fujian cancer registries

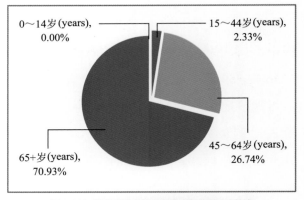

图 4-20f 福建省农村地区胆囊癌年龄别死亡构成
Figure 4-20f Distribution of age-specific mortality of gallbladder cancer in rural areas of Fujian cancer registries

第二十一节　喉

2019 年福建省肿瘤登记地区喉癌发病率为 1.68/10 万，中标率为 1.14/10 万，世标率为 1.16/10 万，占全部恶性肿瘤发病的 0.55%，居发病第 21 位。其中男性发病率为 3.16/10 万，女性发病率为 0.12/10 万，男性是女性的 26.33 倍。城市地区发病率为 1.86/10 万，农村地区发病率为 1.55/10 万，城市地区比农村地区高 20.00%，年龄标化后高 16.82%。2019 年全省估计新发喉癌 658 例，其中男性 633 例，女性 25 例。

同期肿瘤登记地区喉癌死亡率为 1.04/10 万，中标率为 0.67/10 万，世标率为 0.67/10 万，占全部恶性肿瘤死亡的 0.64%，居死亡第 20 位。其中男性死亡率为 1.83/10 万，女性死亡率为 0.20/10 万，男性是女性 9.15 倍。城市地区死亡率为 0.94/10 万，农村地区死亡率为 1.10/10 万，城市地区比农村地区低 14.55%，年龄标化后低 16.67%。2019 年全省估计喉癌死亡 421 例，其中男性 380 例，女性 41 例（表 4-21）。

Section 21　Larynx

Larynx cancer was the 21st most common cancer in the registration areas of Fujian Province in 2019. The crude incidence rate was 1.68 per 100,000 (1.14 per 100,000 for ASR China and 1.16 per 100,000 for ASR World), accounting for 0.55% of all new cancer cases. The crude incidence rate was 3.16 per 100,000 for males and 0.12 per 100,000 for females, 26.33 times higher for males than females. The crude incidence rate was 1.86 per 100,000 in urban areas and 1.55 per 100,000 in rural areas,20.00% higher in urban areas than in rural areas and 16.82% higher after age standardization. There were an estimated 658 new cases diagnosed as larynx cancer in Fujian Province in 2019 (633 males and 25 females).

Larynx cancer was the 20th most common cause of cancer deaths in the registration areas of Fujian Province in 2019. The crude mortality rate was 1.04 per 100,000 (0.67 per 100,000 for ASR China and 0.67 per 100,000 for ASR World), accounting for 0.64% of all cancer deaths. The crude mortality rate was 1.83 per 100,000 for males and 0.20 per 100,000 for females, 9.15 times higher for males than females. The crude mortality rate was 0.94 per 100,000 in urban areas and 1.10 per 100,000 in rural areas,14.55% lower in urban areas than in rural areas and 16.67% lower after age standardization. There were an estimated 421 cases died of larynx cancer in 2019 (380 males and 41 females)(Table 4-21).

表 4-21　2019 年福建省肿瘤登记地区喉癌发病与死亡

Table 4-21　Incidence and mortality of larynx cancer in Fujian cancer registration areas, 2019

地区 Areas	性别 Sex	全省估计病例数 Estimated cases in Fujian Province	肿瘤登记 地区病例数 Cases	粗率 Crude rate （1/10^5）	构成 Freq. （%）	中标率 ASR China （1/10^5）	世标率 ASR world （1/10^5）	累积率 Cum.rate （0~74，%）
发病 Incidence								
全省 All	合计 Both	658	259	1.68	0.55	1.14	1.16	0.16
	男性 Male	633	250	3.16	0.99	2.22	2.26	0.30
	女性 Female	25	9	0.12	0.04	0.08	0.08	0.01
城市 Urban areas	合计 Both	242	120	1.86	0.55	1.25	1.26	0.17
	男性 Male	235	117	3.59	1.02	2.46	2.51	0.34
	女性 Female	7	3	0.09	0.03	0.07	0.06	0.00
农村 Rural areas	合计 Both	416	139	1.55	0.56	1.07	1.09	0.14
	男性 Male	398	133	2.85	0.97	2.04	2.08	0.28
	女性 Female	18	6	0.14	0.05	0.09	0.09	0.01
死亡 Mortality								
全省 All	合计 Both	421	160	1.04	0.64	0.67	0.67	0.08
	男性 Male	380	145	1.83	0.87	1.24	1.26	0.16
	女性 Female	41	15	0.20	0.18	0.11	0.11	0.01
城市 Urban areas	合计 Both	127	61	0.94	0.58	0.60	0.61	0.08
	男性 Male	120	57	1.75	0.82	1.15	1.18	0.15
	女性 Female	7	4	0.12	0.11	0.08	0.07	0.01
农村 Rural areas	合计 Both	294	99	1.10	0.69	0.72	0.72	0.09
	男性 Male	260	88	1.89	0.92	1.31	1.32	0.16
	女性 Female	34	11	0.26	0.23	0.14	0.13	0.01

全省、城市、农村地区喉癌发病病例中，45~64 岁年龄组所占比例最大，分别为 52.51%、51.67% 和 53.24%。在全省、城市、农村地区喉癌死亡病例中，65+ 岁年龄组所占比例最大，分别为 63.13%、63.93% 和 62.63%（图 4-21a~ 图 4-21f）。

The largest proportions of larynx cancer new cases in Fujian Province, urban and rural areas were at the age group of 45-64 years, with 52.51%, 51.67% and 53.24%, respectively. Among the cases of larynx cancer deaths, the largest proportions were at the age group of 65+ years in Fujian Province, urban, and rural areas, with 63.13%, 63.93% and 62.63%, respectively (Figure 4-21a~4-21f).

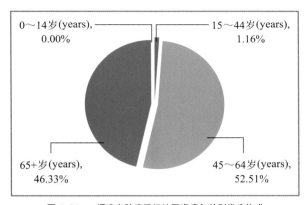

图 4-21a　福建省肿瘤登记地区喉癌年龄别发病构成
Figure 4-21a　Distribution of age-specific incidence of larynx cancer
in Fujian cancer registration areas

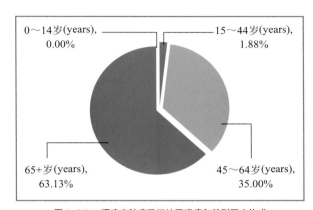

图 4-21b　福建省肿瘤登记地区喉癌年龄别死亡构成
Figure 4-21b　Distribution of age-specific mortality of larynx cancer
in Fujian cancer registration areas

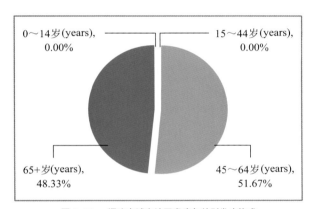

图 4-21c　福建省城市地区喉癌年龄别发病构成
Figure 4-21c　Distribution of age-specific incidence of larynx cancer
in urban areas of Fujian cancer registries

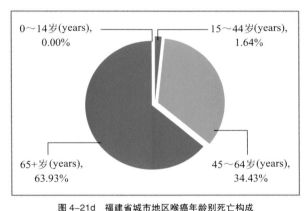

图 4-21d　福建省城市地区喉癌年龄别死亡构成
Figure 4-21d　Distribution of age-specific mortality of larynx cancer
in urban areas of Fujian cancer registries

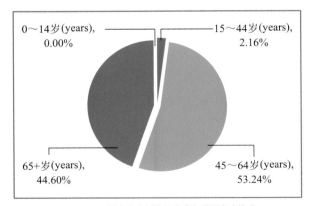

图 4-21e　福建省农村地区喉癌年龄别发病构成
Figure 4-21e　Distribution of age-specific incidence of larynx cancer
in rural areas of Fujian cancer registries

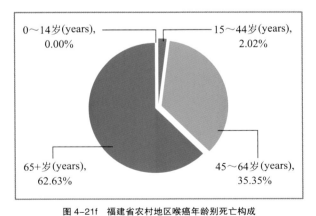

图 4-21f　福建省农村地区喉癌年龄别死亡构成
Figure 4-21f　Distribution of age-specific mortality of larynx cancer
in rural areas of Fujian cancer registries

第二十二节　骨

2019 年福建省肿瘤登记地区骨癌发病率为 0.88/10 万，中标率为 0.76/10 万，世标率为 0.75/10 万，占全部恶性肿瘤发病的 0.29%，居发病第 22 位。其中男性发病率为 0.96/10 万，女性发病率为 0.80/10 万，男性比女性高 20.00%。城市地区发病率为 0.93/10 万，农村地区发病率为 0.85/10 万，城市地区比农村地区高 9.41%，年龄标化后高 12.33%。2019 年全省估计新发骨癌 336 例，其中男性 184 例，女性 152 例。

同期肿瘤登记地区骨癌死亡率为 1.01/10 万，中标率为 0.77/10 万，世标率为 0.76/10 万，占全部恶性肿瘤死亡的 0.63%，居死亡第 21 位。其中男性死亡率为 1.25/10 万，女性死亡率为 0.76/10 万，男性比女性高 64.47%。城市地区死亡率为 1.01/10 万，农村地区死亡率为 1.02/10 万，年龄标化后城市比农村地区高 3.95%。2019 年全省估计骨癌死亡病例 399 例，其中男性 253 例，女性 146 例（表 4-22）。

Section 22　Bone

Bone cancer was the 22nd most common cancer in the registration areas of Fujian Province in 2019. The crude incidence rate was 0.88 per 100,000 (0.76 per 100,000 for ASR China and 0.75 per 100,000 for ASR World), accounting for 0.29% of all new cancer cases. The crude incidence rate was 0.96 per 100,000 for males and 0.80 per 100,000 for females, 20.00% higher for males than females. The crude incidence rate was 0.93 per 100,000 in urban areas and 0.85 per 100,000 in rural areas,9.41% higher in urban areas than in rural areas and 12.33% higher after age standardization. There were an estimated 336 new cases diagnosed as bone cancer in Fujian Province in 2019 (184 males and 152 females).

Bone cancer was the 21st most common cause of cancer deaths in the registration areas of Fujian Province in 2019. The crude mortality rate was 1.01 per 100,000 (0.77 per 100,000 for ASR China and 0.76 per 100,000 for ASR World), accounting for 0.63% of all cancer deaths. The crude mortality rate was 1.25 per 100,000 for males and 0.76 per 100,000 for females, 64.47% higher for males than females. The crude mortality rate was 1.01 per 100,000 in urban areas and 1.02 per 100,000 in rural areas,3.95% higher in urban areas than in rural areas after age standardization. There were an estimated 399 cases died of bone cancer in 2019 (253 males and 146 females)(Table 4-22).

表 4-22 2019 年福建省肿瘤登记地区骨癌发病与死亡

Table 4-22 Incidence and mortality of bone cancer in Fujian cancer registration areas, 2019

地区 Areas	性别 Sex	全省估计病例数 Estimated cases in Fujian Province	肿瘤登记地区病例数 Cases	粗率 Crude rate (1/10^5)	构成 Freq. (%)	中标率 ASR China (1/10^5)	世标率 ASR world (1/10^5)	累积率 Cum.rate (0~74, %)
发病 Incidence								
全省 All	合计 Both	336	136	0.88	0.29	0.76	0.75	0.07
	男性 Male	184	76	0.96	0.30	0.84	0.80	0.07
	女性 Female	152	60	0.80	0.28	0.70	0.70	0.06
城市 Urban areas	合计 Both	120	60	0.93	0.27	0.82	0.77	0.07
	男性 Male	79	39	1.20	0.34	1.05	0.99	0.10
	女性 Female	41	21	0.65	0.20	0.61	0.55	0.04
农村 Rural areas	合计 Both	216	76	0.85	0.30	0.73	0.74	0.06
	男性 Male	105	37	0.79	0.27	0.69	0.66	0.06
	女性 Female	111	39	0.91	0.35	0.78	0.83	0.07
死亡 Mortality								
全省 All	合计 Both	399	156	1.01	0.63	0.77	0.76	0.08
	男性 Male	253	99	1.25	0.60	1.01	0.98	0.10
	女性 Female	146	57	0.76	0.68	0.52	0.54	0.06
城市 Urban areas	合计 Both	131	65	1.01	0.62	0.79	0.76	0.06
	男性 Male	85	42	1.29	0.60	1.07	1.00	0.08
	女性 Female	46	23	0.72	0.65	0.53	0.53	0.05
农村 Rural areas	合计 Both	268	91	1.02	0.63	0.76	0.76	0.09
	男性 Male	168	57	1.22	0.59	0.98	0.97	0.11
	女性 Female	100	34	0.79	0.70	0.52	0.55	0.07

全省、城市、农村地区骨癌发病病例中，45~64 岁年龄组所占比例最大，分别为 38.97%、35.00% 和 42.11%。在全省、城市、农村地区骨癌死亡病例中，65+ 岁年龄组所占比例最大，分别为 50.64%、47.69% 和 52.75%（图 4-22a~ 图 4-22f）。

The largest proportions of bone cancer new cases in Fujian Province, urban and rural areas were at the age group of 45–64 years, with 38.97%, 35.00% and 42.11%, respectively. Among the cases of bone cancer deaths, the largest proportions were at the age group of 65+ years in Fujian Province, urban, and rural areas, with 50.64%, 47.69% and 52.75%, respectively (Figure 4-22a~4-22f).

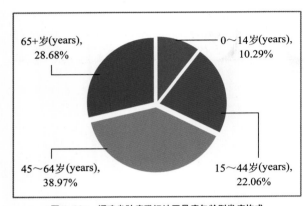

图 4-22a　福建省肿瘤登记地区骨癌年龄别发病构成
Figure 4-22a　Distribution of age-specific incidence of bone cancer in Fujian cancer registration areas

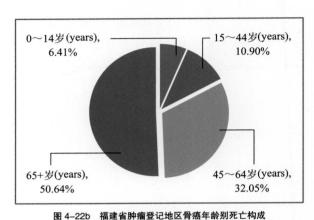

图 4-22b　福建省肿瘤登记地区骨癌年龄别死亡构成
Figure 4-22b　Distribution of age-specific mortality of bone cancer in Fujian cancer registration areas

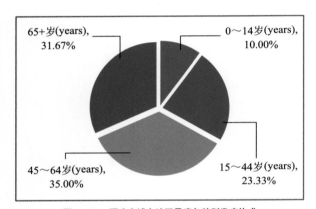

图 4-22c　福建省城市地区骨癌年龄别发病构成
Figure 4-22c　Distribution of age-specific incidence of bone cancer in urban areas of Fujian cancer registries

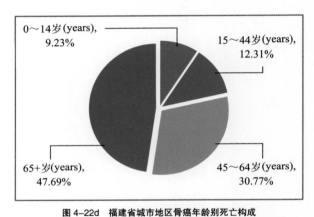

图 4-22d　福建省城市地区骨癌年龄别死亡构成
Figure 4-22d　Distribution of age-specific mortality of bone cancer in urban areas of Fujian cancer registries

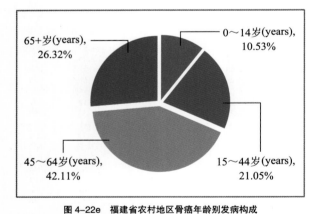

图 4-22e　福建省农村地区骨癌年龄别发病构成
Figure 4-22e　Distribution of age-specific incidence of bone cancer in rural areas of Fujian cancer registries

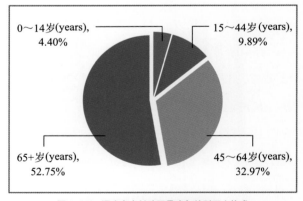

图 4-22f　福建省农村地区骨癌年龄别死亡构成
Figure 4-22f　Distribution of age-specific mortality of bone cancer in rural areas of Fujian cancer registries

附　录
Appendix

附 录 1　2019 年福建省肿瘤登记地区恶性肿瘤发病和死亡结果
Appendix 1　Cancer incidence and mortality in registration areas of Fujian, 2019

附表 1-1　2019 年福建省肿瘤登记地区男女合计发病主要指标

Appendix Table 1-1　Cancer incidence in registration areas of Fujian, both sexes in 2019

ICD10	部位 Site		发病数 Cases	构成 Freq. （%）	粗率 Crude rate （1/10⁵）	中标率 ASR China （1/10⁵）	世标率 ASR world （1/10⁵）	累积率 Cum.rate （0~74,%）
C00	唇	Lip	15	0.03	0.10	0.06	0.07	0.01
C01-C02	舌	Tongue	172	0.37	1.11	0.79	0.78	0.10
C03-C06	口	Mouth	159	0.34	1.03	0.72	0.71	0.09
C07-C08	唾液腺	Salivary glands	97	0.21	0.63	0.49	0.46	0.05
C09	扁桃体	Tonsil	30	0.06	0.19	0.14	0.13	0.01
C10	其他的口咽	Other oropharynx	46	0.10	0.30	0.20	0.20	0.03
C11	鼻咽	Nasopharynx	781	1.66	5.06	4.06	3.72	0.39
C12-C13	喉咽	Hypopharynx	94	0.20	0.61	0.41	0.42	0.05
C14	咽，部位不明	Pharynx unspecified	37	0.08	0.24	0.17	0.16	0.02
C15	食管	Esophagus	2678	5.70	17.36	11.34	11.60	1.49
C16	胃	Stomach	4368	9.30	28.31	19.28	19.13	2.46
C17	小肠	Small intestine	190	0.40	1.23	0.87	0.85	0.10
C18	结肠	Colon	2790	5.94	18.08	12.44	12.13	1.47
C19-C20	直肠	Rectum	2687	5.72	17.42	11.84	11.71	1.45
C21	肛门	Anus	31	0.07	0.20	0.14	0.13	0.02
C22	肝脏	Liver	3852	8.20	24.97	17.72	17.22	2.00
C23-C24	胆囊及其他	Gallbladder etc.	410	0.87	2.66	1.77	1.75	0.21
C25	胰腺	Pancreas	581	1.24	3.77	2.50	2.47	0.31
C30-C31	鼻，鼻窦及其他	Nose, sinuses etc.	54	0.11	0.35	0.24	0.24	0.03
C32	喉	Larynx	259	0.55	1.68	1.14	1.16	0.16
C33-C34	气管，支气管，肺	Trachea, bronchus & lung	8437	17.96	54.69	37.54	37.32	4.77
C37-C38	其他的胸腔器官	Other thoracic organs	141	0.30	0.91	0.69	0.72	0.07
C40-C41	骨	Bone	136	0.29	0.88	0.76	0.75	0.07
C43	皮肤的黑色素瘤	Melanoma of skin	67	0.14	0.43	0.31	0.29	0.04
C44	其他的皮肤	Other skin	373	0.79	2.42	1.59	1.55	0.16
C45	间皮瘤	Mesothelioma	23	0.05	0.15	0.12	0.11	0.02
C46	卡波氏肉瘤	Kaposi sarcoma	1	0.00	0.01	0.00	0.00	0.00
C47;C49	周围神经，其他结缔、软组织	Connective & soft tissue	199	0.42	1.29	1.06	0.98	0.10
C50	乳房	Breast	3105	6.66	41.37	31.56	28.78	2.93
C51	外阴	Vulva	20	0.04	0.27	0.19	0.17	0.02
C52	阴道	Vagina	34	0.07	0.45	0.31	0.31	0.05
C53	子宫颈	Cervix uteri	1509	3.21	20.11	14.66	13.79	1.50
C54	子宫体	Corpus uteri	653	1.39	8.70	6.02	5.89	0.66
C55	子宫，部位不明	Uterus unspecified	107	0.23	1.43	0.96	0.95	0.11
C56	卵巢	Ovary	453	0.96	6.04	4.65	4.46	0.48
C57	其他的女性生殖器	Other female genital organs	26	0.06	0.35	0.26	0.24	0.04
C58	胎盘	Placenta	12	0.03	0.16	0.15	0.12	0.01
C60	阴茎	Penis	46	0.10	0.58	0.42	0.40	0.05
C61	前列腺	Prostate	886	1.89	11.18	7.52	7.39	0.83
C62	睾丸	Testis	52	0.11	0.66	0.73	0.74	0.05
C63	其他的男性生殖器	Other male genital organs	19	0.04	0.24	0.21	0.19	0.02
C64	肾	Kidney	627	1.33	4.06	3.01	2.90	0.34
C65	肾盂	Renal pelvis	62	0.13	0.40	0.27	0.26	0.03
C66	输尿管	Ureter	63	0.13	0.41	0.27	0.27	0.03
C67	膀胱	Bladder	702	1.49	4.55	3.05	3.00	0.35
C68	其他的泌尿器官	Other urinary organs	25	0.05	0.16	0.11	0.11	0.01
C69	眼	Eye	16	0.03	0.10	0.09	0.12	0.01
C70-C72;D32-33;D42-43	脑，神经系统	Brain, nervous system	1340	2.85	8.69	6.88	6.65	0.69
C73	甲状腺	Thyroid	5153	10.97	33.40	29.26	25.43	2.39
C74	肾上腺	Adrenal gland	28	0.06	0.18	0.18	0.18	0.01
C75	其他的内分泌腺	Other endocrine	11	0.02	0.07	0.06	0.06	0.01
C81	霍奇金病	Hodgkin lymphoma	36	0.08	0.23	0.24	0.22	0.02
C82-C85;C96	非霍奇金淋巴瘤	Non-Hodgkin lymphoma	824	1.75	5.34	4.04	3.86	0.44
C88	免疫增生性疾病	Immunoproliferative diseases	12	0.03	0.08	0.05	0.05	0.01
C90	多发性骨髓瘤	Multiple myeloma	244	0.52	1.58	1.07	1.08	0.14
C91	淋巴样白血病	Lymphoid leukemia	201	0.43	1.30	1.18	1.43	0.10
C92-C94; D45-47	髓样白血病	Myeloid leukemia	473	1.01	3.07	2.63	2.58	0.24
C95	白血病，未特指	Leukemia unspecified	111	0.24	0.72	0.59	0.67	0.06
O&U	其他的或未指明部位	Other and unspecified	1394	2.97	9.04	6.53	6.55	0.73
ALL	所有部位合计	All sites	46975	100.00	304.50	221.59	213.81	24.63
ALLbC44	所有部位除外 C44	All sites except C44	46602	99.21	302.08	220.00	212.26	24.48

附表 1-2　2019 年福建省肿瘤登记地区男女合计死亡主要指标
Appendix Table 1-2　Cancer mortality in registration areas of Fujian, both sexes in 2019

ICD10	部位	Site	死亡数 Deaths	构成 Freq. (%)	粗率 Crude rate (1/10⁵)	中标率 ASR China (1/10⁵)	世标率 ASR world (1/10⁵)	累积率 Cum.rate (0~74, %)
C00	唇	Lip	4	0.02	0.03	0.02	0.02	0.00
C01-C02	舌	Tongue	82	0.33	0.53	0.35	0.36	0.04
C03-C06	口	Mouth	91	0.36	0.59	0.39	0.39	0.05
C07-C08	唾液腺	Salivary glands	22	0.09	0.14	0.09	0.09	0.01
C09	扁桃体	Tonsil	19	0.08	0.12	0.08	0.08	0.01
C10	其他的口咽	Other oropharynx	29	0.12	0.19	0.12	0.13	0.01
C11	鼻咽	Nasopharynx	408	1.64	2.64	1.83	1.80	0.21
C12-C13	喉咽	Hypopharynx	48	0.19	0.31	0.21	0.22	0.03
C14	咽，部位不明	Pharynx unspecified	38	0.15	0.25	0.15	0.15	0.01
C15	食管	Esophagus	2400	9.62	15.56	9.70	9.79	1.15
C16	胃	Stomach	3221	12.91	20.88	13.49	13.22	1.54
C17	小肠	Small intestine	99	0.40	0.64	0.41	0.43	0.05
C18	结肠	Colon	1168	4.68	7.57	4.91	4.78	0.53
C19-C20	直肠	Rectum	1185	4.75	7.68	4.86	4.80	0.54
C21	肛门	Anus	26	0.10	0.17	0.11	0.11	0.01
C22	肝脏	Liver	3561	14.27	23.08	15.98	15.53	1.82
C23-C24	胆囊及其他	Gallbladder etc.	310	1.24	2.01	1.27	1.28	0.16
C25	胰腺	Pancreas	572	2.29	3.71	2.41	2.37	0.28
C30-C31	鼻，鼻窦及其他	Nose, sinuses etc.	32	0.13	0.21	0.14	0.14	0.02
C32	喉	Larynx	160	0.64	1.04	0.67	0.67	0.08
C33-C34	气管，支气管，肺	Trachea, bronchus & lung	6043	24.22	39.17	25.59	25.42	3.14
C37-C38	其他的胸腔器官	Other thoracic organs	76	0.30	0.49	0.38	0.37	0.04
C40-C41	骨	Bone	156	0.63	1.01	0.77	0.76	0.08
C43	皮肤的黑色素瘤	Melanoma of skin	42	0.17	0.27	0.18	0.18	0.02
C44	其他的皮肤	Other skin	113	0.45	0.73	0.38	0.40	0.03
C45	间皮瘤	Mesothelioma	14	0.06	0.09	0.06	0.06	0.01
C46	卡波氏肉瘤	Kaposi sarcoma	1	0.00	0.01	0.00	0.00	0.00
C47;C49	周围神经，其他结缔、软组织	Connective & soft tissue	68	0.27	0.44	0.36	0.34	0.04
C50	乳房	Breast	543	2.20	7.23	5.02	4.78	0.52
C51	外阴	Vulva	12	0.05	0.16	0.10	0.09	0.01
C52	阴道	Vagina	13	0.05	0.17	0.11	0.11	0.01
C53	子宫颈	Cervix uteri	415	1.66	5.53	3.75	3.64	0.44
C54	子宫体	Corpus uteri	101	0.40	1.35	0.88	0.87	0.11
C55	子宫，部位不明	Uterus unspecified	70	0.28	0.93	0.60	0.58	0.06
C56	卵巢	Ovary	205	0.82	2.73	1.84	1.82	0.22
C57	其他的女性生殖器	Other female genital organs	14	0.06	0.19	0.12	0.12	0.02
C58	胎盘	Placenta	1	0.00	0.01	0.01	0.01	0.00
C60	阴茎	Penis	22	0.09	0.28	0.19	0.17	0.01
C61	前列腺	Prostate	347	1.39	4.38	2.65	2.68	0.21
C62	睾丸	Testis	7	0.03	0.09	0.09	0.08	0.01
C63	其他的男性生殖器	Other male genital organs	3	0.01	0.04	0.03	0.03	0.00
C64	肾	Kidney	171	0.69	1.11	0.72	0.73	0.09
C65	肾盂	Renal pelvis	26	0.10	0.17	0.11	0.11	0.01
C66	输尿管	Ureter	36	0.14	0.23	0.14	0.14	0.01
C67	膀胱	Bladder	228	0.91	1.48	0.85	0.84	0.08
C68	其他的泌尿器官	Other urinary organs	11	0.04	0.07	0.04	0.04	0.00
C69	眼	Eye	12	0.05	0.08	0.06	0.11	0.01
C70-C72;D32-33;D42-43	脑，神经系统	Brain, nervous system	580	2.32	3.76	2.80	2.78	0.30
C73	甲状腺	Thyroid	108	0.43	0.70	0.46	0.46	0.05
C74	肾上腺	Adrenal gland	21	0.08	0.14	0.10	0.12	0.01
C75	其他的内分泌腺	Other endocrine	5	0.02	0.03	0.02	0.03	0.00
C81	霍奇金病	Hodgkin lymphoma	11	0.04	0.07	0.04	0.05	0.01
C82-C85;C96	非霍奇金淋巴瘤	Non-Hodgkin lymphoma	386	1.55	2.50	1.75	1.71	0.19
C88	免疫增生性疾病	Immunoproliferative diseases	4	0.02	0.03	0.02	0.02	0.00
C90	多发性骨髓瘤	Multiple myeloma	126	0.50	0.82	0.55	0.54	0.07
C91	淋巴样白血病	Lymphoid leukemia	81	0.32	0.53	0.46	0.50	0.04
C92-C94; D45-47	髓样白血病	Myeloid leukemia	266	1.07	1.72	1.33	1.30	0.13
C95	白血病，未特指	Leukemia unspecified	183	0.73	1.19	0.93	0.98	0.09
O&U	其他的或未指明部位	Other and unspecified	951	3.81	6.16	4.24	4.21	0.49
ALL	所有部位合计	All sites	24953	100.00	161.75	107.18	105.99	12.30
ALLbC44	所有部位除外 C44	All sites except C44	24840	99.55	161.01	106.80	105.59	12.28

附表 1-3　2019 年福建省肿瘤登记地区男性发病主要指标

Appendix Table 1-3　Cancer incidence in registration areas of Fujian, male in 2019

ICD10	部位 Site	发病数 Cases	构成 Freq.（%）	粗率 Crude rate（1/10⁵）	中标率 ASR China（1/10⁵）	世标率 ASR world（1/10⁵）	累积率 Cum.rate（0~74,%）
C00	唇 Lip	8	0.03	0.10	0.06	0.07	0.01
C01-C02	舌 Tongue	109	0.43	1.38	1.01	1.00	0.12
C03-C06	口 Mouth	108	0.43	1.36	0.96	0.98	0.13
C07-C08	唾液腺 Salivary glands	58	0.23	0.73	0.57	0.55	0.06
C09	扁桃体 Tonsil	22	0.09	0.28	0.21	0.19	0.02
C10	其他的口咽 Other oropharynx	36	0.14	0.45	0.32	0.32	0.04
C11	鼻咽 Nasopharynx	598	2.37	7.55	6.12	5.64	0.60
C12-C13	喉咽 Hypopharynx	90	0.36	1.14	0.79	0.82	0.11
C14	咽，部位不明 Pharynx unspecified	29	0.11	0.37	0.25	0.25	0.03
C15	食管 Esophagus	1939	7.68	24.48	16.69	17.20	2.16
C16	胃 Stomach	3130	12.39	39.51	27.76	27.85	3.62
C17	小肠 Small intestine	116	0.46	1.46	1.05	1.03	0.12
C18	结肠 Colon	1619	6.41	20.44	14.61	14.35	1.77
C19-C20	直肠 Rectum	1647	6.52	20.79	14.61	14.58	1.81
C21	肛门 Anus	14	0.06	0.18	0.12	0.13	0.02
C22	肝脏 Liver	3097	12.26	39.09	28.79	28.00	3.25
C23-C24	胆囊及其他 Gallbladder etc.	205	0.81	2.59	1.81	1.78	0.21
C25	胰腺 Pancreas	369	1.46	4.66	3.22	3.23	0.40
C30-C31	鼻，鼻窦及其他 Nose, sinuses etc.	37	0.15	0.47	0.34	0.34	0.04
C32	喉 Larynx	250	0.99	3.16	2.22	2.26	0.30
C33-C34	气管，支气管，肺 Trachea, bronchus & lung	5375	21.28	67.85	47.88	47.97	6.26
C37-C38	其他的胸腔器官 Other thoracic organs	83	0.33	1.05	0.82	0.85	0.09
C40-C41	骨 Bone	76	0.30	0.96	0.84	0.80	0.07
C43	皮肤的黑色素瘤 Melanoma of skin	32	0.13	0.40	0.29	0.28	0.03
C44	其他的皮肤 Other skin	167	0.66	2.11	1.50	1.45	0.16
C45	间皮瘤 Mesothelioma	16	0.06	0.20	0.16	0.15	0.02
C46	卡波氏肉瘤 Kaposi sarcoma	1	0.00	0.01	0.01	0.01	0.00
C47;C49	周围神经, 其他结缔、软组织 Connective & soft tissue	109	0.43	1.38	1.16	1.09	0.11
C50	乳房 Breast	23	0.09	0.29	0.22	0.20	0.03
C51	外阴 Vulva	-	-	-	-	-	-
C52	阴道 Vagina	-	-	-	-	-	-
C53	子宫颈 Cervix uteri	-	-	-	-	-	-
C54	子宫体 Corpus uteri	-	-	-	-	-	-
C55	子宫，部位不明 Uterus unspecified	-	-	-	-	-	-
C56	卵巢 Ovary	-	-	-	-	-	-
C57	其他的女性生殖器 Other female genital organs	-	-	-	-	-	-
C58	胎盘 Placenta	-	-	-	-	-	-
C60	阴茎 Penis	46	0.18	0.58	0.42	0.40	0.05
C61	前列腺 Prostate	886	3.51	11.18	7.52	7.39	0.83
C62	睾丸 Testis	52	0.21	0.66	0.73	0.74	0.05
C63	其他的男性生殖器 Other male genital organs	19	0.08	0.24	0.21	0.19	0.02
C64	肾 Kidney	427	1.69	5.39	4.09	3.96	0.46
C65	肾盂 Renal pelvis	40	0.16	0.50	0.35	0.35	0.04
C66	输尿管 Ureter	42	0.17	0.53	0.37	0.37	0.04
C67	膀胱 Bladder	571	2.26	7.21	5.07	4.99	0.58
C68	其他的泌尿器官 Other urinary organs	18	0.07	0.23	0.17	0.16	0.02
C69	眼 Eye	10	0.04	0.13	0.10	0.10	0.01
C70-C72;D32-33;D42-43	脑，神经系统 Brain, nervous system	598	2.37	7.55	6.28	6.11	0.61
C73	甲状腺 Thyroid	1263	5.00	15.94	14.36	12.47	1.18
C74	肾上腺 Adrenal gland	19	0.08	0.24	0.18	0.22	0.02
C75	其他的内分泌腺 Other endocrine	3	0.01	0.04	0.03	0.04	0.00
C81	霍奇金病 Hodgkin lymphoma	26	0.10	0.33	0.33	0.32	0.02
C82-C85;C96	非霍奇金淋巴瘤 Non-Hodgkin lymphoma	485	1.92	6.12	4.77	4.58	0.53
C88	免疫增生性疾病 Immunoproliferative diseases	9	0.04	0.11	0.08	0.08	0.01
C90	多发性骨髓瘤 Multiple myeloma	139	0.55	1.75	1.23	1.25	0.16
C91	淋巴样白血病 Lymphoid leukemia	126	0.50	1.59	1.42	1.69	0.13
C92-C94; D45-47	髓样白血病 Myeloid leukemia	256	1.01	3.23	2.75	2.74	0.26
C95	白血病，未特指 Leukemia unspecified	68	0.27	0.86	0.72	0.79	0.07
O&U	其他的或未指明部位 Other and unspecified	789	3.12	9.96	7.41	7.46	0.83
ALL	所有部位合计 All sites	25255	100.00	318.81	232.99	229.78	27.49
ALLbC44	所有部位除外 C44 All sites except C44	25088	99.34	316.70	231.48	228.32	27.33

113

附表 1-4　2019 年福建省肿瘤登记地区男性死亡主要指标
Appendix Table 1-4　Cancer mortality in registration areas of Fujian, male in 2019

ICD10	部位 Site	死亡数 Deaths	构成 Freq. (%)	粗率 Crude rate (1/10⁵)	中标率 ASR China (1/10⁵)	世标率 ASR world (1/10⁵)	累积率 Cum.rate (0~74,%)
C00	唇 Lip	4	0.02	0.05	0.03	0.04	0.00
C01-C02	舌 Tongue	52	0.31	0.66	0.45	0.47	0.06
C03-C06	口 Mouth	61	0.37	0.77	0.53	0.54	0.07
C07-C08	唾液腺 Salivary glands	15	0.09	0.19	0.13	0.13	0.01
C09	扁桃体 Tonsil	18	0.11	0.23	0.16	0.16	0.02
C10	其他的口咽 Other oropharynx	24	0.14	0.30	0.20	0.21	0.02
C11	鼻咽 Nasopharynx	297	1.79	3.75	2.69	2.67	0.32
C12-C13	喉咽 Hypopharynx	48	0.29	0.61	0.43	0.43	0.06
C14	咽，部位不明 Pharynx unspecified	22	0.13	0.28	0.19	0.20	0.02
C15	食管 Esophagus	1672	10.09	21.11	14.07	14.36	1.69
C16	胃 Stomach	2283	13.77	28.82	19.73	19.44	2.26
C17	小肠 Small intestine	57	0.34	0.72	0.50	0.51	0.06
C18	结肠 Colon	663	4.00	8.37	5.77	5.67	0.62
C19-C20	直肠 Rectum	728	4.39	9.19	6.17	6.14	0.68
C21	肛门 Anus	14	0.08	0.18	0.11	0.12	0.01
C22	肝脏 Liver	2806	16.93	35.42	25.78	25.06	2.94
C23-C24	胆囊及其他 Gallbladder etc.	158	0.95	1.99	1.36	1.37	0.17
C25	胰腺 Pancreas	358	2.16	4.52	3.10	3.08	0.36
C30-C31	鼻，鼻窦及其他 Nose, sinuses etc.	25	0.15	0.32	0.23	0.23	0.03
C32	喉 Larynx	145	0.87	1.83	1.24	1.26	0.16
C33-C34	气管，支气管，肺 Trachea, bronchus & lung	4524	27.29	57.11	39.31	39.21	4.88
C37-C38	其他的胸腔器官 Other thoracic organs	54	0.33	0.68	0.55	0.54	0.06
C40-C41	骨 Bone	99	0.60	1.25	1.01	0.98	0.10
C43	皮肤的黑色素瘤 Melanoma of skin	24	0.14	0.30	0.22	0.22	0.03
C44	其他的皮肤 Other skin	54	0.33	0.68	0.42	0.42	0.04
C45	间皮瘤 Mesothelioma	12	0.07	0.15	0.11	0.10	0.01
C46	卡波氏肉瘤 Kaposi sarcoma	1	0.01	0.01	0.01	0.01	0.00
C47;C49	周围神经,其他结缔、软组织 Connective & soft tissue	44	0.27	0.56	0.47	0.45	0.05
C50	乳房 Breast	6	0.04	0.08	0.05	0.05	0.01
C51	外阴 Vulva	—	—	—	—	—	—
C52	阴道 Vagina	—	—	—	—	—	—
C53	子宫颈 Cervix uteri	—	—	—	—	—	—
C54	子宫体 Corpus uteri	—	—	—	—	—	—
C55	子宫，部位不明 Uterus unspecified	—	—	—	—	—	—
C56	卵巢 Ovary	—	—	—	—	—	—
C57	其他的女性生殖器 Other female genital organs	—	—	—	—	—	—
C58	胎盘 Placenta	—	—	—	—	—	—
C60	阴茎 Penis	22	0.13	0.28	0.19	0.17	0.01
C61	前列腺 Prostate	347	2.09	4.38	2.65	2.68	0.21
C62	睾丸 Testis	7	0.04	0.09	0.09	0.08	0.01
C63	其他的男性生殖器 Other male genital organs	3	0.02	0.04	0.03	0.03	0.00
C64	肾 Kidney	123	0.74	1.55	1.07	1.06	0.13
C65	肾盂 Renal pelvis	18	0.11	0.23	0.15	0.15	0.02
C66	输尿管 Ureter	20	0.12	0.25	0.17	0.15	0.01
C67	膀胱 Bladder	180	1.09	2.27	1.42	1.43	0.14
C68	其他的泌尿器官 Other urinary organs	5	0.03	0.06	0.04	0.04	0.00
C69	眼 Eye	4	0.02	0.05	0.04	0.07	0.00
C70-C72;D32-33;D42-43	脑，神经系统 Brain, nervous system	339	2.05	4.28	3.32	3.30	0.36
C73	甲状腺 Thyroid	50	0.30	0.63	0.45	0.45	0.05
C74	肾上腺 Adrenal gland	9	0.05	0.11	0.08	0.09	0.01
C75	其他的内分泌腺 Other endocrine	3	0.02	0.04	0.03	0.05	0.00
C81	霍奇金病 Hodgkin lymphoma	9	0.05	0.11	0.07	0.08	0.01
C82-C85;C96	非霍奇金淋巴瘤 Non-Hodgkin lymphoma	235	1.42	2.97	2.20	2.12	0.26
C88	免疫增生性疾病 Immunoproliferative diseases	2	0.01	0.03	0.01	0.02	0.00
C90	多发性骨髓瘤 Multiple myeloma	74	0.45	0.93	0.65	0.65	0.08
C91	淋巴样白血病 Lymphoid leukemia	50	0.30	0.63	0.56	0.56	0.05
C92-C94; D45-47	髓样白血病 Myeloid leukemia	148	0.89	1.87	1.48	1.43	0.14
C95	白血病，未特指 Leukemia unspecified	100	0.60	1.26	1.00	1.01	0.10
O&U	其他的或未指明部位 Other and unspecified	559	3.37	7.06	5.09	5.09	0.58
ALL	所有部位合计 All sites	16575	100.00	209.23	145.81	144.83	16.90
ALLbC44	所有部位除外 C44 All sites except C44	16521	99.67	208.55	145.39	144.41	16.86

附表 1-5　2019 年福建省肿瘤登记地区女性发病主要指标

Appendix Table 1-5　Cancer incidence in registration areas of Fujian, female in 2019

ICD10	部位 Site		发病数 Cases	构成 Freq. （%）	粗率 Crude rate （1/10⁵）	中标率 ASR China （1/10⁵）	世标率 ASR world （1/10⁵）	累积率 Cum.rate （0~74，%）
C00	唇	Lip	7	0.03	0.09	0.06	0.06	0.01
C01-C02	舌	Tongue	63	0.29	0.84	0.57	0.56	0.07
C03-C06	口	Mouth	51	0.23	0.68	0.49	0.45	0.05
C07-C08	唾液腺	Salivary glands	39	0.18	0.52	0.42	0.38	0.04
C09	扁桃体	Tonsil	8	0.04	0.11	0.07	0.07	0.01
C10	其他的口咽	Other oropharynx	10	0.05	0.13	0.09	0.09	0.01
C11	鼻咽	Nasopharynx	183	0.84	2.44	1.99	1.79	0.19
C12-C13	喉咽	Hypopharynx	4	0.02	0.05	0.04	0.04	0.00
C14	咽，部位不明	Pharynx unspecified	8	0.04	0.11	0.08	0.07	0.01
C15	食管	Esophagus	739	3.40	9.85	6.09	6.12	0.81
C16	胃	Stomach	1238	5.70	16.49	11.04	10.68	1.30
C17	小肠	Small intestine	74	0.34	0.99	0.70	0.68	0.08
C18	结肠	Colon	1171	5.39	15.60	10.33	9.97	1.18
C19-C20	直肠	Rectum	1040	4.79	13.86	9.16	8.93	1.11
C21	肛门	Anus	17	0.08	0.23	0.15	0.13	0.01
C22	肝脏	Liver	755	3.48	10.06	6.74	6.53	0.75
C23-C24	胆囊及其他	Gallbladder etc.	205	0.94	2.73	1.73	1.73	0.21
C25	胰腺	Pancreas	212	0.98	2.82	1.80	1.75	0.22
C30-C31	鼻，鼻窦及其他	Nose, sinuses etc.	17	0.08	0.23	0.15	0.14	0.02
C32	喉	Larynx	9	0.04	0.12	0.08	0.08	0.01
C33-C34	气管，支气管，肺	Trachea, bronchus & lung	3062	14.10	40.80	27.54	26.99	3.29
C37-C38	其他的胸腔器官	Other thoracic organs	58	0.27	0.77	0.56	0.57	0.06
C40-C41	骨	Bone	60	0.28	0.80	0.70	0.70	0.06
C43	皮肤的黑色素瘤	Melanoma of skin	35	0.16	0.47	0.32	0.31	0.04
C44	其他的皮肤	Other skin	206	0.95	2.74	1.66	1.64	0.16
C45	间皮瘤	Mesothelioma	7	0.03	0.09	0.08	0.07	0.01
C46	卡波氏肉瘤	Kaposi sarcoma	0	0.00	0.00	0.00	0.00	0.00
C47;C49	周围神经，其他结缔、软组织	Connective & soft tissue	90	0.41	1.20	0.95	0.86	0.10
C50	乳房	Breast	3105	14.30	41.37	31.56	28.78	2.93
C51	外阴	Vulva	20	0.09	0.27	0.19	0.17	0.02
C52	阴道	Vagina	34	0.16	0.45	0.31	0.31	0.05
C53	子宫颈	Cervix uteri	1509	6.95	20.11	14.66	13.79	1.50
C54	子宫体	Corpus uteri	653	3.01	8.70	6.02	5.89	0.66
C55	子宫，部位不明	Uterus unspecified	107	0.49	1.43	0.96	0.95	0.11
C56	卵巢	Ovary	453	2.09	6.04	4.65	4.46	0.48
C57	其他的女性生殖器	Other female genital organs	26	0.12	0.35	0.26	0.24	0.04
C58	胎盘	Placenta	12	0.06	0.16	0.15	0.12	0.01
C60	阴茎	Penis	-	-	-	-	-	-
C61	前列腺	Prostate	-	-	-	-	-	-
C62	睾丸	Testis	-	-	-	-	-	-
C63	其他的男性生殖器	Other male genital organs	-	-	-	-	-	-
C64	肾	Kidney	200	0.92	2.66	1.93	1.85	0.21
C65	肾盂	Renal pelvis	22	0.10	0.29	0.19	0.19	0.03
C66	输尿管	Ureter	21	0.10	0.28	0.17	0.17	0.02
C67	膀胱	Bladder	131	0.60	1.75	1.08	1.07	0.13
C68	其他的泌尿器官	Other urinary organs	7	0.03	0.09	0.05	0.05	0.00
C69	眼	Eye	6	0.03	0.08	0.08	0.14	0.01
C70-C72;D32-33;D42-43	脑，神经系统	Brain, nervous system	742	3.42	9.89	7.46	7.16	0.77
C73	甲状腺	Thyroid	3890	17.91	51.83	44.54	38.72	3.61
C74	肾上腺	Adrenal gland	9	0.04	0.12	0.09	0.14	0.01
C75	其他的内分泌腺	Other endocrine	8	0.04	0.11	0.09	0.08	0.01
C81	霍奇金病	Hodgkin lymphoma	10	0.05	0.13	0.15	0.13	0.01
C82-C85;C96	非霍奇金淋巴瘤	Non-Hodgkin lymphoma	339	1.56	4.52	3.30	3.14	0.36
C88	免疫增生性疾病	Immunoproliferative diseases	3	0.01	0.04	0.03	0.03	0.00
C90	多发性骨髓瘤	Multiple myeloma	105	0.48	1.40	0.92	0.92	0.12
C91	淋巴样白血病	Lymphoid leukemia	75	0.35	1.00	0.92	1.14	0.08
C92-C94;D45-47	髓样白血病	Myeloid leukemia	217	1.00	2.89	2.51	2.41	0.21
C95	白血病，未特指	Leukemia unspecified	43	0.20	0.57	0.46	0.55	0.05
O&U	其他的或未指明部位	Other and unspecified	605	2.79	8.06	5.67	5.67	0.63
ALL	所有部位合计	All sites	21720	100.00	289.39	211.99	199.68	21.84
ALLbC44	所有部位除外 C44	All sites except C44	21514	99.05	286.65	210.33	198.04	21.68

附表 1-6　2019 年福建省肿瘤登记地区女性死亡主要指标

Appendix Table 1-6　Cancer mortality in registration areas of Fujian, female in 2019

ICD10	部位 Site		死亡数 Deaths	构成 Freq. （%）	粗率 Crude rate （1/10⁵）	中标率 ASR China （1/10⁵）	世标率 ASR world （1/10⁵）	累积率 Cum.rate （0~74,%）
C00	唇	Lip	0	0.00	0.00	0.00	0.00	0.00
C01-C02	舌	Tongue	30	0.36	0.40	0.25	0.25	0.03
C03-C06	口	Mouth	30	0.36	0.40	0.24	0.23	0.03
C07-C08	唾液腺	Salivary glands	7	0.08	0.09	0.04	0.04	0.00
C09	扁桃体	Tonsil	1	0.01	0.01	0.01	0.01	0.00
C10	其他的口咽	Other oropharynx	5	0.06	0.07	0.04	0.04	0.00
C11	鼻咽	Nasopharynx	111	1.32	1.48	0.98	0.94	0.11
C12-C13	喉咽	Hypopharynx	0	0.00	0.00	0.00	0.00	0.00
C14	咽，部位不明	Pharynx unspecified	16	0.19	0.21	0.10	0.10	0.01
C15	食管	Esophagus	728	8.69	9.70	5.46	5.39	0.61
C16	胃	Stomach	938	11.20	12.50	7.53	7.31	0.82
C17	小肠	Small intestine	42	0.50	0.56	0.32	0.35	0.04
C18	结肠	Colon	505	6.03	6.73	4.07	3.94	0.44
C19-C20	直肠	Rectum	457	5.45	6.09	3.62	3.53	0.40
C21	肛门	Anus	12	0.14	0.16	0.10	0.10	0.01
C22	肝脏	Liver	755	9.01	10.06	6.27	6.11	0.70
C23-C24	胆囊及其他	Gallbladder etc.	152	1.81	2.03	1.18	1.21	0.15
C25	胰腺	Pancreas	214	2.55	2.85	1.75	1.68	0.19
C30-C31	鼻，鼻窦及其他	Nose, sinuses etc.	7	0.08	0.09	0.06	0.06	0.01
C32	喉	Larynx	15	0.18	0.20	0.11	0.11	0.01
C33-C34	气管，支气管，肺	Trachea, bronchus & lung	1519	18.13	20.24	12.34	12.14	1.41
C37-C38	其他的胸腔器官	Other thoracic organs	22	0.26	0.29	0.19	0.19	0.02
C40-C41	骨	Bone	57	0.68	0.76	0.52	0.54	0.06
C43	皮肤的黑色素瘤	Melanoma of skin	18	0.21	0.24	0.15	0.15	0.02
C44	其他的皮肤	Other skin	59	0.70	0.79	0.34	0.37	0.02
C45	间皮瘤	Mesothelioma	2	0.02	0.03	0.02	0.02	0.00
C46	卡波氏肉瘤	Kaposi sarcoma	0	0.00	0.00	0.00	0.00	0.00
C47;C49	周围神经,其它结缔、软组织	Connective & soft tissue	24	0.29	0.32	0.25	0.23	0.02
C50	乳房	Breast	543	6.48	7.23	5.02	4.78	0.52
C51	外阴	Vulva	12	0.14	0.16	0.10	0.09	0.01
C52	阴道	Vagina	13	0.16	0.17	0.11	0.11	0.01
C53	子宫颈	Cervix uteri	415	4.95	5.53	3.75	3.64	0.44
C54	子宫体	Corpus uteri	101	1.21	1.35	0.88	0.87	0.11
C55	子宫，部位不明	Uterus unspecified	70	0.84	0.93	0.60	0.58	0.06
C56	卵巢	Ovary	205	2.45	2.73	1.84	1.82	0.22
C57	其他的女性生殖器	Other female genital organs	14	0.17	0.19	0.12	0.12	0.02
C58	胎盘	Placenta	1	0.01	0.01	0.01	0.01	0.00
C60	阴茎	Penis	-	-	-	-	-	-
C61	前列腺	Prostate	-	-	-	-	-	-
C62	睾丸	Testis	-	-	-	-	-	-
C63	其他的男性生殖器	Other male genital organs	-	-	-	-	-	-
C64	肾	Kidney	48	0.57	0.64	0.40	0.41	0.05
C65	肾盂	Renal pelvis	8	0.10	0.11	0.06	0.06	0.01
C66	输尿管	Ureter	16	0.19	0.21	0.12	0.12	0.02
C67	膀胱	Bladder	48	0.57	0.64	0.33	0.32	0.02
C68	其他的泌尿器官	Other urinary organs	6	0.07	0.08	0.04	0.04	0.00
C69	眼	Eye	8	0.10	0.11	0.09	0.15	0.01
C70-C72;D32-33;D42-43	脑，神经系统	Brain, nervous system	241	2.88	3.21	2.29	2.26	0.24
C73	甲状腺	Thyroid	58	0.69	0.77	0.47	0.47	0.05
C74	肾上腺	Adrenal gland	12	0.14	0.16	0.12	0.15	0.01
C75	其他的内分泌腺	Other endocrine	2	0.02	0.03	0.01	0.01	0.00
C81	霍奇金病	Hodgkin lymphoma	2	0.02	0.03	0.02	0.02	0.01
C82-C85;C96	非霍奇金淋巴瘤	Non-Hodgkin lymphoma	151	1.80	2.01	1.30	1.29	0.13
C88	免疫增生性疾病	Immunoproliferative diseases	2	0.02	0.03	0.02	0.02	0.00
C90	多发性骨髓瘤	Multiple myeloma	52	0.62	0.69	0.44	0.43	0.05
C91	淋巴样白血病	Lymphoid leukemia	31	0.37	0.41	0.36	0.39	0.03
C92-C94;D45-47	髓样白血病	Myeloid leukemia	118	1.41	1.57	1.18	1.16	0.12
C95	白血病，未特指	Leukemia unspecified	83	0.99	1.11	0.88	0.98	0.08
O&U	其他的或未指明部位	Other and unspecified	392	4.68	5.22	3.39	3.34	0.39
ALL	所有部位合计	All sites	8378	100.00	111.63	69.90	68.68	7.73
ALLbC44	所有部位除外 C44	All sites except C44	8319	99.30	110.84	69.56	68.32	7.71

附表 1-7　2019 年福建省城市肿瘤登记地区男女合计发病主要指标

Appendix Table 1-7　Cancer incidence in urban registration areas of Fujian, both sexes in 2019

ICD10	部位 Site		发病数 Cases	构成 Freq. (%)	粗率 Crude rate (1/10^5)	中标率 ASR China (1/10^5)	世标率 ASR world (1/10^5)	累积率 Cum.rate (0~74, %)
C00	唇	Lip	5	0.02	0.08	0.05	0.05	0.01
C01-C02	舌	Tongue	95	0.43	1.47	1.03	1.00	0.12
C03-C06	口	Mouth	74	0.34	1.14	0.81	0.80	0.11
C07-C08	唾液腺	Salivary glands	45	0.21	0.70	0.52	0.49	0.05
C09	扁桃体	Tonsil	15	0.07	0.23	0.16	0.15	0.01
C10	其他的口咽	Other oropharynx	27	0.12	0.42	0.28	0.29	0.04
C11	鼻咽	Nasopharynx	285	1.30	4.41	3.46	3.23	0.36
C12-C13	喉咽	Hypopharynx	37	0.17	0.57	0.39	0.40	0.05
C14	咽,部位不明	Pharynx unspecified	19	0.09	0.29	0.19	0.19	0.02
C15	食管	Esophagus	1141	5.20	17.65	11.42	11.61	1.45
C16	胃	Stomach	1853	8.45	28.67	19.01	18.97	2.42
C17	小肠	Small intestine	87	0.40	1.35	0.96	0.92	0.11
C18	结肠	Colon	1364	6.22	21.10	14.18	13.86	1.68
C19-C20	直肠	Rectum	1217	5.55	18.83	12.55	12.44	1.51
C21	肛门	Anus	15	0.07	0.23	0.15	0.15	0.02
C22	肝脏	Liver	1726	7.87	26.70	18.54	18.11	2.08
C23-C24	胆囊及其他	Gallbladder etc.	173	0.79	2.68	1.74	1.73	0.22
C25	胰腺	Pancreas	272	1.24	4.21	2.76	2.71	0.33
C30-C31	鼻,鼻窦及其他	Nose, sinuses etc.	27	0.12	0.42	0.29	0.28	0.03
C32	喉	Larynx	120	0.55	1.86	1.25	1.26	0.17
C33-C34	气管,支气管,肺	Trachea, bronchus & lung	3990	18.19	61.73	41.80	41.45	5.26
C37-C38	其他的胸腔器官	Other thoracic organs	71	0.32	1.10	0.84	0.86	0.09
C40-C41	骨	Bone	60	0.27	0.93	0.82	0.77	0.07
C43	皮肤的黑色素瘤	Melanoma of skin	32	0.15	0.50	0.34	0.34	0.04
C44	其他的皮肤	Other skin	170	0.77	2.63	1.75	1.73	0.18
C45	间皮瘤	Mesothelioma	12	0.05	0.19	0.15	0.14	0.02
C46	卡波氏肉瘤	Kaposi sarcoma	1	0.00	0.02	0.00	0.01	0.00
C47;C49	周围神经,其他结缔、软组织	Connective & soft tissue	79	0.36	1.22	0.98	0.91	0.10
C50	乳房	Breast	1594	7.31	49.67	37.39	34.32	3.53
C51	外阴	Vulva	6	0.03	0.19	0.12	0.11	0.01
C52	阴道	Vagina	15	0.07	0.47	0.32	0.32	0.06
C53	子宫颈	Cervix uteri	583	2.66	18.17	13.48	12.48	1.34
C54	子宫体	Corpus uteri	287	1.31	8.94	6.26	6.14	0.72
C55	子宫,部位不明	Uterus unspecified	62	0.28	1.93	1.29	1.29	0.15
C56	卵巢	Ovary	206	0.94	6.42	4.94	4.73	0.49
C57	其他的女性生殖器	Other female genital organs	10	0.05	0.31	0.22	0.21	0.03
C58	胎盘	Placenta	5	0.02	0.16	0.14	0.12	0.01
C60	阴茎	Penis	17	0.08	0.52	0.38	0.36	0.04
C61	前列腺	Prostate	445	2.03	13.67	8.89	8.70	0.96
C62	睾丸	Testis	27	0.12	0.83	0.96	0.99	0.06
C63	其他的男性生殖器	Other male genital organs	11	0.05	0.34	0.30	0.27	0.02
C64	肾	Kidney	314	1.43	4.86	3.54	3.39	0.37
C65	肾盂	Renal pelvis	27	0.12	0.42	0.27	0.26	0.03
C66	输尿管	Ureter	31	0.14	0.48	0.31	0.30	0.03
C67	膀胱	Bladder	334	1.52	5.17	3.40	3.34	0.39
C68	其他的泌尿器官	Other urinary organs	12	0.05	0.19	0.12	0.12	0.01
C69	眼	Eye	6	0.03	0.09	0.07	0.08	0.01
C70-C72;D32-33;D42-43	脑,神经系统	Brain, nervous system	640	2.92	9.90	7.76	7.49	0.79
C73	甲状腺	Thyroid	2819	12.85	43.61	37.91	33.06	3.10
C74	肾上腺	Adrenal gland	13	0.06	0.20	0.14	0.16	0.01
C75	其他的内分泌腺	Other endocrine	8	0.04	0.12	0.11	0.11	0.01
C81	霍奇金病	Hodgkin lymphoma	22	0.10	0.34	0.38	0.34	0.02
C82-C85;C96	非霍奇金淋巴瘤	Non-Hodgkin lymphoma	386	1.76	5.97	4.39	4.26	0.50
C88	免疫增生性疾病	Immunoproliferative diseases	5	0.02	0.08	0.05	0.05	0.01
C90	多发性骨髓瘤	Multiple myeloma	139	0.63	2.15	1.43	1.43	0.16
C91	淋巴样白血病	Lymphoid leukemia	99	0.45	1.53	1.35	1.56	0.12
C92-C94; D45-47	髓样白血病	Myeloid leukemia	202	0.92	3.12	2.64	2.61	0.26
C95	白血病,未特指	Leukemia unspecified	51	0.23	0.79	0.60	0.68	0.07
O&U	其他的或未指明部位	Other and unspecified	541	2.47	8.37	5.87	5.88	0.66
ALL	所有部位合计	All sites	21939	100.00	339.40	244.36	235.16	26.82
ALLbC44	所有部位除外 C44	All sites except C44	21769	99.23	336.77	242.61	233.43	26.64

附表 1-8　2019 年福建省城市肿瘤登记地区男女合计死亡主要指标

Appendix Table 1-8　Cancer mortality in urban registration areas of Fujian, both sexes in 2019

ICD10	部位 Site	死亡数 Deaths	构成 Freq.（%）	粗率 Crude rate（1/10⁵）	中标率 ASR China（1/10⁵）	世标率 ASR world（1/10⁵）	累积率 Cum.rate（0~74,%）
C00	唇 Lip	0	0.00	0.00	0.00	0.00	0.00
C01-C02	舌 Tongue	44	0.42	0.68	0.44	0.45	0.05
C03-C06	口 Mouth	39	0.37	0.60	0.39	0.40	0.05
C07-C08	唾液腺 Salivary glands	14	0.13	0.22	0.13	0.13	0.01
C09	扁桃体 Tonsil	9	0.09	0.14	0.09	0.09	0.01
C10	其他的口咽 Other oropharynx	16	0.15	0.25	0.16	0.17	0.02
C11	鼻咽 Nasopharynx	173	1.64	2.68	1.82	1.82	0.22
C12-C13	喉咽 Hypopharynx	29	0.28	0.45	0.31	0.31	0.04
C14	咽，部位不明 Pharynx unspecified	20	0.19	0.31	0.18	0.18	0.01
C15	食管 Esophagus	898	8.53	13.89	8.56	8.71	1.04
C16	胃 Stomach	1295	12.31	20.03	12.73	12.44	1.43
C17	小肠 Small intestine	53	0.50	0.82	0.51	0.54	0.07
C18	结肠 Colon	545	5.18	8.43	5.21	5.16	0.58
C19-C20	直肠 Rectum	507	4.82	7.84	4.87	4.79	0.53
C21	肛门 Anus	10	0.10	0.15	0.09	0.10	0.01
C22	肝脏 Liver	1445	13.73	22.35	15.15	14.80	1.72
C23-C24	胆囊及其他 Gallbladder etc.	138	1.31	2.13	1.34	1.36	0.17
C25	胰腺 Pancreas	253	2.40	3.91	2.51	2.47	0.29
C30-C31	鼻，鼻窦及其他 Nose, sinuses etc.	13	0.12	0.20	0.14	0.14	0.02
C32	喉 Larynx	61	0.58	0.94	0.60	0.61	0.08
C33-C34	气管，支气管，肺 Trachea, bronchus & lung	2528	24.02	39.11	25.01	24.86	3.04
C37-C38	其他的胸腔器官 Other thoracic organs	44	0.42	0.68	0.51	0.49	0.05
C40-C41	骨 Bone	65	0.62	1.01	0.79	0.76	0.06
C43	皮肤的黑色素瘤 Melanoma of skin	26	0.25	0.40	0.28	0.27	0.04
C44	其他的皮肤 Other skin	43	0.41	0.67	0.32	0.35	0.02
C45	间皮瘤 Mesothelioma	9	0.09	0.14	0.08	0.09	0.01
C46	卡波氏肉瘤 Kaposi sarcoma	0	0.00	0.00	0.00	0.00	0.00
C47;C49	周围神经，其他结缔、软组织 Connective & soft tissue	28	0.27	0.43	0.38	0.35	0.04
C50	乳房 Breast	277	2.66	8.63	5.90	5.64	0.60
C51	外阴 Vulva	7	0.07	0.22	0.13	0.12	0.01
C52	阴道 Vagina	4	0.04	0.12	0.09	0.08	0.01
C53	子宫颈 Cervix uteri	142	1.35	4.43	3.10	2.95	0.35
C54	子宫体 Corpus uteri	43	0.41	1.34	0.89	0.89	0.12
C55	子宫，部位不明 Uterus unspecified	22	0.21	0.69	0.40	0.40	0.04
C56	卵巢 Ovary	93	0.88	2.90	1.93	1.89	0.23
C57	其他的女性生殖器 Other female genital organs	9	0.09	0.28	0.18	0.18	0.02
C58	胎盘 Placenta	0	0.00	0.00	0.00	0.00	0.00
C60	阴茎 Penis	8	0.08	0.25	0.17	0.14	0.01
C61	前列腺 Prostate	164	1.56	5.04	2.83	2.92	0.21
C62	睾丸 Testis	3	0.03	0.09	0.11	0.11	0.01
C63	其他的男性生殖器 Other male genital organs	1	0.01	0.03	0.03	0.02	0.00
C64	肾 Kidney	95	0.90	1.47	0.93	0.93	0.10
C65	肾盂 Renal pelvis	15	0.14	0.23	0.14	0.14	0.02
C66	输尿管 Ureter	25	0.24	0.39	0.23	0.22	0.02
C67	膀胱 Bladder	110	1.05	1.70	0.94	0.95	0.09
C68	其他的泌尿器官 Other urinary organs	4	0.04	0.06	0.02	0.03	0.00
C69	眼 Eye	4	0.04	0.06	0.04	0.04	0.00
C70-C72;D32-33;D42-43	脑，神经系统 Brain, nervous system	227	2.16	3.51	2.55	2.49	0.26
C73	甲状腺 Thyroid	55	0.52	0.85	0.54	0.55	0.07
C74	肾上腺 Adrenal gland	12	0.11	0.19	0.13	0.14	0.01
C75	其他的内分泌腺 Other endocrine	1	0.01	0.02	0.00	0.01	0.00
C81	霍奇金病 Hodgkin lymphoma	9	0.09	0.14	0.08	0.09	0.01
C82-C85;C96	非霍奇金淋巴瘤 Non-Hodgkin lymphoma	184	1.75	2.85	1.91	1.84	0.19
C88	免疫增生性疾病 Immunoproliferative diseases	2	0.02	0.03	0.02	0.02	0.00
C90	多发性骨髓瘤 Multiple myeloma	66	0.63	1.02	0.66	0.65	0.07
C91	淋巴样白血病 Lymphoid leukemia	38	0.36	0.59	0.49	0.56	0.04
C92-C94; D45-47	髓样白血病 Myeloid leukemia	122	1.16	1.89	1.40	1.43	0.15
C95	白血病，未特指 Leukemia unspecified	76	0.72	1.18	0.92	0.93	0.09
O&U	其他的或未指明部位 Other and unspecified	398	3.78	6.16	4.07	4.09	0.45
ALL	所有部位合计 All sites	10524	100.00	162.81	105.57	104.62	12.00
ALLbC44	所有部位除外 C44 All sites except C44	10481	99.59	162.14	105.25	104.27	11.98

附表 1-9 2019 年福建省城市肿瘤登记地区男性发病主要指标

Appendix Table 1-9 Cancer incidence in urban registration areas of Fujian, male in 2019

ICD10	部位	Site	发病数 Cases	构成 Freq. (%)	粗率 Crude rate (1/10⁵)	中标率 ASR China (1/10⁵)	世标率 ASR world (1/10⁵)	累积率 Cum.rate (0~74, %)
C00	唇	Lip	3	0.03	0.09	0.05	0.06	0.01
C01-C02	舌	Tongue	62	0.54	1.90	1.38	1.32	0.16
C03-C06	口	Mouth	48	0.42	1.47	1.04	1.07	0.15
C07-C08	唾液腺	Salivary glands	24	0.21	0.74	0.57	0.54	0.06
C09	扁桃体	Tonsil	10	0.09	0.31	0.23	0.21	0.02
C10	其他的口咽	Other oropharynx	21	0.18	0.65	0.44	0.45	0.06
C11	鼻咽	Nasopharynx	220	1.92	6.76	5.35	5.02	0.56
C12-C13	喉咽	Hypopharynx	36	0.31	1.11	0.77	0.78	0.10
C14	咽，部位不明	Pharynx unspecified	15	0.13	0.46	0.30	0.30	0.04
C15	食管	Esophagus	870	7.58	26.73	17.92	18.35	2.26
C16	胃	Stomach	1316	11.47	40.43	27.39	27.64	3.57
C17	小肠	Small intestine	54	0.47	1.66	1.22	1.14	0.13
C18	结肠	Colon	793	6.91	24.36	16.94	16.60	2.03
C19-C20	直肠	Rectum	753	6.56	23.13	15.77	15.78	1.91
C21	肛门	Anus	7	0.06	0.22	0.15	0.16	0.02
C22	肝脏	Liver	1370	11.94	42.09	30.16	29.49	3.40
C23-C24	胆囊及其他	Gallbladder etc.	86	0.75	2.64	1.81	1.79	0.23
C25	胰腺	Pancreas	167	1.46	5.13	3.45	3.45	0.40
C30-C31	鼻，鼻窦及其他	Nose, sinuses etc.	18	0.16	0.55	0.38	0.39	0.04
C32	喉	Larynx	117	1.02	3.59	2.46	2.51	0.34
C33-C34	气管，支气管，肺	Trachea, bronchus & lung	2383	20.77	73.21	50.26	50.35	6.53
C37-C38	其他的胸腔器官	Other thoracic organs	37	0.32	1.14	0.89	0.95	0.10
C40-C41	骨	Bone	39	0.34	1.20	1.05	0.99	0.10
C43	皮肤的黑色素瘤	Melanoma of skin	18	0.16	0.55	0.37	0.38	0.05
C44	其他的皮肤	Other skin	74	0.64	2.27	1.65	1.62	0.18
C45	间皮瘤	Mesothelioma	8	0.07	0.25	0.19	0.18	0.04
C46	卡波氏肉瘤	Kaposi sarcoma	1	0.01	0.03	0.01	0.02	0.00
C47;C49	周围神经,其他结缔、软组织	Connective & soft tissue	45	0.39	1.38	1.20	1.10	0.11
C50	乳房	Breast	10	0.09	0.31	0.22	0.19	0.02
C51	外阴	Vulva	–	–	–	–	–	–
C52	阴道	Vagina	–	–	–	–	–	–
C53	子宫颈	Cervix uteri	–	–	–	–	–	–
C54	子宫体	Corpus uteri	–	–	–	–	–	–
C55	子宫，部位不明	Uterus unspecified	–	–	–	–	–	–
C56	卵巢	Ovary	–	–	–	–	–	–
C57	其他的女性殖器	Other female genital organs	–	–	–	–	–	–
C58	胎盘	Placenta	–	–	–	–	–	–
C60	阴茎	Penis	17	0.15	0.52	0.38	0.36	0.04
C61	前列腺	Prostate	445	3.88	13.67	8.89	8.70	0.96
C62	睾丸	Testis	27	0.24	0.83	0.96	0.99	0.06
C63	其他的男性殖器	Other male genital organs	11	0.10	0.34	0.30	0.27	0.02
C64	肾	Kidney	220	1.92	6.76	5.03	4.82	0.52
C65	肾盂	Renal pelvis	18	0.16	0.55	0.37	0.37	0.04
C66	输尿管	Ureter	20	0.17	0.61	0.42	0.42	0.05
C67	膀胱	Bladder	269	2.34	8.26	5.67	5.59	0.64
C68	其他的泌尿器官	Other urinary organs	8	0.07	0.25	0.18	0.18	0.03
C69	眼	Eye	4	0.03	0.12	0.11	0.09	0.01
C70-C72;D32-33;D42-43	脑，神经系统	Brain, nervous system	270	2.35	8.29	6.61	6.44	0.67
C73	甲状腺	Thyroid	722	6.29	22.18	19.70	17.25	1.64
C74	肾上腺	Adrenal gland	9	0.08	0.28	0.20	0.19	0.02
C75	其他的内分泌腺	Other endocrine	3	0.03	0.09	0.07	0.09	0.01
C81	霍奇金病	Hodgkin lymphoma	15	0.13	0.46	0.49	0.46	0.03
C82-C85;C96	非霍奇金淋巴瘤	Non-Hodgkin lymphoma	226	1.97	6.94	5.29	5.15	0.61
C88	免疫增生性疾病	Immunoproliferative diseases	5	0.04	0.15	0.11	0.10	0.01
C90	多发性骨髓瘤	Multiple myeloma	80	0.70	2.46	1.67	1.68	0.19
C91	淋巴样白血病	Lymphoid leukemia	62	0.54	1.90	1.73	1.89	0.16
C92-C94; 45-47	髓样白血病	Myeloid leukemia	105	0.92	3.23	2.75	2.75	0.28
C95	白血病，未特指	Leukemia unspecified	28	0.24	0.86	0.65	0.70	0.06
O&U	其他的或未指明部位	Other and unspecified	305	2.66	9.37	6.68	6.75	0.76
ALL	所有部位合计	All sites	11474	100.00	352.50	251.86	248.08	29.41
ALLbC44	所有部位除外 C44	All sites except C44	11400	99.36	350.23	250.20	246.46	29.24

附表 1-10　2019 年福建省城市肿瘤登记地区男性死亡主要指标

Appendix Table 1-10　Cancer mortality in urban registration areas of Fujian, male in 2019

ICD10	部位	Site	死亡数 Deaths	构成 Freq. (%)	粗率 Crude rate (1/10^5)	中标率 ASR China (1/10^5)	世标率 ASR world (1/10^5)	累积率 Cum.rate (0~74, %)
C00	唇	Lip	0	0.00	0.00	0.00	0.00	0.00
C01-C02	舌	Tongue	29	0.42	0.89	0.59	0.61	0.07
C03-C06	口	Mouth	24	0.34	0.74	0.49	0.52	0.07
C07-C08	唾液腺	Salivary glands	9	0.13	0.28	0.19	0.19	0.02
C09	扁桃体	Tonsil	8	0.11	0.25	0.16	0.17	0.02
C10	其他的口咽	Other oropharynx	15	0.21	0.46	0.30	0.32	0.04
C11	鼻咽	Nasopharynx	120	1.72	3.69	2.56	2.60	0.32
C12-C13	喉咽	Hypopharynx	29	0.42	0.89	0.62	0.62	0.08
C14	咽，部位不明	Pharynx unspecified	11	0.16	0.34	0.23	0.24	0.02
C15	食管	Esophagus	693	9.93	21.29	13.83	14.24	1.70
C16	胃	Stomach	934	13.39	28.69	19.02	18.67	2.11
C17	小肠	Small intestine	29	0.42	0.89	0.62	0.64	0.09
C18	结肠	Colon	313	4.49	9.62	6.25	6.22	0.67
C19-C20	直肠	Rectum	323	4.63	9.92	6.47	6.49	0.72
C21	肛门	Anus	3	0.04	0.09	0.06	0.06	0.01
C22	肝脏	Liver	1136	16.28	34.90	24.59	24.06	2.78
C23-C24	胆囊及其他	Gallbladder etc.	73	1.05	2.24	1.51	1.51	0.19
C25	胰腺	Pancreas	153	2.19	4.70	3.16	3.14	0.37
C30-C31	鼻，鼻窦及其他	Nose, sinuses etc.	11	0.16	0.34	0.25	0.24	0.03
C32	喉	Larynx	57	0.82	1.75	1.15	1.18	0.15
C33-C34	气管，支气管，肺	Trachea, bronchus & lung	1867	26.76	57.36	38.37	38.33	4.79
C37-C38	其他的胸腔器官	Other thoracic organs	30	0.43	0.92	0.68	0.67	0.07
C40-C41	骨	Bone	42	0.60	1.29	1.07	1.00	0.08
C43	皮肤的黑色素瘤	Melanoma of skin	16	0.23	0.49	0.35	0.34	0.05
C44	其他的皮肤	Other skin	21	0.30	0.65	0.35	0.37	0.02
C45	间皮瘤	Mesothelioma	7	0.10	0.22	0.13	0.15	0.02
C46	卡波氏肉瘤	Kaposi sarcoma	0	0.00	0.00	0.00	0.00	0.00
C47;C49	周围神经，其他结缔、软组织	Connective & soft tissue	14	0.20	0.43	0.39	0.35	0.03
C50	乳房	Breast	3	0.04	0.09	0.06	0.07	0.01
C51	外阴	Vulva	–	–	–	–	–	–
C52	阴道	Vagina	–	–	–	–	–	–
C53	子宫颈	Cervix uteri	–	–	–	–	–	–
C54	子宫体	Corpus uteri	–	–	–	–	–	–
C55	子宫，部位不明	Uterus unspecified	–	–	–	–	–	–
C56	卵巢	Ovary	–	–	–	–	–	–
C57	其他的女性生殖器	Other female genital organs	–	–	–	–	–	–
C58	胎盘	Placenta	–	–	–	–	–	–
C60	阴茎	Penis	8	0.11	0.25	0.17	0.14	0.01
C61	前列腺	Prostate	164	2.35	5.04	2.83	2.92	0.21
C62	睾丸	Testis	3	0.04	0.09	0.11	0.11	0.01
C63	其他的男性生殖器	Other male genital organs	1	0.01	0.03	0.03	0.02	0.00
C64	肾	Kidney	67	0.96	2.06	1.36	1.32	0.14
C65	肾盂	Renal pelvis	10	0.14	0.31	0.20	0.20	0.02
C66	输尿管	Ureter	13	0.19	0.40	0.26	0.24	0.02
C67	膀胱	Bladder	83	1.19	2.55	1.55	1.57	0.17
C68	其他的泌尿器官	Other urinary organs	1	0.01	0.03	0.01	0.02	0.00
C69	眼	Eye	0	0.00	0.00	0.00	0.00	0.00
C70-C72;D32-33;D42-43	脑，神经系统	Brain, nervous system	133	1.91	4.09	3.09	3.04	0.33
C73	甲状腺	Thyroid	22	0.32	0.68	0.46	0.48	0.06
C74	肾上腺	Adrenal gland	5	0.07	0.15	0.10	0.11	0.02
C75	其他的内分泌腺	Other endocrine	0	0.00	0.00	0.00	0.00	0.00
C81	霍奇金病	Hodgkin lymphoma	7	0.10	0.22	0.12	0.14	0.01
C82-C85;C96	非霍奇金淋巴瘤	Non-Hodgkin lymphoma	100	1.43	3.07	2.19	2.07	0.23
C88	免疫增生性疾病	Immunoproliferative diseases	2	0.03	0.06	0.03	0.04	0.00
C90	多发性骨髓瘤	Multiple myeloma	34	0.49	1.04	0.70	0.69	0.07
C91	淋巴样白血病	Lymphoid leukemia	23	0.33	0.71	0.55	0.64	0.04
C92-C94; D45-47	髓样白血病	Myeloid leukemia	64	0.92	1.97	1.49	1.51	0.15
C95	白血病，未特指	Leukemia unspecified	40	0.57	1.23	0.87	0.88	0.08
O&U	其他的或未指明部位	Other and unspecified	227	3.25	6.97	4.82	4.87	0.52
ALL	所有部位合计	All sites	6977	100.00	214.35	144.37	143.98	16.63
ALLbC44	所有部位除外 C44	All sites except C44	6956	99.70	213.70	144.02	143.61	16.61

附表 1-11　2019 年福建省城市肿瘤登记地区女性发病主要指标

Appendix Table 1-11　Cancer incidence in urban registration areas of Fujian, female in 2019

ICD10	部位	Site	发病数 Cases	构成 Freq.（%）	粗率 Crude rate（1/10⁵）	中标率 ASR China（1/10⁵）	世标率 ASR world（1/10⁵）	累积率 Cum.rate（0~74，%）
C00	唇	Lip	2	0.02	0.06	0.05	0.04	0.01
C01-C02	舌	Tongue	33	0.32	1.03	0.69	0.69	0.08
C03-C06	口	Mouth	26	0.25	0.81	0.59	0.54	0.07
C07-C08	唾液腺	Salivary glands	21	0.20	0.65	0.47	0.44	0.05
C09	扁桃体	Tonsil	5	0.05	0.16	0.10	0.10	0.01
C10	其他的口咽	Other oropharynx	6	0.06	0.19	0.13	0.13	0.02
C11	鼻咽	Nasopharynx	65	0.62	2.03	1.61	1.47	0.16
C12-C13	喉咽	Hypopharynx	1	0.01	0.03	0.02	0.02	0.00
C14	咽，部位不明	Pharynx unspecified	4	0.04	0.12	0.08	0.07	0.01
C15	食管	Esophagus	271	2.59	8.44	5.13	5.10	0.66
C16	胃	Stomach	537	5.13	16.73	11.06	10.76	1.29
C17	小肠	Small intestine	33	0.32	1.03	0.71	0.70	0.09
C18	结肠	Colon	571	5.46	17.79	11.55	11.24	1.33
C19-C20	直肠	Rectum	464	4.43	14.46	9.51	9.30	1.12
C21	肛门	Anus	8	0.08	0.25	0.16	0.14	0.01
C22	肝脏	Liver	356	3.40	11.09	7.30	7.12	0.80
C23-C24	胆囊及其他	Gallbladder etc.	87	0.83	2.71	1.68	1.69	0.21
C25	胰腺	Pancreas	105	1.00	3.27	2.12	2.02	0.25
C30-C31	鼻，鼻窦及其他	Nose, sinuses etc.	9	0.09	0.28	0.19	0.18	0.02
C32	喉	Larynx	3	0.03	0.09	0.07	0.06	0.00
C33-C34	气管，支气管，肺	Trachea, bronchus & lung	1607	15.36	50.08	33.81	33.05	4.03
C37-C38	其他的胸腔器官	Other thoracic organs	34	0.32	1.06	0.79	0.75	0.08
C40-C41	骨	Bone	21	0.20	0.65	0.61	0.55	0.04
C43	皮肤的黑色素瘤	Melanoma of skin	14	0.13	0.44	0.31	0.29	0.03
C44	其他的皮肤	Other skin	96	0.92	2.99	1.83	1.82	0.18
C45	间皮瘤	Mesothelioma	4	0.04	0.12	0.10	0.09	0.01
C46	卡波氏肉瘤	Kaposi sarcoma	0	0.00	0.00	0.00	0.00	0.00
C47;C49	周围神经,其他结缔、软组织	Connective & soft tissue	34	0.32	1.06	0.76	0.71	0.08
C50	乳房	Breast	1594	15.23	49.67	37.39	34.32	3.53
C51	外阴	Vulva	6	0.06	0.19	0.12	0.11	0.01
C52	阴道	Vagina	15	0.14	0.47	0.32	0.32	0.06
C53	子宫颈	Cervix uteri	583	5.57	18.17	13.48	12.48	1.34
C54	子宫体	Corpus uteri	287	2.74	8.94	6.26	6.14	0.72
C55	子宫，部位不明	Uterus unspecified	62	0.59	1.93	1.29	1.29	0.15
C56	卵巢	Ovary	206	1.97	6.42	4.94	4.73	0.49
C57	其他的女性生殖器	Other female genital organs	10	0.10	0.31	0.22	0.21	0.03
C58	胎盘	Placenta	5	0.05	0.16	0.14	0.12	0.01
C60	阴茎	Penis	–	–	–	–	–	–
C61	前列腺	Prostate	–	–	–	–	–	–
C62	睾丸	Testis	–	–	–	–	–	–
C63	其他的男性生殖器	Other male genital organs	–	–	–	–	–	–
C64	肾	Kidney	94	0.90	2.93	2.09	1.97	0.22
C65	肾盂	Renal pelvis	9	0.09	0.28	0.17	0.16	0.01
C66	输尿管	Ureter	11	0.11	0.34	0.20	0.19	0.02
C67	膀胱	Bladder	65	0.62	2.03	1.23	1.22	0.15
C68	其他的泌尿器官	Other urinary organs	4	0.04	0.12	0.06	0.06	0.00
C69	眼	Eye	2	0.02	0.06	0.04	0.08	0.01
C70-C72;D32-33;D42-43	脑，神经系统	Brain, nervous system	370	3.54	11.53	8.89	8.55	0.90
C73	甲状腺	Thyroid	2097	20.04	65.35	55.86	48.70	4.54
C74	肾上腺	Adrenal gland	4	0.04	0.12	0.09	0.15	0.01
C75	其他的内分泌腺	Other endocrine	5	0.05	0.16	0.14	0.12	0.01
C81	霍奇金病	Hodgkin lymphoma	7	0.07	0.22	0.26	0.21	0.02
C82-C85;C96	非霍奇金淋巴瘤	Non-Hodgkin lymphoma	160	1.53	4.99	3.50	3.38	0.40
C88	免疫增生性疾病	Immunoproliferative diseases	0	0.00	0.00	0.00	0.00	0.00
C90	多发性骨髓瘤	Multiple myeloma	59	0.56	1.84	1.22	1.19	0.14
C91	淋巴样白血病	Lymphoid leukemia	37	0.35	1.15	0.96	1.25	0.09
C92-C94; D45-47	髓样白血病	Myeloid leukemia	97	0.93	3.02	2.52	2.47	0.23
C95	白血病，未特指	Leukemia unspecified	23	0.22	0.72	0.56	0.70	0.07
O&U	其他的或未指明部位	Other and unspecified	236	2.26	7.35	5.10	5.07	0.55
ALL	所有部位合计	All sites	10465	100.00	326.11	238.50	224.27	24.34
ALLbC44	所有部位除外 C44	All sites except C44	10369	99.08	323.12	236.67	222.45	24.16

附表 1-12　2019 年福建省城市肿瘤登记地区女性死亡主要指标

Appendix Table 1-12　Cancer mortality in urban registration areas of Fujian, female in 2019

ICD10	部位	Site	死亡数 Deaths	构成 Freq.（%）	粗率 Crude rate（1/10⁵）	中标率 ASR China（1/10⁵）	世标率 ASR world（1/10⁵）	累积率 Cum.rate（0~74,%）
C00	唇	Lip	0	0.00	0.00	0.00	0.00	0.00
C01-C02	舌	Tongue	15	0.42	0.47	0.31	0.30	0.03
C03-C06	口	Mouth	15	0.42	0.47	0.29	0.28	0.04
C07-C08	唾液腺	Salivary glands	5	0.14	0.16	0.07	0.08	0.00
C09	扁桃体	Tonsil	1	0.03	0.03	0.02	0.02	0.00
C10	其他的口咽	Other oropharynx	1	0.03	0.03	0.02	0.02	0.00
C11	鼻咽	Nasopharynx	53	1.49	1.65	1.11	1.06	0.12
C12-C13	喉咽	Hypopharynx	0	0.00	0.00	0.00	0.00	0.00
C14	咽，部位不明	Pharynx unspecified	9	0.25	0.28	0.12	0.11	0.00
C15	食管	Esophagus	205	5.78	6.39	3.55	3.48	0.40
C16	胃	Stomach	361	10.18	11.25	6.85	6.67	0.77
C17	小肠	Small intestine	24	0.68	0.75	0.39	0.43	0.05
C18	结肠	Colon	232	6.54	7.23	4.26	4.19	0.48
C19-C20	直肠	Rectum	184	5.19	5.73	3.35	3.21	0.35
C21	肛门	Anus	7	0.20	0.22	0.12	0.12	0.01
C22	肝脏	Liver	309	8.71	9.63	6.05	5.90	0.69
C23-C24	胆囊及其他	Gallbladder etc.	65	1.83	2.03	1.19	1.24	0.16
C25	胰腺	Pancreas	100	2.82	3.12	1.90	1.84	0.21
C30-C31	鼻，鼻窦及其他	Nose, sinuses etc.	2	0.06	0.06	0.04	0.04	0.01
C32	喉	Larynx	4	0.11	0.12	0.08	0.07	0.01
C33-C34	气管，支气管，肺	Trachea, bronchus & lung	661	18.64	20.60	12.37	12.17	1.35
C37-C38	其他的胸腔器官	Other thoracic organs	14	0.39	0.44	0.33	0.33	0.03
C40-C41	骨	Bone	23	0.65	0.72	0.53	0.53	0.05
C43	皮肤的黑色素瘤	Melanoma of skin	10	0.28	0.31	0.21	0.20	0.03
C44	其他的皮肤	Other skin	22	0.62	0.69	0.30	0.33	0.02
C45	间皮瘤	Mesothelioma	2	0.06	0.06	0.04	0.05	0.01
C46	卡波氏肉瘤	Kaposi sarcoma	0	0.00	0.00	0.00	0.00	0.00
C47;C49	周围神经,其它结缔、软组织	Connective & soft tissue	14	0.39	0.44	0.37	0.35	0.04
C50	乳房	Breast	277	7.81	8.63	5.90	5.64	0.60
C51	外阴	Vulva	7	0.20	0.22	0.13	0.12	0.01
C52	阴道	Vagina	4	0.11	0.12	0.09	0.08	0.01
C53	子宫颈	Cervix uteri	142	4.00	4.43	3.10	2.95	0.35
C54	子宫体	Corpus uteri	43	1.21	1.34	0.89	0.89	0.12
C55	子宫,部位不明	Uterus unspecified	22	0.62	0.69	0.40	0.40	0.04
C56	卵巢	Ovary	93	2.62	2.90	1.93	1.89	0.23
C57	其他的女性生殖器	Other female genital organs	9	0.25	0.28	0.18	0.18	0.02
C58	胎盘	Placenta	0	0.00	0.00	0.00	0.00	0.00
C60	阴茎	Penis	-	-	-	-	-	-
C61	前列腺	Prostate	-	-	-	-	-	-
C62	睾丸	Testis	-	-	-	-	-	-
C63	其他的男性生殖器	Other male genital organs	-	-	-	-	-	-
C64	肾	Kidney	28	0.79	0.87	0.54	0.57	0.05
C65	肾盂	Renal pelvis	5	0.14	0.16	0.09	0.09	0.01
C66	输尿管	Ureter	12	0.34	0.37	0.20	0.20	0.02
C67	膀胱	Bladder	27	0.76	0.84	0.40	0.40	0.02
C68	其他的泌尿器官	Other urinary organs	3	0.08	0.09	0.03	0.03	0.00
C69	眼	Eye	4	0.11	0.12	0.09	0.15	0.01
C70-C72;D32-33;D42-43	脑，神经系统	Brain, nervous system	94	2.65	2.93	2.02	1.95	0.19
C73	甲状腺	Thyroid	33	0.93	1.03	0.60	0.61	0.08
C74	肾上腺	Adrenal gland	7	0.20	0.22	0.15	0.17	0.01
C75	其他的内分泌腺	Other endocrine	1	0.03	0.03	0.01	0.01	0.00
C81	霍奇金病	Hodgkin lymphoma	2	0.06	0.06	0.05	0.05	0.01
C82-C85;C96	非霍奇金淋巴瘤	Non-Hodgkin lymphoma	84	2.37	2.62	1.63	1.60	0.15
C88	免疫增生性疾病	Immunoproliferative diseases	0	0.00	0.00	0.00	0.00	0.00
C90	多发性骨髓瘤	Multiple myeloma	32	0.90	1.00	0.62	0.60	0.06
C91	淋巴样白血病	Lymphoid leukemia	15	0.42	0.47	0.46	0.50	0.04
C92-C94; D45-47	髓样白血病	Myeloid leukemia	58	1.64	1.81	1.32	1.35	0.15
C95	白血病，未特指	Leukemia unspecified	36	1.01	1.12	1.00	1.04	0.10
O&U	其他的或未指明部位	Other and unspecified	171	4.82	5.33	3.35	3.33	0.38
ALL	所有部位合计	All sites	3547	100.00	110.53	69.05	67.80	7.51
ALLbC44	所有部位除外 C44	All sites except C44	3525	99.38	109.85	68.76	67.48	7.49

附表 1-13　2019 年福建省农村肿瘤登记地区男女合计发病主要指标

Appendix Table 1-13　Cancer incidence in rural registration areas of Fujian, both sexes in 2019

ICD10	部位	Site	发病数 Cases	构成 Freq. (%)	粗率 Crude rate (1/10⁵)	中标率 ASR China (1/10⁵)	世标率 ASR world (1/10⁵)	累积率 Cum.rate (0~74,%)
C00	唇	Lip	10	0.04	0.11	0.07	0.08	0.01
C01-C02	舌	Tongue	77	0.31	0.86	0.61	0.62	0.08
C03-C06	口	Mouth	85	0.34	0.95	0.65	0.64	0.07
C07-C08	唾液腺	Salivary glands	52	0.21	0.58	0.47	0.44	0.04
C09	扁桃体	Tonsil	15	0.06	0.17	0.12	0.11	0.01
C10	其他的口咽	Other oropharynx	19	0.08	0.21	0.14	0.14	0.02
C11	鼻咽	Nasopharynx	496	1.98	5.53	4.51	4.08	0.42
C12-C13	喉咽	Hypopharynx	57	0.23	0.64	0.43	0.44	0.06
C14	咽,部位不明	Pharynx unspecified	18	0.07	0.20	0.15	0.14	0.02
C15	食管	Esophagus	1537	6.14	17.15	11.29	11.61	1.51
C16	胃	Stomach	2515	10.05	28.06	19.48	19.26	2.49
C17	小肠	Small intestine	103	0.41	1.15	0.80	0.80	0.10
C18	结肠	Colon	1426	5.70	15.91	11.15	10.85	1.32
C19-C20	直肠	Rectum	1470	5.87	16.40	11.32	11.17	1.41
C21	肛门	Anus	16	0.06	0.18	0.12	0.12	0.01
C22	肝脏	Liver	2126	8.49	23.72	17.13	16.55	1.94
C23-C24	胆囊及其他	Gallbladder etc.	237	0.95	2.64	1.78	1.76	0.21
C25	胰腺	Pancreas	309	1.23	3.45	2.30	2.29	0.29
C30-C31	鼻,鼻窦及其他	Nose, sinuses etc.	27	0.11	0.30	0.21	0.21	0.02
C32	喉	Larynx	139	0.56	1.55	1.07	1.09	0.14
C33-C34	气管,支气管,肺	Trachea, bronchus & lung	4447	17.76	49.61	34.36	34.24	4.41
C37-C38	其他的胸腔器官	Other thoracic organs	70	0.28	0.78	0.58	0.60	0.06
C40-C41	骨	Bone	76	0.30	0.85	0.73	0.74	0.06
C43	皮肤的黑色素瘤	Melanoma of skin	35	0.14	0.39	0.28	0.26	0.03
C44	其他的皮肤	Other skin	203	0.81	2.26	1.47	1.43	0.14
C45	间皮瘤	Mesothelioma	11	0.04	0.12	0.09	0.09	0.01
C46	卡波氏肉瘤	Kaposi sarcoma	0	0.00	0.00	0.00	0.00	0.00
C47;C49	周围神经,其他结缔、软组织	Connective & soft tissue	120	0.48	1.34	1.12	1.04	0.11
C50	乳房	Breast	1511	6.09	35.17	27.14	24.61	2.48
C51	外阴	Vulva	14	0.06	0.33	0.24	0.21	0.03
C52	阴道	Vagina	19	0.08	0.44	0.30	0.30	0.04
C53	子宫颈	Cervix uteri	926	3.70	21.55	15.49	14.73	1.62
C54	子宫体	Corpus uteri	366	1.46	8.52	5.83	5.69	0.62
C55	子宫,部位不明	Uterus unspecified	45	0.18	1.05	0.70	0.69	0.07
C56	卵巢	Ovary	247	0.99	5.75	4.42	4.25	0.47
C57	其他的女性生殖器	Other female genital organs	16	0.06	0.37	0.29	0.27	0.05
C58	胎盘	Placenta	7	0.03	0.16	0.16	0.13	0.01
C60	阴茎	Penis	29	0.12	0.62	0.46	0.44	0.06
C61	前列腺	Prostate	441	1.76	9.45	6.51	6.42	0.74
C62	睾丸	Testis	25	0.10	0.54	0.59	0.58	0.04
C63	其他的男性生殖器	Other male genital organs	8	0.03	0.17	0.14	0.14	0.02
C64	肾	Kidney	313	1.25	3.49	2.62	2.55	0.31
C65	肾盂	Renal pelvis	35	0.14	0.39	0.27	0.27	0.04
C66	输尿管	Ureter	32	0.13	0.36	0.24	0.24	0.03
C67	膀胱	Bladder	368	1.47	4.11	2.78	2.74	0.32
C68	其他的泌尿器官	Other urinary organs	13	0.05	0.15	0.10	0.10	0.02
C69	眼	Eye	10	0.04	0.11	0.10	0.15	0.01
C70-C72;D32-33;D42-43	脑,神经系统	Brain, nervous system	700	2.80	7.81	6.27	6.05	0.62
C73	甲状腺	Thyroid	2334	9.32	26.04	22.96	19.92	1.87
C74	肾上腺	Adrenal gland	15	0.06	0.17	0.14	0.20	0.01
C75	其他的内分泌腺	Other endocrine	3	0.01	0.03	0.02	0.02	0.00
C81	霍奇金病	Hodgkin lymphoma	14	0.06	0.16	0.15	0.15	0.01
C82-C85;C96	非霍奇金淋巴瘤	Non-Hodgkin lymphoma	438	1.75	4.89	3.78	3.57	0.40
C88	免疫增生性疾病	Immunoproliferative diseases	7	0.03	0.08	0.05	0.06	0.01
C90	多发性骨髓瘤	Multiple myeloma	105	0.42	1.17	0.81	0.83	0.12
C91	淋巴样白血病	Lymphoid leukemia	102	0.41	1.14	1.06	1.33	0.09
C92-C94; D45-47	髓样白血病	Myeloid leukemia	271	1.08	3.02	2.63	2.55	0.22
C95	白血病,未特指	Leukemia unspecified	60	0.24	0.67	0.58	0.66	0.05
O&U	其他的或未指明部位	Other and unspecified	853	3.41	9.52	7.00	7.03	0.78
ALL	所有部位合计	All sites	25036	100.00	279.32	204.80	198.17	23.02
ALLbC44	所有部位除外 C44	All sites except C44	24833	99.19	277.06	203.33	196.74	22.88

附表 1-14　　2019 年福建省农村肿瘤登记地区男女合计死亡主要指标

Appendix Table 1-14　　Cancer mortality in rural registration areas of Fujian, both sexes in 2019

ICD10	部位	Site	死亡数 Deaths	构成 Freq. (%)	粗率 Crude rate (1/10⁵)	中标率 ASR China (1/10⁵)	世标率 ASR world (1/10⁵)	累积率 Cum.rate (0~74,%)
C00	唇	Lip	4	0.03	0.04	0.03	0.03	0.00
C01-C02	舌	Tongue	38	0.26	0.42	0.27	0.29	0.04
C03-C06	口	Mouth	52	0.36	0.58	0.38	0.38	0.05
C07-C08	唾液腺	Salivary glands	8	0.06	0.09	0.06	0.05	0.00
C09	扁桃体	Tonsil	10	0.07	0.11	0.08	0.08	0.01
C10	其他的口咽	Other oropharynx	13	0.09	0.15	0.10	0.09	0.01
C11	鼻咽	Nasopharynx	235	1.63	2.62	1.84	1.79	0.21
C12-C13	喉咽	Hypopharynx	19	0.13	0.21	0.15	0.15	0.02
C14	咽，部位不明	Pharynx unspecified	18	0.12	0.20	0.13	0.13	0.01
C15	食管	Esophagus	1502	10.41	16.76	10.55	10.60	1.22
C16	胃	Stomach	1926	13.35	21.49	14.06	13.81	1.62
C17	小肠	Small intestine	46	0.32	0.51	0.34	0.36	0.04
C18	结肠	Colon	623	4.32	6.95	4.67	4.50	0.50
C19-C20	直肠	Rectum	678	4.70	7.56	4.87	4.81	0.55
C21	肛门	Anus	16	0.11	0.18	0.11	0.12	0.02
C22	肝脏	Liver	2116	14.66	23.61	16.60	16.07	1.89
C23-C24	胆囊及其他	Gallbladder etc.	172	1.19	1.92	1.22	1.22	0.15
C25	胰腺	Pancreas	319	2.21	3.56	2.34	2.29	0.27
C30-C31	鼻，鼻窦及其他	Nose, sinuses etc.	19	0.13	0.21	0.15	0.14	0.02
C32	喉	Larynx	99	0.69	1.10	0.72	0.72	0.09
C33-C34	气管，支气管，肺	Trachea, bronchus & lung	3515	24.36	39.22	26.00	25.82	3.22
C37-C38	其他的胸腔器官	Other thoracic organs	32	0.22	0.36	0.28	0.28	0.03
C40-C41	骨	Bone	91	0.63	1.02	0.76	0.76	0.09
C43	皮肤的黑色素瘤	Melanoma of skin	16	0.11	0.18	0.12	0.12	0.02
C44	其他的皮肤	Other skin	70	0.49	0.78	0.42	0.44	0.04
C45	间皮瘤	Mesothelioma	5	0.03	0.06	0.04	0.04	0.01
C46	卡波氏肉瘤	Kaposi sarcoma	1	0.01	0.01	0.01	0.01	0.00
C47;C49	周围神经,其它结缔、软组织	Connective & soft tissue	40	0.28	0.45	0.35	0.34	0.04
C50	乳房	Breast	266	1.86	6.19	4.37	4.15	0.46
C51	外阴	Vulva	5	0.03	0.12	0.07	0.07	0.01
C52	阴道	Vagina	9	0.06	0.21	0.12	0.13	0.01
C53	子宫颈	Cervix uteri	273	1.89	6.35	4.22	4.16	0.51
C54	子宫体	Corpus uteri	58	0.40	1.35	0.86	0.85	0.10
C55	子宫，部位不明	Uterus unspecified	48	0.33	1.12	0.75	0.71	0.08
C56	卵巢	Ovary	112	0.78	2.61	1.76	1.75	0.21
C57	其他的女性生殖器	Other female genital organs	5	0.03	0.12	0.08	0.08	0.01
C58	胎盘	Placenta	1	0.01	0.02	0.02	0.02	0.00
C60	阴茎	Penis	14	0.10	0.30	0.21	0.20	0.01
C61	前列腺	Prostate	183	1.27	3.92	2.51	2.50	0.21
C62	睾丸	Testis	4	0.03	0.09	0.09	0.07	0.01
C63	其他的男性生殖器	Other male genital organs	2	0.01	0.04	0.02	0.03	0.00
C64	肾	Kidney	76	0.53	0.85	0.57	0.58	0.08
C65	肾盂	Renal pelvis	11	0.08	0.12	0.08	0.08	0.01
C66	输尿管	Ureter	11	0.08	0.12	0.08	0.08	0.01
C67	膀胱	Bladder	118	0.82	1.32	0.78	0.76	0.07
C68	其他的泌尿器官	Other urinary organs	7	0.05	0.08	0.05	0.05	0.01
C69	眼	Eye	8	0.06	0.09	0.08	0.14	0.01
C70-C72;D32-33;D42-43	脑，神经系统	Brain, nervous system	353	2.45	3.94	2.99	3.00	0.33
C73	甲状腺	Thyroid	53	0.37	0.59	0.41	0.40	0.04
C74	肾上腺	Adrenal gland	9	0.06	0.10	0.07	0.10	0.01
C75	其他的内分泌腺	Other endocrine	4	0.03	0.04	0.04	0.06	0.01
C81	霍奇金病	Hodgkin lymphoma	2	0.01	0.02	0.01	0.02	0.00
C82-C85;C96	非霍奇金淋巴瘤	Non-Hodgkin lymphoma	202	1.40	2.25	1.63	1.61	0.20
C88	免疫增生性疾病	Immunoproliferative diseases	2	0.01	0.02	0.02	0.01	0.00
C90	多发性骨髓瘤	Multiple myeloma	60	0.42	0.67	0.47	0.46	0.06
C91	淋巴样白血病	Lymphoid leukemia	43	0.30	0.48	0.44	0.45	0.04
C92-C94; D45-47	髓样白血病	Myeloid leukemia	144	1.00	1.61	1.26	1.18	0.12
C95	白血病，未特指	Leukemia unspecified	107	0.74	1.19	0.96	1.05	0.09
O&U	其他的或未指明部位	Other and unspecified	553	3.83	6.17	4.35	4.28	0.51
ALL	所有部位合计	All sites	14429	100.00	160.98	108.39	107.03	12.53
ALLbC44	所有部位除外 C44	All sites except C44	14359	99.51	160.20	107.96	106.59	12.50

附表 1-15　2019 年福建省农村肿瘤登记地区男性发病主要指标

Appendix Table 1-15　Cancer incidence in rural registration areas of Fujian, male in 2019

ICD10	部位 Site		发病数 Cases	构成 Freq. (%)	粗率 Crude rate (1/10⁵)	中标率 ASR China (1/10⁵)	世标率 ASR world (1/10⁵)	累积率 Cum.rate (0~74,%)
C00	唇	Lip	5	0.04	0.11	0.07	0.08	0.01
C01-C02	舌	Tongue	47	0.34	1.01	0.74	0.76	0.09
C03-C06	口	Mouth	60	0.44	1.29	0.90	0.92	0.11
C07-C08	唾液腺	Salivary glands	34	0.25	0.73	0.57	0.55	0.06
C09	扁桃体	Tonsil	12	0.09	0.26	0.20	0.18	0.02
C10	其他的口咽	Other oropharynx	15	0.11	0.32	0.23	0.23	0.02
C11	鼻咽	Nasopharynx	378	2.74	8.10	6.67	6.07	0.63
C12-C13	喉咽	Hypopharynx	54	0.39	1.16	0.81	0.84	0.11
C14	咽,部位不明	Pharynx unspecified	14	0.10	0.30	0.21	0.21	0.02
C15	食管	Esophagus	1069	7.76	22.91	15.83	16.38	2.09
C16	胃	Stomach	1814	13.16	38.87	28.01	27.99	3.65
C17	小肠	Small intestine	62	0.45	1.33	0.92	0.95	0.11
C18	结肠	Colon	826	5.99	17.70	12.90	12.70	1.58
C19-C20	直肠	Rectum	894	6.49	19.16	13.77	13.71	1.73
C21	肛门	Anus	7	0.05	0.15	0.11	0.11	0.02
C22	肝脏	Liver	1727	12.53	37.01	27.79	26.91	3.14
C23-C24	胆囊及其他	Gallbladder etc.	119	0.86	2.55	1.81	1.78	0.20
C25	胰腺	Pancreas	202	1.47	4.33	3.05	3.06	0.39
C30-C31	鼻,鼻窦及其他	Nose, sinuses etc.	19	0.14	0.41	0.31	0.30	0.03
C32	喉	Larynx	133	0.97	2.85	2.04	2.08	0.28
C33-C34	气管,支气管,肺	Trachea, bronchus & lung	2992	21.71	64.11	46.10	46.20	6.06
C37-C38	其他的胸腔器官	Other thoracic organs	46	0.33	0.99	0.76	0.77	0.09
C40-C41	骨	Bone	37	0.27	0.79	0.69	0.66	0.06
C43	皮肤的黑色素瘤	Melanoma of skin	14	0.10	0.30	0.23	0.20	0.01
C44	其他的皮肤	Other skin	93	0.67	1.99	1.41	1.35	0.14
C45	间皮瘤	Mesothelioma	8	0.06	0.17	0.13	0.13	0.02
C46	卡波氏肉瘤	Kaposi sarcoma	0	0.00	0.00	0.00	0.00	0.00
C47;C49	周围神经,其它结缔、软组织	Connective & soft tissue	64	0.46	1.37	1.13	1.09	0.12
C50	乳房	Breast	13	0.09	0.28	0.22	0.21	0.03
C51	外阴	Vulva	-	-	-	-	-	-
C52	阴道	Vagina	-	-	-	-	-	-
C53	子宫颈	Cervix uteri	-	-	-	-	-	-
C54	子宫体	Corpus uteri	-	-	-	-	-	-
C55	子宫,部位不明	Uterus unspecified	-	-	-	-	-	-
C56	卵巢	Ovary	-	-	-	-	-	-
C57	其他的女性生殖器	Other female genital organs	-	-	-	-	-	-
C58	胎盘	Placenta	-	-	-	-	-	-
C60	阴茎	Penis	29	0.21	0.62	0.46	0.44	0.06
C61	前列腺	Prostate	441	3.20	9.45	6.51	6.42	0.74
C62	睾丸	Testis	25	0.18	0.54	0.59	0.58	0.04
C63	其他的男性生殖器	Other male genital organs	8	0.06	0.17	0.14	0.14	0.02
C64	肾	Kidney	207	1.50	4.44	3.40	3.34	0.41
C65	肾盂	Renal pelvis	22	0.16	0.47	0.33	0.33	0.04
C66	输尿管	Ureter	22	0.16	0.47	0.34	0.33	0.04
C67	膀胱	Bladder	302	2.19	6.47	4.63	4.55	0.53
C68	其他的泌尿器官	Other urinary organs	10	0.07	0.21	0.16	0.16	0.02
C69	眼	Eye	6	0.04	0.13	0.09	0.11	0.01
C70-C72;D32-33;D42-43	脑,神经系统	Brain, nervous system	328	2.38	7.03	6.04	5.87	0.56
C73	甲状腺	Thyroid	541	3.93	11.59	10.61	9.13	0.86
C74	肾上腺	Adrenal gland	10	0.07	0.21	0.18	0.26	0.01
C75	其他的内分泌腺	Other endocrine	0	0.00	0.00	0.00	0.00	0.00
C81	霍奇金病	Hodgkin lymphoma	11	0.08	0.24	0.23	0.22	0.02
C82-C85;C96	非霍奇金淋巴瘤	Non-Hodgkin lymphoma	259	1.88	5.55	4.40	4.19	0.47
C88	免疫增生性疾病	Immunoproliferative diseases	4	0.03	0.09	0.06	0.07	0.01
C90	多发性骨髓瘤	Multiple myeloma	59	0.43	1.26	0.92	0.94	0.13
C91	淋巴样白血病	Lymphoid leukemia	64	0.46	1.37	1.22	1.58	0.11
C92-C94; D45-47	髓样白血病	Myeloid leukemia	151	1.10	3.24	2.76	2.73	0.25
C95	白血病,未特指	Leukemia unspecified	40	0.29	0.86	0.76	0.87	0.07
O&U	其他的或未指明部位	Other and unspecified	484	3.51	10.37	7.90	7.95	0.87
ALL	所有部位合计	All sites	13781	100.00	295.30	219.37	216.62	26.09
ALLbC44	所有部位除外 C44	All sites except C44	13688	99.33	293.31	217.96	215.28	25.95

附表 1-16　2019 年福建省农村肿瘤登记地区男性死亡主要指标

Appendix Table 1-16　Cancer mortality in rural registration areas of Fujian, male in 2019

ICD10	部位 Site		死亡数 Deaths	构成 Freq. （%）	粗率 Crude rate （1/10⁵）	中标率 ASR China （1/10⁵）	世标率 ASR world （1/10⁵）	累积率 Cum.rate （0~74，%）
C00	唇	Lip	4	0.04	0.09	0.06	0.06	0.01
C01-C02	舌	Tongue	23	0.24	0.49	0.35	0.36	0.05
C03-C06	口	Mouth	37	0.39	0.79	0.56	0.56	0.07
C07-C08	唾液腺	Salivary glands	6	0.06	0.13	0.09	0.08	0.01
C09	扁桃体	Tonsil	10	0.10	0.21	0.16	0.15	0.02
C10	其他的口咽	Other oropharynx	9	0.09	0.19	0.13	0.13	0.01
C11	鼻咽	Nasopharynx	177	1.84	3.79	2.79	2.72	0.32
C12-C13	喉咽	Hypopharynx	19	0.20	0.41	0.29	0.30	0.04
C14	咽，部位不明	Pharynx unspecified	11	0.11	0.24	0.17	0.17	0.02
C15	食管	Esophagus	979	10.20	20.98	14.27	14.46	1.68
C16	胃	Stomach	1349	14.06	28.91	20.24	19.99	2.37
C17	小肠	Small intestine	28	0.29	0.60	0.40	0.42	0.04
C18	结肠	Colon	350	3.65	7.50	5.41	5.25	0.58
C19-C20	直肠	Rectum	405	4.22	8.68	5.97	5.90	0.65
C21	肛门	Anus	11	0.11	0.24	0.15	0.16	0.02
C22	肝脏	Liver	1670	17.40	35.79	26.62	25.77	3.05
C23-C24	胆囊及其他	Gallbladder etc.	85	0.89	1.82	1.26	1.27	0.15
C25	胰腺	Pancreas	205	2.14	4.39	3.05	3.04	0.36
C30-C31	鼻，鼻窦及其他	Nose, sinuses etc.	14	0.15	0.30	0.22	0.22	0.03
C32	喉	Larynx	88	0.92	1.89	1.31	1.32	0.16
C33-C34	气管，支气管，肺	Trachea, bronchus & lung	2657	27.68	56.93	39.99	39.84	4.94
C37-C38	其他的胸腔器官	Other thoracic organs	24	0.25	0.51	0.46	0.45	0.04
C40-C41	骨	Bone	57	0.59	1.22	0.98	0.97	0.11
C43	皮肤的黑色素瘤	Melanoma of skin	8	0.08	0.17	0.12	0.13	0.02
C44	其他的皮肤	Other skin	33	0.34	0.71	0.47	0.46	0.05
C45	间皮瘤	Mesothelioma	5	0.05	0.11	0.09	0.08	0.01
C46	卡波氏肉瘤	Kaposi sarcoma	1	0.01	0.02	0.01	0.02	0.00
C47;C49	周围神经，其他结缔、软组织	Connective & soft tissue	30	0.31	0.64	0.53	0.52	0.06
C50	乳房	Breast	3	0.03	0.06	0.03	0.04	0.00
C51	外阴	Vulva	-	-	-	-	-	-
C52	阴道	Vagina	-	-	-	-	-	-
C53	子宫颈	Cervix uteri	-	-	-	-	-	-
C54	子宫体	Corpus uteri	-	-	-	-	-	-
C55	子宫，部位不明	Uterus unspecified	-	-	-	-	-	-
C56	卵巢	Ovary	-	-	-	-	-	-
C57	其他的女性生殖器	Other female genital organs	-	-	-	-	-	-
C58	胎盘	Placenta	-	-	-	-	-	-
C60	阴茎	Penis	14	0.15	0.30	0.21	0.20	0.01
C61	前列腺	Prostate	183	1.91	3.92	2.51	2.50	0.21
C62	睾丸	Testis	4	0.04	0.09	0.09	0.07	0.01
C63	其他的男性生殖器	Other male genital organs	2	0.02	0.04	0.02	0.03	0.00
C64	肾	Kidney	56	0.58	1.20	0.86	0.87	0.12
C65	肾盂	Renal pelvis	8	0.08	0.17	0.12	0.12	0.02
C66	输尿管	Ureter	7	0.07	0.15	0.10	0.09	0.01
C67	膀胱	Bladder	97	1.01	2.08	1.33	1.33	0.12
C68	其他的泌尿器官	Other urinary organs	4	0.04	0.09	0.06	0.06	0.01
C69	眼	Eye	4	0.04	0.09	0.07	0.13	0.01
C70-C72;D32-33;D42-43	脑，神经系统	Brain, nervous system	206	2.15	4.41	3.50	3.50	0.39
C73	甲状腺	Thyroid	28	0.29	0.60	0.44	0.43	0.05
C74	肾上腺	Adrenal gland	4	0.04	0.09	0.06	0.08	0.01
C75	其他的内分泌腺	Other endocrine	3	0.03	0.06	0.05	0.09	0.01
C81	霍奇金病	Hodgkin lymphoma	2	0.02	0.04	0.03	0.03	0.00
C82-C85;C96	非霍奇金淋巴瘤	Non-Hodgkin lymphoma	135	1.41	2.89	2.20	2.16	0.28
C88	免疫增生性疾病	Immunoproliferative diseases	0	0.00	0.00	0.00	0.00	0.00
C90	多发性骨髓瘤	Multiple myeloma	40	0.42	0.86	0.62	0.61	0.09
C91	淋巴样白血病	Lymphoid leukemia	27	0.28	0.58	0.56	0.55	0.05
C92-C94;D45-47	髓样白血病	Myeloid leukemia	84	0.88	1.80	1.46	1.36	0.13
C95	白血病，未特指	Leukemia unspecified	60	0.63	1.29	1.10	1.13	0.11
O&U	其他的或未指明部位	Other and unspecified	332	3.46	7.11	5.26	5.21	0.62
ALL	所有部位合计	All sites	9598	100.00	205.67	146.80	145.40	17.10
ALLbC44	所有部位除外 C44	All sites except C44	9565	99.66	204.96	146.34	144.94	17.04

附表 1-17　2019 年福建省农村肿瘤登记地区女性发病主要指标

Appendix Table 1-17　Cancer incidence in rural registration areas of Fujian, female in 2019

ICD10	部位 Site	发病数 Cases	构成 Freq. （%）	粗率 Crude rate （1/10^5）	中标率 ASR China （1/10^5）	世标率 ASR world （1/10^5）	累积率 Cum.rate （0~74，%）
C00	唇	Lip	5	0.04	0.12	0.08	0.08	0.01
C01-C02	舌	Tongue	30	0.27	0.70	0.48	0.47	0.06
C03-C06	口	Mouth	25	0.22	0.58	0.41	0.37	0.04
C07-C08	唾液腺	Salivary glands	18	0.16	0.42	0.38	0.34	0.03
C09	扁桃体	Tonsil	3	0.03	0.07	0.04	0.05	0.01
C10	其他的口咽	Other oropharynx	4	0.04	0.09	0.06	0.06	0.01
C11	鼻咽	Nasopharynx	118	1.05	2.75	2.29	2.04	0.21
C12-C13	喉咽	Hypopharynx	3	0.03	0.07	0.05	0.05	0.01
C14	咽，部位不明	Pharynx unspecified	4	0.04	0.09	0.08	0.07	0.01
C15	食管	Esophagus	468	4.16	10.89	6.81	6.90	0.92
C16	胃	Stomach	701	6.23	16.32	11.03	10.61	1.31
C17	小肠	Small intestine	41	0.36	0.95	0.69	0.66	0.08
C18	结肠	Colon	600	5.33	13.97	9.42	9.02	1.06
C19-C20	直肠	Rectum	576	5.12	13.41	8.89	8.65	1.10
C21	肛门	Anus	9	0.08	0.21	0.14	0.13	0.01
C22	肝脏	Liver	399	3.55	9.29	6.32	6.09	0.71
C23-C24	胆囊及其他	Gallbladder etc.	118	1.05	2.75	1.77	1.76	0.22
C25	胰腺	Pancreas	107	0.95	2.49	1.56	1.54	0.19
C30-C31	鼻，鼻窦及其他	Nose, sinuses etc.	8	0.07	0.19	0.12	0.11	0.01
C32	喉	Larynx	6	0.05	0.14	0.09	0.09	0.01
C33-C34	气管，支气管，肺	Trachea, bronchus & lung	1455	12.93	33.87	22.76	22.40	2.73
C37-C38	其他的胸腔器官	Other thoracic organs	24	0.21	0.56	0.39	0.44	0.04
C40-C41	骨	Bone	39	0.35	0.91	0.78	0.83	0.07
C43	皮肤的黑色素瘤	Melanoma of skin	21	0.19	0.49	0.33	0.33	0.05
C44	其他的皮肤	Other skin	110	0.98	2.56	1.54	1.52	0.14
C45	间皮瘤	Mesothelioma	3	0.03	0.07	0.06	0.05	0.00
C46	卡波氏肉瘤	Kaposi sarcoma	0	0.00	0.00	0.00	0.00	0.00
C47;C49	周围神经,其他结缔、软组织	Connective & soft tissue	56	0.50	1.30	1.10	0.99	0.11
C50	乳房	Breast	1511	13.43	35.17	27.14	24.61	2.48
C51	外阴	Vulva	14	0.12	0.33	0.24	0.21	0.03
C52	阴道	Vagina	19	0.17	0.44	0.30	0.30	0.04
C53	子宫颈	Cervix uteri	926	8.23	21.55	15.49	14.73	1.62
C54	子宫体	Corpus uteri	366	3.25	8.52	5.83	5.69	0.62
C55	子宫，部位不明	Uterus unspecified	45	0.40	1.05	0.70	0.69	0.07
C56	卵巢	Ovary	247	2.19	5.75	4.42	4.25	0.47
C57	其他的女性生殖器	Other female genital organs	16	0.14	0.37	0.29	0.27	0.05
C58	胎盘	Placenta	7	0.06	0.16	0.16	0.13	0.01
C60	阴茎	Penis	—	—	—	—	—	—
C61	前列腺	Prostate	—	—	—	—	—	—
C62	睾丸	Testis	—	—	—	—	—	—
C63	其他的男性生殖器	Other male genital organs	—	—	—	—	—	—
C64	肾	Kidney	106	0.94	2.47	1.81	1.75	0.21
C65	肾盂	Renal pelvis	13	0.12	0.30	0.21	0.21	0.04
C66	输尿管	Ureter	10	0.09	0.23	0.15	0.15	0.03
C67	膀胱	Bladder	66	0.59	1.54	0.95	0.95	0.11
C68	其他的泌尿器官	Other urinary organs	3	0.03	0.07	0.05	0.05	0.01
C69	眼	Eye	4	0.04	0.09	0.13	0.21	Cum.rate
C70-C72;D32-33;D42-43	脑，神经系统	Brain, nervous system	372	3.31	8.66	6.43	6.17	0.67
C73	甲状腺	Thyroid	1793	15.93	41.73	36.00	31.29	2.92
C74	肾上腺	Adrenal gland	5	0.04	0.12	0.10	0.13	0.01
C75	其他的内分泌腺	Other endocrine	3	0.03	0.07	0.04	0.05	0.01
C81	霍奇金病	Hodgkin lymphoma	3	0.03	0.07	0.07	0.07	0.01
C82-C85;C96	非霍奇金淋巴瘤	Non-Hodgkin lymphoma	179	1.59	4.17	3.14	2.96	0.33
C88	免疫增生性疾病	Immunoproliferative diseases	3	0.03	0.07	0.04	0.05	0.00
C90	多发性骨髓瘤	Multiple myeloma	46	0.41	1.07	0.70	0.72	0.10
C91	淋巴样白血病	Lymphoid leukemia	38	0.34	0.88	0.88	1.04	0.07
C92-C94; D45-47	髓样白血病	Myeloid leukemia	120	1.07	2.79	2.52	2.38	0.20
C95	白血病，未特指	Leukemia unspecified	20	0.18	0.47	0.37	0.42	0.03
O&U	其他的或未指明部位	Other and unspecified	369	3.28	8.59	6.09	6.11	0.68
ALL	所有部位合计	All sites	11255	100.00	261.96	191.92	181.22	19.95
ALLbC44	所有部位除外 C44	All sites except C44	11145	99.02	259.40	190.38	179.70	19.81

附表 1-18　2019 年福建省农村肿瘤登记地区女性死亡主要指标

Appendix Table 1-18　Cancer mortality in rural registration areas of Fujian, female in 2019

ICD10	部位 Site	死亡数 Deaths	构成 Freq. (%)	粗率 Crude rate (1/10⁵)	中标率 ASR China (1/10⁵)	世标率 ASR world (1/10⁵)	累积率 Cum.rate (0~74, %)
C00	唇 Lip	0	0.00	0.00	0.00	0.00	0.00
C01-C02	舌 Tongue	15	0.31	0.35	0.20	0.22	0.03
C03-C06	口 Mouth	15	0.31	0.35	0.20	0.19	0.03
C07-C08	唾液腺 Salivary glands	2	0.04	0.05	0.02	0.02	0.00
C09	扁桃体 Tonsil	0	0.00	0.00	0.00	0.00	0.00
C10	其他的口咽 Other oropharynx	4	0.08	0.09	0.06	0.05	0.00
C11	鼻咽 Nasopharynx	58	1.20	1.35	0.88	0.85	0.10
C12-C13	喉咽 Hypopharynx	0	0.00	0.00	0.00	0.00	0.00
C14	咽，部位不明 Pharynx unspecified	7	0.14	0.16	0.09	0.09	0.01
C15	食管 Esophagus	523	10.83	12.17	6.90	6.83	0.76
C16	胃 Stomach	577	11.94	13.43	8.04	7.81	0.86
C17	小肠 Small intestine	18	0.37	0.42	0.28	0.30	0.04
C18	结肠 Colon	273	5.65	6.35	3.94	3.75	0.41
C19-C20	直肠 Rectum	273	5.65	6.35	3.83	3.78	0.44
C21	肛门 Anus	5	0.10	0.12	0.08	0.08	0.02
C22	肝脏 Liver	446	9.23	10.38	6.44	6.27	0.71
C23-C24	胆囊及其他 Gallbladder etc.	87	1.80	2.02	1.17	1.18	0.15
C25	胰腺 Pancreas	114	2.36	2.65	1.65	1.57	0.18
C30-C31	鼻，鼻窦及其他 Nose, sinuses etc.	5	0.10	0.12	0.07	0.07	0.01
C32	喉 Larynx	11	0.23	0.26	0.14	0.13	0.01
C33-C34	气管，支气管，肺 Trachea, bronchus & lung	858	17.76	19.97	12.30	12.12	1.47
C37-C38	其他的胸腔器官 Other thoracic organs	8	0.17	0.19	0.08	0.10	0.01
C40-C41	骨 Bone	34	0.70	0.79	0.52	0.55	0.07
C43	皮肤的黑色素瘤 Melanoma of skin	8	0.17	0.19	0.11	0.11	0.02
C44	其他的皮肤 Other skin	37	0.77	0.86	0.37	0.39	0.02
C45	间皮瘤 Mesothelioma	0	0.00	0.00	0.00	0.00	0.00
C46	卡波氏肉瘤 Kaposi sarcoma	0	0.00	0.00	0.00	0.00	0.00
C47;C49	周围神经,其他结缔、软组织 Connective & soft tissue	10	0.21	0.23	0.16	0.14	0.01
C50	乳房 Breast	266	5.51	6.19	4.37	4.15	0.46
C51	外阴 Vulva	5	0.10	0.12	0.07	0.07	0.01
C52	阴道 Vagina	9	0.19	0.21	0.12	0.13	0.01
C53	子宫颈 Cervix uteri	273	5.65	6.35	4.22	4.16	0.51
C54	子宫体 Corpus uteri	58	1.20	1.35	0.86	0.85	0.10
C55	子宫，部位不明 Uterus unspecified	48	0.99	1.12	0.75	0.71	0.08
C56	卵巢 Ovary	112	2.32	2.61	1.76	1.75	0.21
C57	其他的女性生殖器 Other female genital organs	5	0.10	0.12	0.08	0.08	0.01
C58	胎盘 Placenta	1	0.02	0.02	0.02	0.02	0.00
C60	阴茎 Penis	—	—	—	—	—	—
C61	前列腺 Prostate	—	—	—	—	—	—
C62	睾丸 Testis	—	—	—	—	—	—
C63	其他的男性生殖器 Other male genital organs	—	—	—	—	—	—
C64	肾 Kidney	20	0.41	0.47	0.29	0.30	0.05
C65	肾盂 Renal pelvis	3	0.06	0.07	0.04	0.04	0.00
C66	输尿管 Ureter	4	0.08	0.09	0.07	0.07	0.01
C67	膀胱 Bladder	21	0.43	0.49	0.28	0.26	0.02
C68	其他的泌尿器官 Other urinary organs	3	0.06	0.07	0.05	0.05	0.01
C69	眼 Eye	4	0.08	0.09	0.09	0.16	0.01
C70-C72;D32-33;D42-43	脑，神经系统 Brain, nervous system	147	3.04	3.42	2.49	2.49	0.27
C73	甲状腺 Thyroid	25	0.52	0.58	0.36	0.36	0.03
C74	肾上腺 Adrenal gland	5	0.10	0.12	0.09	0.13	0.01
C75	其他的内分泌腺 Other endocrine	1	0.02	0.02	0.01	0.02	0.00
C81	霍奇金病 Hodgkin lymphoma	0	0.00	0.00	0.00	0.00	0.00
C82-C85;C96	非霍奇金淋巴瘤 Non-Hodgkin lymphoma	67	1.39	1.56	1.05	1.04	0.12
C88	免疫增生性疾病 Immunoproliferative diseases	2	0.04	0.05	0.03	0.03	0.00
C90	多发性骨髓瘤 Multiple myeloma	20	0.41	0.47	0.31	0.30	0.04
C91	淋巴样白血病 Lymphoid leukemia	16	0.33	0.37	0.30	0.33	0.02
C92-C94; D45-47	髓样白血病 Myeloid leukemia	60	1.24	1.40	1.06	1.01	0.10
C95	白血病，未特指 Leukemia unspecified	47	0.97	1.09	0.81	0.96	0.07
O&U	其他的或未指明部位 Other and unspecified	221	4.57	5.14	3.42	3.35	0.40
ALL	所有部位合计 All sites	4831	100.00	112.44	70.57	69.41	7.90
ALLbC44	所有部位除外 C44 All sites except C44	4794	99.23	111.58	70.20	69.02	7.88

附录 2　2019 年福建省 24 个肿瘤登记地区恶性肿瘤发病和死亡结果
Appendix 2　Cancer incidence and mortality in 24 registration areas of Fujian, 2019

附表 2-1　2019 年长乐区恶性肿瘤发病主要指标

Appendix Table 2-1　Cancer incidence in Changle, 2019

ICD10	部位 Site		发病数 Cases	构成 Freq. （%）	粗率 Crude rate （1/10⁵）	中标率 ASR China （1/10⁵）	世标率 ASR world （1/10⁵）	累积率 Cum.rate （0~74,%）
C00-10, C12-14	口腔和咽喉（除外鼻咽）	Oral Cavity & Pharynx but Nasopharynx	21	0.87	2.77	1.96	1.86	0.22
C11	鼻咽	Nasopharynx	40	1.67	5.28	4.19	3.84	0.38
C15	食管	Esophagus	71	2.96	9.38	5.88	5.74	0.68
C16	胃	Stomach	359	14.95	47.43	29.58	29.43	3.84
C18-21	结直肠肛门	Colon, Rectum & Anus	202	8.41	26.69	16.89	16.54	2.02
C22	肝脏	Liver	223	9.28	29.46	20.51	19.73	2.32
C23-C24	胆囊及其他	Gallbladder	21	0.87	2.77	1.60	1.62	0.20
C25	胰腺	Pancreas	38	1.58	5.02	3.07	3.05	0.40
C32	喉	Larynx	6	0.25	0.79	0.46	0.49	0.07
C33-C34	气管，支气管，肺	Trachea, Bronchus & Lung	438	18.23	57.86	38.02	37.57	4.97
C37-C38	其他的胸腔器官	Other thoracic organs	6	0.25	0.79	0.66	0.59	0.06
C40-C41	骨	Bone	11	0.46	1.45	1.12	1.08	0.09
C43	皮肤的黑色素瘤	Melanoma of skin	1	0.04	0.13	0.08	0.08	0.01
C50	乳房	Breast	142	5.91	39.33	29.41	26.43	2.67
C53	子宫颈	Cervix	57	2.37	15.79	11.42	10.39	1.03
C54-55	子宫体及子宫部位不明	Corpus Uterus & Unspectified	32	1.33	8.86	5.81	5.67	0.69
C56	卵巢	Ovary	14	0.58	3.88	2.61	2.48	0.32
C61	前列腺	Prostate	43	1.79	10.86	6.63	6.95	0.87
C62	睾丸	Testis	3	0.12	0.76	0.80	1.36	0.09
C64-66, 68	肾及泌尿系统不明	Kidney & Unspecified Urinary Organs	37	1.54	4.89	3.26	3.16	0.37
C67	膀胱	Bladder	43	1.79	5.68	3.63	3.54	0.43
C70-C72;D32-33; D42-43	脑，神经系统	Brain & Central Nervous System	66	2.75	8.72	6.42	6.11	0.71
C73	甲状腺	Thyroid	377	15.70	49.80	39.79	36.14	3.66
C81-85, 88,90,96	淋巴瘤	Lymphoma	51	2.12	6.74	4.64	4.55	0.48
C91-C95; D45-47	白血病	Leukaemia	36	1.50	4.76	3.85	4.27	0.40
Other	其他	Other	64	2.66	8.45	5.45	5.48	0.62
ALL	所有部位合计	All sites	2402	100.00	317.31	218.92	211.16	24.75
ALLbC44	所有部位除外 C44	All sites except C44	2387	99.38	315.33	217.64	209.94	24.61

附表 2-2　2019 年长乐区恶性肿瘤死亡主要指标
Appendix Table 2-2　Cancer mortality in Changle, 2019

ICD10	部位 Site	死亡数 Deaths	构成 Freq.（%）	粗率 Crude rate（1/10⁵）	中标率 ASR China（1/10⁵）	世标率 ASR world（1/10⁵）	累积率 Cum.rate（0~74,%）
C00-10, C12-14	口腔和咽喉（除外鼻咽）Oral Cavity & Pharynx but asopharynx	10	0.87	1.32	0.90	0.79	0.05
C11	鼻咽 Nasopharynx	23	2.00	3.04	1.92	1.95	0.21
C15	食管 Esophagus	56	4.86	7.40	4.30	4.18	0.42
C16	胃 Stomach	259	22.48	34.21	20.95	20.11	2.20
C18-21	结直肠肛门 Colon, Rectum & Anus	96	8.33	12.68	7.92	7.50	0.74
C22	肝脏 Liver	165	14.32	21.80	14.59	14.19	1.66
C23-C24	胆囊及其他 Gallbladder	19	1.65	2.51	1.50	1.51	0.20
C25	胰腺 Pancreas	30	2.60	3.96	2.55	2.37	0.26
C32	喉 Larynx	3	0.26	0.40	0.25	0.25	0.02
C33-C34	气管,支气管,肺 Trachea, Bronchus & Lung	242	21.01	31.97	19.96	19.55	2.23
C37-C38	其他的胸腔器官 Other thoracic organs	1	0.09	0.13	0.13	0.09	0.01
C40-C41	骨 Bone	12	1.04	1.59	1.30	1.26	0.12
C43	皮肤的黑色素瘤 Melanoma of skin	0	0.00	0.00	0.00	0.00	0.00
C50	乳房 Breast	26	2.26	7.20	4.78	4.57	0.45
C53	子宫颈 Cervix	20	1.74	5.54	3.74	3.48	0.37
C54-55	子宫体及子宫部位不明 Corpus Uterus & Unspectified	5	0.43	1.38	0.75	0.85	0.11
C56	卵巢 Ovary	5	0.43	1.38	0.73	0.82	0.08
C61	前列腺 Prostate	15	1.30	3.79	2.38	2.26	0.20
C62	睾九 Testis	1	0.09	0.25	0.37	0.39	0.02
C64-66, 68	肾及泌尿系统不明 Kidney & Unspecified Urinary Organs	15	1.30	1.98	1.17	1.10	0.10
C67	膀胱 Bladder	10	0.87	1.32	0.87	0.77	0.04
C70-C72; D32-33;D42-43	脑,神经系统 Brain & Central Nervous System	20	1.74	2.64	1.70	1.67	0.20
C73	甲状腺 Thyroid	12	1.04	1.59	0.99	0.97	0.11
C81-85, 88,90,96	淋巴瘤 Lymphoma	22	1.91	2.91	1.82	1.79	0.21
C91-C95; D45-47	白血病 Leukaemia	29	2.52	3.83	2.77	3.09	0.32
Other	其他 Other	56	4.86	7.40	4.33	4.30	0.41
ALL	所有部位合计 All sites	1152	100.00	152.18	96.31	93.66	10.16
ALLbC44	所有部位除外 C44 All sites except C44	1144	99.31	151.13	95.79	93.13	10.14

附表 2-3　2019 年福清市恶性肿瘤发病主要指标
Appendix Table 2-3　Cancer incidence in Fuqing, 2019

ICD10	部位	Site	发病数 Cases	构成 Freq. (%)	粗率 Crude rate (1/10⁵)	中标率 ASR China (1/10⁵)	世标率 ASR world (1/10⁵)	累积率 Cum.rate (0~74,%)
C00-10, C12-14	口腔和咽喉（除外鼻咽）	Oral Cavity & Pharynx but Nasopharynx	46	0.96	3.32	2.23	2.23	0.24
C11	鼻咽	Nasopharynx	61	1.28	4.40	3.54	3.36	0.36
C15	食管	Esophagus	214	4.49	15.43	9.48	9.61	1.14
C16	胃	Stomach	462	9.69	33.30	22.64	22.30	2.80
C18-21	结直肠肛门	Colon, Rectum & Anus	362	7.59	26.09	18.10	17.77	2.22
C22	肝脏	Liver	542	11.37	39.07	29.08	27.78	3.21
C23-C24	胆囊及其他	Gallbladder	44	0.92	3.17	2.10	2.05	0.25
C25	胰腺	Pancreas	69	1.45	4.97	3.21	3.15	0.36
C32	喉	Larynx	15	0.31	1.08	0.73	0.76	0.11
C33-C34	气管，支气管，肺	Trachea, Bronchus & Lung	871	18.26	62.78	43.90	43.48	5.55
C37-C38	其他的胸腔器官	Other thoracic organs	14	0.29	1.01	0.70	0.68	0.06
C40-C41	骨	Bone	11	0.23	0.79	0.76	0.76	0.06
C43	皮肤的黑色素瘤	Melanoma of skin	1	0.02	0.07	0.05	0.05	0.01
C50	乳房	Breast	274	5.83	40.74	32.31	29.28	2.95
C53	子宫颈	Cervix	113	2.37	16.80	12.23	11.67	1.22
C54-55	子宫体及子宫部位不明	Corpus Uterus & Unspectified	48	1.01	7.14	5.19	5.03	0.52
C56	卵巢	Ovary	31	0.65	4.61	3.50	3.39	0.41
C61	前列腺	Prostate	67	1.40	9.37	6.02	6.02	0.71
C62	睾丸	Testis	3	0.06	0.42	0.41	0.41	0.03
C64-66, 68	肾及泌尿系统不明	Kidney & Unspecified Urinary Organs	82	1.72	5.91	4.40	4.23	0.53
C67	膀胱	Bladder	56	1.17	4.04	2.81	2.64	0.29
C70-C72; D32-33;D42-43	脑，神经系统	Brain & Central Nervous System	127	2.66	9.15	7.05	6.69	0.73
C73	甲状腺	Thyroid	825	17.30	59.47	51.81	45.84	4.41
C81-85, 88,90,96	淋巴瘤	Lymphoma	108	2.26	7.78	6.08	5.78	0.59
C91-C95; D45-47	白血病	Leukaemia	75	1.57	5.41	4.61	4.98	0.35
Other	其他	Other	244	5.12	17.59	12.73	12.81	1.50
ALL	所有部位合计	All sites	4769	100.00	343.76	255.89	244.95	27.73
ALLbC44	所有部位除外 C44	All sites except C44	4737	99.33	341.45	254.41	243.54	27.57

附表 2-4　2019 年福清市恶性肿瘤死亡主要指标

Appendix Table 2-4　Cancer mortality in Fuqing, 2019

ICD10	部位 Site	死亡数 Deaths	构成 Freq.（%）	粗率 Crude rate（1/10⁵）	中标率 ASR China（1/10⁵）	世标率 ASR world（1/10⁵）	累积率 Cum.rate（0~74,%）
C00-10, C12-14	口腔和咽喉（除外鼻咽） Oral Cavity & Pharynx but Nasopharynx	16	0.70	1.15	0.69	0.69	0.08
C11	鼻咽 Nasopharynx	33	1.45	2.38	1.74	1.63	0.20
C15	食管 Esophagus	199	8.77	14.34	8.11	8.14	0.82
C16	胃 Stomach	308	13.57	22.20	13.58	13.22	1.40
C18-21	结直肠肛门 Colon, Rectum & Anus	157	6.92	11.32	7.24	6.90	0.69
C22	肝脏 Liver	433	19.07	31.21	22.27	21.43	2.50
C23-C24	胆囊及其他 Gallbladder	35	1.54	2.52	1.53	1.58	0.20
C25	胰腺 Pancreas	66	2.91	4.76	2.96	2.88	0.28
C32	喉 Larynx	10	0.44	0.72	0.47	0.48	0.07
C33-C34	气管，支气管，肺 Trachea, Bronchus & Lung	494	21.76	35.61	23.11	22.78	2.79
C37-C38	其他的胸腔器官 Other thoracic organs	6	0.26	0.43	0.36	0.33	0.02
C40-C41	骨 Bone	14	0.62	1.01	0.74	0.75	0.11
C43	皮肤的黑色素瘤 Melanoma of skin	3	0.13	0.22	0.10	0.11	0.01
C50	乳房 Breast	43	1.94	6.39	4.55	4.22	0.43
C53	子宫颈 Cervix	31	1.37	4.61	3.25	3.17	0.36
C54-55	子宫体及子宫部位不明 Corpus Uterus & Unspectified	16	0.70	2.38	1.75	1.64	0.21
C56	卵巢 Ovary	20	0.88	2.97	2.11	2.00	0.24
C61	前列腺 Prostate	39	1.72	5.46	3.22	3.25	0.34
C62	睾丸 Testis	0	0.00	0.00	0.00	0.00	0.00
C64-66, 68	肾及泌尿系统不明 Kidney & Unspecified Urinary Organs	18	0.79	1.30	0.86	0.84	0.09
C67	膀胱 Bladder	19	0.84	1.37	0.76	0.70	0.05
C70-C72; D32-33; D42-43	脑，神经系统 Brain & Central Nervous System	68	3.00	4.90	3.73	3.70	0.43
C73	甲状腺 Thyroid	22	0.97	1.59	1.09	1.07	0.12
C81-85, 88,90,96	淋巴瘤 Lymphoma	32	1.41	2.31	1.66	1.62	0.20
C91-C95; D45-47	白血病 Leukaemia	35	1.54	2.52	1.91	1.77	0.13
Other	其他 Other	152	6.70	10.96	7.26	7.44	0.74
ALL	所有部位合计 All sites	2270	100.00	163.63	107.57	105.20	11.73
ALLbC44	所有部位除外 C44 All sites except C44	2261	99.60	162.98	107.24	104.88	11.71

附表 2-5　2019 年永泰县恶性肿瘤发病主要指标
Appendix Table 2-5　Cancer incidence in Yongtai, 2019

ICD10	部位 Site		发病数 Cases	构成 Freq. (%)	粗率 Crude rate (1/10⁵)	中标率 ASR China (1/10⁵)	世标率 ASR world (1/10⁵)	累积率 Cum.rate (0~74, %)
C00-10, C12-14	口腔和咽喉（除外鼻咽）	Oral Cavity & Pharynx but Nasopharynx	7	0.67	1.81	1.36	1.15	0.09
C11	鼻咽	Nasopharynx	23	2.19	5.96	4.23	4.22	0.45
C15	食管	Esophagus	37	3.52	9.59	5.95	6.03	0.63
C16	胃	Stomach	105	10.00	27.22	19.14	18.56	2.41
C18-21	结直肠肛门	Colon, Rectum & Anus	138	13.14	35.77	24.68	23.79	3.10
C22	肝脏	Liver	79	7.52	20.48	13.85	13.65	1.44
C23-C24	胆囊及其他	Gallbladder	10	0.95	2.59	1.65	1.68	0.16
C25	胰腺	Pancreas	9	0.86	2.33	1.47	1.51	0.22
C32	喉	Larynx	7	0.67	1.81	1.12	1.21	0.20
C33-C34	气管，支气管，肺	Trachea, Bronchus & Lung	221	21.05	57.29	38.71	38.40	4.98
C37-C38	其他的胸腔器官	Other thoracic organs	4	0.38	1.04	0.74	0.72	0.10
C40-C41	骨	Bone	6	0.57	1.56	1.10	1.34	0.13
C43	皮肤的黑色素瘤	Melanoma of skin	2	0.19	0.52	0.36	0.35	0.02
C50	乳房	Breast	53	5.05	29.27	21.36	19.83	2.03
C53	子宫颈	Cervix	46	4.38	25.40	17.47	16.87	1.87
C54-55	子宫体及子宫部位不明	Corpus Uterus & Unspectified	24	2.29	13.25	9.25	9.00	0.92
C56	卵巢	Ovary	4	0.38	2.21	1.43	1.45	0.18
C61	前列腺	Prostate	15	1.43	7.33	4.63	4.71	0.56
C62	睾丸	Testis	1	0.10	0.49	0.55	0.47	0.03
C64-66, 68	肾及泌尿系统不明	Kidney & Unspecified Urinary Organs	13	1.24	3.37	2.44	2.42	0.36
C67	膀胱	Bladder	19	1.81	4.93	3.15	3.15	0.32
C70-C72; D32-33; D42-43	脑，神经系统	Brain & Central Nervous System	28	2.67	7.26	5.50	5.23	0.53
C73	甲状腺	Thyroid	110	10.48	28.51	24.50	21.06	1.94
C81-85, 88,90,96	淋巴瘤	Lymphoma	18	1.71	4.67	3.85	3.85	0.45
C91-C95; D45-47	白血病	Leukaemia	17	1.62	4.41	3.50	3.85	0.38
Other	其他	Other	54	5.14	14.00	10.63	10.84	1.02
ALL	所有部位合计	All sites	1050	100.00	272.19	194.47	188.49	21.68
ALLbC44	所有部位除外 C44	All sites except C44	1041	99.14	269.86	192.91	187.11	21.54

附表 2-6　2019 年永泰县恶性肿瘤死亡主要指标

Appendix Table 2-6　Cancer mortality in Yongtai, 2019

ICD10	部位 Site		死亡数 Deaths	构成 Freq. （%）	粗率 Crude rate （1/10⁵）	中标率 ASR China （1/10⁵）	世标率 ASR world （1/10⁵）	累积率 Cum.rate （0~74，%）
C00-10,C12-14	口腔和咽喉（除外鼻咽）	Oral Cavity & Pharynx but Nasopharynx	4	0.76	1.04	0.73	0.65	0.05
C11	鼻咽	Nasopharynx	8	1.53	2.07	1.43	1.41	0.18
C15	食管	Esophagus	28	5.35	7.26	4.66	4.47	0.47
C16	胃	Stomach	80	15.30	20.74	13.63	13.30	1.72
C18-21	结直肠肛门	Colon, Rectum & Anus	49	9.37	12.70	8.55	8.17	1.00
C22	肝脏	Liver	69	13.19	17.89	12.42	12.03	1.36
C23-C24	胆囊及其他	Gallbladder	5	0.96	1.30	0.71	0.74	0.07
C25	胰腺	Pancreas	8	1.53	2.07	1.44	1.38	0.20
C32	喉	Larynx	3	0.57	0.78	0.49	0.54	0.08
C33-C34	气管，支气管，肺	Trachea, Bronchus & Lung	147	28.11	38.11	24.84	24.43	3.34
C37-C38	其他的胸腔器官	Other thoracic organs	0	0.00	0.00	0.00	0.00	0.00
C40-C41	骨	Bone	6	1.15	1.56	1.13	1.16	0.07
C43	皮肤的黑色素瘤	Melanoma of skin	0	0.00	0.00	0.00	0.00	0.00
C50	乳房	Breast	7	1.53	3.87	3.18	2.68	0.34
C53	子宫颈	Cervix	14	2.68	7.73	5.05	4.84	0.42
C54-55	子宫体及子宫部位不明	Corpus Uterus & Unspectified	6	1.15	3.31	2.20	2.06	0.20
C56	卵巢	Ovary	0	0.00	0.00	0.00	0.00	0.00
C61	前列腺	Prostate	7	1.34	3.42	2.16	1.91	0.06
C62	睾丸	Testis	0	0.00	0.00	0.00	0.00	0.00
C64-66，68	肾及泌尿系统不明	Kidney & Unspecified Urinary Organs	5	0.96	1.30	0.79	0.86	0.15
C67	膀胱	Bladder	4	0.76	1.04	0.54	0.61	0.10
C70-C72; D32-33;D42-43	脑，神经系统	Brain & Central Nervous System	12	2.29	3.11	2.23	2.05	0.18
C73	甲状腺	Thyroid	1	0.19	0.26	0.16	0.17	0.03
C81-85, 88,90,96	淋巴瘤	Lymphoma	10	1.91	2.59	1.72	1.76	0.23
C91-C95; D45-47	白血病	Leukaemia	11	2.10	2.85	2.38	2.72	0.27
Other	其他	Other	38	7.27	9.85	7.41	7.76	0.84
ALL	所有部位合计	All sites	523	100.00	135.58	91.44	89.90	10.80
ALLbC44	所有部位除外 C44	All sites except C44	520	99.43	134.80	91.10	89.49	10.76

附表 2-7　2019 年厦门市区恶性肿瘤发病主要指标

Appendix Table 2-7　Cancer incidence in Xiamen, 2019

ICD10	部位 Site	发病数 Cases	构成 Freq. （%）	粗率 Crude rate （1/10⁵）	中标率 ASR China （1/10⁵）	世标率 ASR world （1/10⁵）	累积率 Cum.rate （0~74，%）
C00-10, C12-14	口腔和咽喉（除外鼻咽） Oral Cavity & Pharynx but Nasopharynx	100	1.60	5.71	4.43	4.42	0.55
C11	鼻咽 Nasopharynx	55	0.88	3.14	2.48	2.45	0.29
C15	食管 Esophagus	289	4.62	16.51	12.24	12.45	1.50
C16	胃 Stomach	377	6.03	21.53	16.41	16.37	1.99
C18-21	结直肠肛门 Colon, Rectum & Anus	834	13.33	47.63	36.39	35.96	4.22
C22	肝脏 Liver	420	6.71	23.99	18.13	18.19	2.14
C23-C24	胆囊及其他 Gallbladder	48	0.77	2.74	2.01	1.99	0.23
C25	胰腺 Pancreas	80	1.28	4.57	3.51	3.43	0.38
C32	喉 Larynx	42	0.67	2.40	1.91	1.92	0.26
C33-C34	气管，支气管，肺 Trachea, Bronchus & Lung	1129	18.05	64.48	49.87	49.57	6.28
C37-C38	其他的胸腔器官 Other thoracic organs	17	0.27	0.97	0.79	0.80	0.08
C40-C41	骨 Bone	13	0.21	0.74	0.74	0.66	0.06
C43	皮肤的黑色素瘤 Melanoma of skin	11	0.18	0.63	0.48	0.47	0.06
C50	乳房 Breast	582	9.38	65.13	52.10	48.72	5.14
C53	子宫颈 Cervix	120	1.92	13.43	10.72	9.88	1.07
C54-55	子宫体及子宫部位不明 Corpus Uterus & Unspectified	114	1.82	12.76	9.99	9.93	1.20
C56	卵巢 Ovary	59	0.94	6.60	5.86	5.57	0.53
C61	前列腺 Prostate	116	1.85	13.53	10.11	9.89	1.10
C62	睾丸 Testis	13	0.21	1.52	1.48	1.35	0.08
C64-66，68	肾及泌尿系统不明 Kidney & Unspecified Urinary Organs	130	2.08	7.43	5.99	5.76	0.60
C67	膀胱 Bladder	91	1.45	5.20	3.87	3.75	0.38
C70-C72; D32-33;D42-43	脑，神经系统 Brain & Central Nervous System	178	2.85	10.17	8.64	8.46	0.86
C73	甲状腺 Thyroid	865	13.83	49.41	44.11	38.04	3.56
C81-85, 88,90,96	淋巴瘤 Lymphoma	178	2.85	10.17	8.36	8.15	0.92
C91-C95; D45-47	白血病 Leukaemia	112	1.79	6.40	5.50	5.96	0.55
Other	其他 Other	278	4.44	15.88	12.70	12.34	1.36
ALL	所有部位合计 All sites	6256	100.00	357.32	285.17	275.15	30.98
ALLbC44	所有部位除外 C44 All sites except C44	6206	99.20	354.46	282.96	273.01	30.76

附表 2-8　2019 年厦门市区恶性肿瘤死亡主要指标

Appendix Table 2-8　Cancer mortality in Xiamen, 2019

ICD10	部位 Site	死亡数 Deaths	构成 Freq.（%）	粗率 Crude rate（1/10⁵）	中标率 ASR China（1/10⁵）	世标率 ASR world（1/10⁵）	累积率 Cum.rate（0~74，%）
C00-10, C12-14	口腔和咽喉（除外鼻咽） Oral Cavity & Pharynx but Nasopharynx	53	2.03	3.03	2.31	2.36	0.28
C11	鼻咽 Nasopharynx	31	1.19	1.77	1.33	1.41	0.20
C15	食管 Esophagus	192	7.36	10.97	7.76	7.98	0.89
C16	胃 Stomach	238	9.13	13.59	10.03	9.85	1.14
C18-21	结直肠肛门 Colon, Rectum & Anus	320	12.27	18.28	12.84	12.86	1.34
C22	肝脏 Liver	301	11.54	17.19	12.59	12.55	1.36
C23-C24	胆囊及其他 Gallbladder	32	1.23	1.83	1.31	1.33	0.16
C25	胰腺 Pancreas	79	3.03	4.51	3.45	3.35	0.41
C32	喉 Larynx	18	0.69	1.03	0.78	0.79	0.11
C33-C34	气管，支气管，肺 Trachea, Bronchus & Lung	605	23.20	34.56	25.10	25.22	2.92
C37-C38	其他的胸腔器官 Other thoracic organs	20	0.77	1.14	0.96	0.96	0.09
C40-C41	骨 Bone	8	0.31	0.46	0.49	0.44	0.05
C43	皮肤的黑色素瘤 Melanoma of skin	8	0.31	0.46	0.38	0.35	0.04
C50	乳房 Breast	105	4.03	11.75	8.53	8.43	0.87
C53	子宫颈 Cervix	28	1.07	3.13	2.57	2.45	0.27
C54-55	子宫体及子宫部位不明 Corpus Uterus & Unspectified	14	0.54	1.57	1.13	1.09	0.10
C56	卵巢 Ovary	28	1.07	3.13	2.40	2.28	0.30
C61	前列腺 Prostate	62	2.38	7.23	4.57	4.76	0.26
C62	睾丸 Testis	1	0.04	0.12	0.14	0.11	0.01
C64-66, 68	肾及泌尿系统不明 Kidney & Unspecified Urinary Organs	53	2.03	3.03	2.25	2.24	0.25
C67	膀胱 Bladder	36	1.38	2.06	1.34	1.38	0.13
C70-C72; D32-33;D42-43	脑，神经系统 Brain & Central Nervous System	51	1.96	2.91	2.52	2.47	0.18
C73	甲状腺 Thyroid	13	0.50	0.74	0.51	0.52	0.04
C81-85, 88,90,96	淋巴瘤 Lymphoma	90	3.45	5.14	3.73	3.64	0.33
C91-C95; D45-47	白血病 Leukaemia	73	2.80	4.17	3.22	3.44	0.33
Other	其他 Other	149	5.71	8.51	6.20	6.32	0.58
ALL	所有部位合计 All sites	2608	100.00	148.96	108.90	109.10	11.76
ALLbC44	所有部位除外 C44 All sites except C44	2594	99.46	148.16	108.43	108.59	11.73

附表 2-9　2019 年翔安区恶性肿瘤发病主要指标

Appendix Table 2-9　Cancer incidence in Xiang'an, 2019

ICD10	部位 Site	发病数 Cases	构成 Freq. （%）	粗率 Crude rate （1/10^5）	中标率 ASR China （1/10^5）	世标率 ASR world （1/10^5）	累积率 Cum.rate （0~74，%）
C00-10, C12-14	口腔和咽喉（除外鼻咽）	Oral Cavity & Pharynx but Nasopharynx	27	2.15	7.31	5.14	5.18	0.57
C11	鼻咽	Nasopharynx	18	1.44	4.87	4.51	4.03	0.43
C15	食管	Esophagus	156	12.45	42.23	30.14	30.60	3.87
C16	胃	Stomach	84	6.70	22.74	16.79	16.65	2.03
C18-21	结直肠肛门	Colon, Rectum & Anus	131	10.45	35.47	27.68	27.03	3.45
C22	肝脏	Liver	147	11.73	39.80	30.50	29.25	3.24
C23-C24	胆囊及其他	Gallbladder	5	0.40	1.35	1.04	0.96	0.11
C25	胰腺	Pancreas	11	0.88	2.98	2.23	2.22	0.33
C32	喉	Larynx	8	0.64	2.17	1.67	1.63	0.20
C33-C34	气管，支气管，肺	Trachea, Bronchus & Lung	221	17.64	59.83	43.35	43.24	5.16
C37-C38	其他的胸腔器官	Other thoracic organs	6	0.48	1.62	1.21	1.21	0.13
C40-C41	骨	Bone	2	0.16	0.54	0.52	0.50	0.03
C43	皮肤的黑色素瘤	Melanoma of skin	2	0.16	0.54	0.41	0.44	0.08
C50	乳房	Breast	79	6.30	42.79	33.96	30.71	2.95
C53	子宫颈	Cervix	36	2.87	19.50	16.41	14.08	1.28
C54-55	子宫体及子宫部位不明	Corpus Uterus & Unspectified	15	1.20	8.12	6.02	5.89	0.65
C56	卵巢	Ovary	5	0.40	2.71	2.16	2.04	0.22
C61	前列腺	Prostate	15	1.20	8.12	7.36	6.66	0.53
C62	睾丸	Testis	1	0.08	0.54	0.61	0.51	0.03
C64-66，68	肾及泌尿系统不明	Kidney & Unspecified Urinary Organs	16	1.28	4.33	3.35	3.24	0.43
C67	膀胱	Bladder	17	1.36	4.60	3.28	3.23	0.36
C70-C72; D32-33;D42-43	脑，神经系统	Brain & Central Nervous System	36	2.87	9.75	8.03	7.52	0.85
C73	甲状腺	Thyroid	112	8.94	30.32	26.94	22.94	2.18
C81-85, 88,90,96	淋巴瘤	Lymphoma	30	2.39	8.12	6.48	6.06	0.74
C91-C95; D45-47	白血病	Leukaemia	8	0.64	2.17	2.10	2.43	0.15
Other	其他	Other	65	5.19	17.60	13.59	13.83	1.55
ALL	所有部位合计	All sites	1253	100.00	339.23	262.37	252.26	28.74
ALLbC44	所有部位除外 C44	All sites except C44	1244	99.28	336.80	260.84	250.67	28.59

附表 2-10　2019 年翔安区恶性肿瘤死亡主要指标

Appendix Table 2-10　Cancer mortality in Xiang'an, 2019

ICD10	部位 Site		死亡数 Deaths	构成 Freq. （%）	粗率 Crude rate （1/10^5）	中标率 ASR China （1/10^5）	世标率 ASR world （1/10^5）	累积率 Cum.rate （0~74，%）
C00-10, C12-14	口腔和咽喉（除外鼻咽）	Oral Cavity & Pharynx but Nasopharynx	17	2.73	4.60	3.28	3.36	0.42
C11	鼻咽	Nasopharynx	7	1.13	1.90	1.35	1.40	0.16
C15	食管	Esophagus	102	16.40	27.62	19.85	19.90	2.48
C16	胃	Stomach	49	7.88	13.27	9.52	9.42	1.01
C18-21	结直肠肛门	Colon, Rectum & Anus	34	5.47	9.21	6.57	6.36	0.69
C22	肝脏	Liver	128	20.58	34.65	26.23	25.59	3.15
C23-C24	胆囊及其他	Gallbladder	4	0.64	1.08	0.81	0.80	0.14
C25	胰腺	Pancreas	8	1.29	2.17	1.68	1.61	0.20
C32	喉	Larynx	5	0.80	1.35	0.97	1.02	0.14
C33-C34	气管，支气管，肺	Trachea, Bronchus & Lung	150	24.12	40.61	29.70	29.17	3.77
C37-C38	其他的胸腔器官	Other thoracic organs	3	0.48	0.81	0.58	0.62	0.11
C40-C41	骨	Bone	2	0.32	0.54	0.34	0.37	0.05
C43	皮肤的黑色素瘤	Melanoma of skin	0	0.00	0.00	0.00	0.00	0.00
C50	乳房	Breast	17	2.89	9.21	6.93	6.61	0.75
C53	子宫颈	Cervix	11	1.77	5.96	4.61	4.34	0.51
C54-55	子宫体及子宫部位不明	Corpus Uterus & Unspectified	3	0.48	1.62	1.25	1.24	0.19
C56	卵巢	Ovary	4	0.64	2.17	1.52	1.62	0.20
C61	前列腺	Prostate	4	0.64	2.17	1.96	1.75	0.20
C62	睾丸	Testis	0	0.00	0.00	0.00	0.00	0.00
C64-66, 68	肾及泌尿系统不明	Kidney & Unspecified Urinary Organs	5	0.80	1.35	1.01	0.89	0.09
C67	膀胱	Bladder	6	0.96	1.62	1.08	1.06	0.13
C70-C72;D32-33;D42-43	脑，神经系统	Brain & Central Nervous System	16	2.57	4.33	3.59	3.48	0.40
C73	甲状腺	Thyroid	2	0.32	0.54	0.41	0.44	0.08
C81-85, 88,90,96	淋巴瘤	Lymphoma	3	0.48	0.81	0.54	0.52	0.02
C91-C95; D45-47	白血病	Leukaemia	8	1.29	2.17	2.25	2.45	0.19
Other	其他	Other	33	5.31	8.93	6.75	6.83	0.73
ALL	所有部位合计	All sites	622	100.00	168.40	124.98	123.36	14.97
ALLbC44	所有部位除外 C44	All sites except C44	620	99.68	167.86	124.64	123.04	14.97

附表 2-11　2019 年涵江区恶性肿瘤发病主要指标
Appendix Table 2-11　Cancer incidence in Hanjiang, 2019

ICD10		部位 Site	发病数 Cases	构成 Freq. （%）	粗率 Crude rate （1/10⁵）	中标率 ASR China （1/10⁵）	世标率 ASR world （1/10⁵）	累积率 Cum.rate （0~74，%）
C00-10, C12-14	口腔和咽喉（除外鼻咽）	Oral Cavity & Pharynx but Nasopharynx	25	1.30	5.56	3.30	3.09	0.38
C11	鼻咽	Nasopharynx	25	1.30	5.56	4.62	4.09	0.38
C15	食管	Esophagus	154	8.01	34.22	18.46	18.86	2.50
C16	胃	Stomach	373	19.41	82.89	46.54	46.64	5.97
C18-21	结直肠肛门	Colon, Rectum & Anus	162	8.43	36.00	21.04	20.74	2.55
C22	肝脏	Liver	166	8.64	36.89	21.72	21.42	2.53
C23-C24	胆囊及其他	Gallbladder	12	0.62	2.67	1.61	1.70	0.21
C25	胰腺	Pancreas	21	1.09	4.67	2.65	2.54	0.29
C32	喉	Larynx	4	0.21	0.89	0.51	0.54	0.10
C33-C34	气管，支气管，肺	Trachea, Bronchus & Lung	337	17.53	74.89	42.57	42.82	5.56
C37-C38	其他的胸腔器官	Other thoracic organs	10	0.52	2.22	1.64	1.97	0.17
C40-C41	骨	Bone	7	0.36	1.56	1.75	1.56	0.14
C43	皮肤的黑色素瘤	Melanoma of skin	4	0.21	0.89	0.49	0.51	0.05
C50	乳房	Breast	93	4.89	41.07	28.51	26.22	2.77
C53	子宫颈	Cervix	41	2.13	18.10	12.40	11.65	1.22
C54-55	子宫体及子宫部位不明	Corpus Uterus & Unspectified	30	1.56	13.25	7.95	7.73	0.96
C56	卵巢	Ovary	18	0.94	7.95	5.34	5.10	0.59
C61	前列腺	Prostate	31	1.61	13.87	7.96	7.78	0.92
C62	睾丸	Testis	1	0.05	0.45	0.63	0.66	0.04
C64-66, 68	肾及泌尿系统不明	Kidney & Unspecified Urinary Organs	30	1.56	6.67	4.11	4.37	0.48
C67	膀胱	Bladder	21	1.09	4.67	3.11	2.83	0.31
C70-C72; D32-33;D42-43	脑，神经系统	Brain & Central Nervous System	29	1.51	6.44	5.24	5.38	0.50
C73	甲状腺	Thyroid	202	10.51	44.89	35.91	32.37	3.11
C81-85, 88,90,96	淋巴瘤	Lymphoma	40	2.08	8.89	5.76	5.56	0.71
C91-C95; D45-47	白血病	Leukaemia	20	1.04	4.44	2.90	3.27	0.38
Other	其他	Other	65	3.38	14.44	8.99	8.51	1.02
ALL	所有部位合计	All sites	1922	100.00	427.11	264.81	258.85	30.66
ALLbC44	所有部位除外 C44	All sites except C44	1913	99.53	425.11	263.65	257.79	30.56

附表 2-12　2019 年涵江区恶性肿瘤死亡主要指标

Appendix Table 2-12　Cancer mortality in Hanjiang, 2019

ICD10	部位 Site		死亡数 Deaths	构成 Freq. （%）	粗率 Crude rate （1/10⁵）	中标率 ASR China （1/10⁵）	世标率 ASR world （1/10⁵）	累积率 Cum.rate （0~74，%）
C00-10, C12-14	口腔和咽喉（除外鼻咽）	Oral Cavity & Pharynx but Nasopharynx	7	0.74	1.56	0.62	0.70	0.06
C11	鼻咽	Nasopharynx	10	1.06	2.22	1.51	1.49	0.19
C15	食管	Esophagus	115	12.14	25.56	13.44	13.48	1.58
C16	胃	Stomach	264	27.88	58.67	31.72	31.25	3.98
C18-21	结直肠肛门	Colon, Rectum & Anus	60	6.34	13.33	7.23	7.29	0.93
C22	肝脏	Liver	143	15.10	31.78	19.11	18.64	2.32
C23-C24	胆囊及其他	Gallbladder	5	0.53	1.11	0.56	0.56	0.09
C25	胰腺	Pancreas	11	1.16	2.44	1.33	1.32	0.15
C32	喉	Larynx	0	0.00	0.00	0.00	0.00	0.00
C33-C34	气管，支气管，肺	Trachea, Bronchus & Lung	172	18.16	38.22	20.56	20.65	2.63
C37-C38	其他的胸腔器官	Other thoracic organs	2	0.21	0.44	0.32	0.27	0.01
C40-C41	骨	Bone	5	0.53	1.11	0.89	0.98	0.05
C43	皮肤的黑色素瘤	Melanoma of skin	1	0.11	0.22	0.12	0.13	0.02
C50	乳房	Breast	20	2.22	8.83	5.34	5.21	0.55
C53	子宫颈	Cervix	11	1.16	4.86	3.19	2.91	0.31
C54-55	子宫体及子宫部位不明	Corpus Uterus & Unspectified	6	0.63	2.65	1.41	1.49	0.19
C56	卵巢	Ovary	7	0.74	3.09	1.91	1.75	0.13
C61	前列腺	Prostate	8	0.84	3.58	1.99	1.93	0.21
C62	睾丸	Testis	0	0.00	0.00	0.00	0.00	0.00
C64-66，68	肾及泌尿系统不明	Kidney & Unspecified Urinary Organs	6	0.63	1.33	0.79	1.03	0.09
C67	膀胱	Bladder	7	0.74	1.56	0.82	0.77	0.07
C70-C72; D32-33;D42-43	脑，神经系统	Brain & Central Nervous System	19	2.01	4.22	2.93	2.57	0.26
C73	甲状腺	Thyroid	11	1.16	2.44	1.47	1.51	0.21
C81-85, 88,90,96	淋巴瘤	Lymphoma	10	1.06	2.22	1.39	1.30	0.13
C91-C95; D45-47	白血病	Leukaemia	13	1.37	2.89	2.28	2.44	0.23
Other	其他	Other	33	3.48	7.33	4.79	4.34	0.50
ALL	所有部位合计	All sites	947	100.00	210.45	119.04	117.61	14.21
ALLbC44	所有部位除外 C44	All sites except C44	946	99.89	210.22	118.94	117.53	14.21

附表 2-13　2019 年仙游县恶性肿瘤发病主要指标
Appendix Table 2-13　Cancer incidence in Xianyou, 2019

ICD10	部位 Site		发病数 Cases	构成 Freq. （%）	粗率 Crude rate （1/10⁵）	中标率 ASR China （1/10⁵）	世标率 ASR world （1/10⁵）	累积率 Cum.rate （0~74，%）
C00-10, C12-14	口腔和咽喉（除外鼻咽）	Oral Cavity & Pharynx but Nasopharynx	31	0.95	2.64	1.98	1.89	0.19
C11	鼻咽	Nasopharynx	41	1.25	3.49	2.93	2.63	0.26
C15	食管	Esophagus	330	10.09	28.09	19.57	20.04	2.80
C16	胃	Stomach	521	15.93	44.34	31.66	31.76	4.24
C18-21	结直肠肛门	Colon, Rectum & Anus	312	9.54	26.55	19.56	18.94	2.34
C22	肝脏	Liver	222	6.79	18.89	14.32	13.92	1.71
C23-C24	胆囊及其他	Gallbladder	13	0.40	1.11	0.78	0.77	0.11
C25	胰腺	Pancreas	24	0.73	2.04	1.44	1.44	0.17
C32	喉	Larynx	8	0.24	0.68	0.47	0.48	0.06
C33-C34	气管，支气管，肺	Trachea, Bronchus & Lung	528	16.14	44.94	32.43	32.53	4.43
C37-C38	其他的胸腔器官	Other thoracic organs	15	0.46	1.28	1.01	1.10	0.12
C40-C41	骨	Bone	5	0.15	0.43	0.43	0.37	0.03
C43	皮肤的黑色素瘤	Melanoma of skin	6	0.18	0.51	0.40	0.35	0.03
C50	乳房	Breast	221	6.85	38.91	29.91	27.59	2.89
C53	子宫颈	Cervix	98	3.00	17.25	13.02	12.20	1.30
C54-55	子宫体及子宫部位不明	Corpus Uterus & Unspectified	41	1.25	7.22	5.28	5.03	0.51
C56	卵巢	Ovary	35	1.07	6.16	4.59	4.18	0.37
C61	前列腺	Prostate	32	0.98	5.27	3.84	3.81	0.45
C62	睾丸	Testis	4	0.12	0.66	0.69	0.76	0.07
C64-66，68	肾及泌尿系统不明	Kidney & Unspecified Urinary Organs	47	1.44	4.00	2.93	2.86	0.34
C67	膀胱	Bladder	44	1.35	3.74	2.53	2.60	0.29
C70-C72; D32-33;D42-43	脑，神经系统	Brain & Central Nervous System	78	2.38	6.64	5.48	5.07	0.52
C73	甲状腺	Thyroid	344	10.52	29.28	25.80	22.58	2.15
C81-85, 88,90,96	淋巴瘤	Lymphoma	72	2.20	6.13	4.65	4.61	0.55
C91-C95; D45-47	白血病	Leukaemia	62	1.90	5.28	4.81	5.31	0.41
Other	其他	Other	134	4.10	11.40	8.58	8.99	0.93
ALL	所有部位合计	All sites	3271	100.00	278.38	210.54	205.16	24.51
ALLbC44	所有部位除外 C44	All sites except C44	3251	99.39	276.68	209.49	204.02	24.38

附表 2-14　2019 年仙游县恶性肿瘤死亡主要指标

Appendix Table 2-14　Cancer mortality in Xianyou, 2019

ICD10	部位 Site		死亡数 Deaths	构成 Freq. （%）	粗率 Crude rate （1/10⁵）	中标率 ASR China （1/10⁵）	世标率 ASR world （1/10⁵）	累积率 Cum.rate （0~74，%）
C00-10,C12-14	口腔和咽喉（除外鼻咽）	Oral Cavity & Pharynx but Nasopharynx	13	0.66	1.11	0.81	0.76	0.08
C11	鼻咽	Nasopharynx	25	1.26	2.13	1.44	1.47	0.15
C15	食管	Esophagus	315	15.91	26.81	17.62	17.66	2.07
C16	胃	Stomach	435	21.97	37.02	25.35	25.18	3.15
C18-21	结直肠肛门	Colon, Rectum & Anus	130	6.57	11.06	7.67	7.71	0.97
C22	肝脏	Liver	298	15.05	25.36	18.33	17.91	2.18
C23-C24	胆囊及其他	Gallbladder	12	0.61	1.02	0.66	0.68	0.09
C25	胰腺	Pancreas	29	1.46	2.47	1.79	1.63	0.16
C32	喉	Larynx	6	0.30	0.51	0.35	0.35	0.05
C33-C34	气管，支气管，肺	Trachea, Bronchus & Lung	409	20.66	34.81	23.62	23.80	2.93
C37-C38	其他的胸腔器官	Other thoracic organs	1	0.05	0.09	0.06	0.06	0.01
C40-C41	骨	Bone	13	0.66	1.11	0.87	0.87	0.11
C43	皮肤的黑色素瘤	Melanoma of skin	1	0.05	0.09	0.07	0.05	0.00
C50	乳房	Breast	25	1.26	4.40	3.15	3.14	0.41
C53	子宫颈	Cervix	34	1.72	5.99	4.12	4.10	0.54
C54-55	子宫体及子宫部位不明	Corpus Uterus & Unspectified	7	0.35	1.23	0.85	0.80	0.08
C56	卵巢	Ovary	12	0.61	2.11	1.44	1.41	0.15
C61	前列腺	Prostate	16	0.81	2.64	1.93	1.75	0.18
C62	睾丸	Testis	1	0.05	0.16	0.15	0.14	0.04
C64-66，68	肾及泌尿系统不明	Kidney & Unspecified Urinary Organs	9	0.45	0.77	0.50	0.53	0.07
C67	膀胱	Bladder	11	0.56	0.94	0.62	0.64	0.09
C70-C72; D32-33;D42-43	脑，神经系统	Brain & Central Nervous System	40	2.02	3.40	2.47	2.53	0.32
C73	甲状腺	Thyroid	11	0.56	0.94	0.65	0.67	0.09
C81-85, 88,90,96	淋巴瘤	Lymphoma	31	1.57	2.64	1.97	2.02	0.25
C91-C95; D45-47	白血病	Leukaemia	40	2.02	3.40	2.83	2.90	0.27
Other	其他	Other	56	2.83	4.77	3.43	3.52	0.36
ALL	所有部位合计	All sites	1980	100.00	168.51	116.88	116.57	14.08
ALLbC44	所有部位除外 C44	All sites except C44	1972	99.60	167.83	116.48	116.17	14.04

附表 2-15　2019 年泉港区恶性肿瘤发病主要指标
Appendix Table 2-15　Cancer incidence in Quangang, 2019

ICD10	部位 Site	发病数 Cases	构成 Freq. （%）	粗率 Crude rate （1/10⁵）	中标率 ASR China （1/10⁵）	世标率 ASR world （1/10⁵）	累积率 Cum.rate （0~74，%）
C00-10, C12-14	口腔和咽喉（除外鼻咽） Oral Cavity & Pharynx but Nasopharynx	28	2.15	6.64	5.45	5.38	0.68
C11	鼻咽 Nasopharynx	15	1.15	3.56	3.17	2.96	0.30
C15	食管 Esophagus	252	19.33	59.75	45.45	45.87	5.50
C16	胃 Stomach	111	8.51	26.32	19.44	19.85	2.52
C18-21	结直肠肛门 Colon, Rectum & Anus	108	8.28	25.61	19.24	19.16	2.21
C22	肝脏 Liver	123	9.43	29.16	23.71	22.66	2.62
C23-C24	胆囊及其他 Gallbladder	10	0.77	2.37	1.78	1.74	0.15
C25	胰腺 Pancreas	9	0.69	2.13	1.43	1.55	0.19
C32	喉 Larynx	12	0.92	2.85	2.11	2.22	0.27
C33-C34	气管，支气管，肺 Trachea, Bronchus & Lung	202	15.49	47.90	37.01	37.15	4.61
C37-C38	其他的胸腔器官 Other thoracic organs	4	0.31	0.95	0.71	0.74	0.08
C40-C41	骨 Bone	2	0.15	0.47	0.40	0.37	0.03
C43	皮肤的黑色素瘤 Melanoma of skin	0	0.00	0.00	0.00	0.00	0.00
C50	乳房 Breast	74	5.67	36.10	30.20	26.86	2.54
C53	子宫颈 Cervix	45	3.45	21.95	17.50	16.30	1.67
C54-55	子宫体及子宫部位不明 Corpus Uterus & Unspectified	20	1.53	9.76	7.53	7.42	0.74
C56	卵巢 Ovary	14	1.07	6.83	5.45	5.17	0.46
C61	前列腺 Prostate	13	1.00	6.00	5.13	5.34	0.75
C62	睾丸 Testis	0	0.00	0.00	0.00	0.00	0.00
C64-66，68	肾及泌尿系统不明 Kidney & Unspecified Urinary Organs	23	1.76	5.45	4.33	4.23	0.39
C67	膀胱 Bladder	14	1.07	3.32	2.51	2.56	0.34
C70-C72; D32-33;D42-43	脑，神经系统 Brain & Central Nervous System	36	2.76	8.54	7.05	6.80	0.63
C73	甲状腺 Thyroid	87	6.67	20.63	18.56	16.71	1.62
C81-85, 88,90,96	淋巴瘤 Lymphoma	18	1.38	4.27	3.60	3.44	0.37
C91-C95; D45-47	白血病 Leukaemia	12	0.92	2.85	2.86	2.98	0.27
Other	其他 Other	72	5.52	17.07	14.09	14.32	1.52
ALL	所有部位合计 All sites	1304	100.00	309.20	245.38	240.88	27.34
ALLbC44	所有部位除外 C44 All sites except C44	1297	99.46	307.54	243.97	239.45	27.21

附表 2-16　2019 年泉港区恶性肿瘤死亡主要指标

Appendix Table 2-16　Cancer mortality in Quangang, 2019

ICD10	部位 Site		死亡数 Deaths	构成 Freq. （%）	粗率 Crude rate （1/10⁵）	中标率 ASR China （1/10⁵）	世标率 ASR world （1/10⁵）	累积率 Cum.rate （0~74，%）
C00-10, C12-14	口腔和咽喉（除外鼻咽）	Oral Cavity & Pharynx but Nasopharynx	14	1.64	3.32	2.22	2.34	0.26
C11	鼻咽	Nasopharynx	9	1.05	2.13	1.70	1.61	0.15
C15	食管	Esophagus	222	25.93	52.64	37.19	37.57	4.30
C16	胃	Stomach	76	8.88	18.02	13.99	13.86	1.73
C18-21	结直肠肛门	Colon, Rectum & Anus	46	5.37	10.91	8.04	7.84	0.92
C22	肝脏	Liver	128	14.95	30.35	23.85	23.16	2.79
C23-C24	胆囊及其他	Gallbladder	4	0.47	0.95	0.70	0.73	0.07
C25	胰腺	Pancreas	16	1.87	3.79	2.86	2.97	0.40
C32	喉	Larynx	10	1.17	2.37	1.65	1.72	0.19
C33-C34	气管，支气管，肺	Trachea, Bronchus & Lung	178	20.79	42.21	32.43	31.97	3.94
C37-C38	其他的胸腔器官	Other thoracic organs	3	0.35	0.71	0.58	0.57	0.07
C40-C41	骨	Bone	10	1.17	2.37	1.79	1.69	0.18
C43	皮肤的黑色素瘤	Melanoma of skin	2	0.23	0.47	0.35	0.38	0.06
C50	乳房	Breast	12	1.40	5.85	4.64	4.40	0.52
C53	子宫颈	Cervix	7	0.82	3.41	2.64	2.53	0.33
C54-55	子宫体及子宫部位不明	Corpus Uterus & Unspectified	3	0.35	1.46	1.16	1.15	0.16
C56	卵巢	Ovary	4	0.47	1.95	1.33	1.43	0.19
C61	前列腺	Prostate	7	0.82	3.23	2.30	2.31	0.16
C62	睾丸	Testis	0	0.00	0.00	0.00	0.00	0.00
C64-66, 68	肾及泌尿系统不明	Kidney & Unspecified Urinary Organs	5	0.58	1.19	0.50	0.60	0.02
C67	膀胱	Bladder	8	0.93	1.90	1.06	0.98	0.06
C70-C72; D32-33;D42-43	脑，神经系统	Brain & Central Nervous System	18	2.10	4.27	3.52	3.32	0.53
C73	甲状腺	Thyroid	2	0.23	0.47	0.30	0.28	0.02
C81-85, 88,90,96	淋巴瘤	Lymphoma	9	1.05	2.13	1.78	1.77	0.16
C91-C95; D45-47	白血病	Leukaemia	18	2.10	4.27	3.72	3.64	0.38
Other	其他	Other	45	5.26	10.67	7.87	8.31	0.93
ALL	所有部位合计	All sites	856	100.00	202.97	152.03	151.09	17.86
ALLbC44	所有部位除外 C44	All sites except C44	852	99.53	202.02	151.58	150.51	17.81

附表 2-17　2019 年安溪县恶性肿瘤发病主要指标

Appendix Table 2-17　Cancer incidence in Anxi, 2019

ICD10	部位 Site		发病数 Cases	构成 Freq. （%）	粗率 Crude rate （1/10^5）	中标率 ASR China （1/10^5）	世标率 ASR world （1/10^5）	累积率 Cum.rate （0~74，%）
C00-10, C12-14	口腔和咽喉（除外鼻咽）	Oral Cavity & Pharynx but Nasopharynx	47	1.76	3.87	3.42	3.28	0.44
C11	鼻咽	Nasopharynx	55	2.06	4.53	4.00	3.63	0.34
C15	食管	Esophagus	343	12.85	28.23	22.69	23.26	3.07
C16	胃	Stomach	344	12.89	28.31	23.29	23.20	2.99
C18-21	结直肠肛门	Colon, Rectum & Anus	330	12.36	27.16	22.33	21.85	2.75
C22	肝脏	Liver	193	7.23	15.88	12.90	12.62	1.42
C23-C24	胆囊及其他	Gallbladder	14	0.52	1.15	0.88	0.86	0.08
C25	胰腺	Pancreas	15	0.56	1.23	1.03	1.05	0.16
C32	喉	Larynx	13	0.49	1.07	0.89	0.89	0.12
C33-C34	气管，支气管，肺	Trachea, Bronchus & Lung	371	13.90	30.53	25.27	25.33	3.30
C37-C38	其他的胸腔器官	Other thoracic organs	5	0.19	0.41	0.43	0.41	0.03
C40-C41	骨	Bone	7	0.26	0.58	0.51	0.46	0.05
C43	皮肤的黑色素瘤	Melanoma of skin	7	0.26	0.58	0.50	0.49	0.08
C50	乳房	Breast	140	5.25	24.66	20.18	18.46	1.86
C53	子宫颈	Cervix	159	5.96	28.00	22.18	21.04	2.36
C54-55	子宫体及子宫部位不明	Corpus Uterus & Unspecified	42	1.57	7.40	5.59	5.49	0.60
C56	卵巢	Ovary	32	1.20	5.64	4.82	4.50	0.53
C61	前列腺	Prostate	38	1.42	5.87	5.37	5.14	0.54
C62	睾丸	Testis	4	0.15	0.62	0.78	0.76	0.05
C64-66，68	肾及泌尿系统不明	Kidney & Unspecified Urinary Organs	32	1.20	2.63	2.29	2.22	0.31
C67	膀胱	Bladder	26	0.97	2.14	1.83	1.84	0.29
C70-C72; D32-33;D42-43	脑，神经系统	Brain & Central Nervous System	77	2.88	6.34	5.75	5.98	0.55
C73	甲状腺	Thyroid	123	4.61	10.12	9.64	8.13	0.69
C81-85, 88,90,96	淋巴瘤	Lymphoma	67	2.51	5.51	4.71	4.64	0.57
C91-C95; D45-47	白血病	Leukaemia	50	1.87	4.11	3.91	4.19	0.31
Other	其他	Other	135	5.06	11.11	9.93	9.67	1.10
ALL	所有部位合计	All sites	2669	100.00	219.63	185.22	181.31	21.59
ALLbC44	所有部位除外 C44	All sites except C44	2653	99.40	218.31	184.14	180.22	21.50

附表 2-18　2019 年安溪县恶性肿瘤死亡主要指标
Appendix Table 2-18　Cancer mortality in Anxi, 2019

ICD10	部位 Site		死亡数 Deaths	构成 Freq. （%）	粗率 Crude rate （1/10⁵）	中标率 ASR China （1/10⁵）	世标率 ASR world （1/10⁵）	累积率 Cum.rate （0~74，%）
C00-10, C12-14	口腔和咽喉（除外鼻咽）	Oral Cavity & Pharynx but Nasopharynx	29	1.55	2.39	1.92	1.95	0.25
C11	鼻咽	Nasopharynx	28	1.49	2.30	2.00	1.82	0.19
C15	食管	Esophagus	388	20.72	31.93	25.60	25.55	3.03
C16	胃	Stomach	239	12.76	19.67	16.25	15.95	1.88
C18-21	结直肠肛门	Colon, Rectum & Anus	148	7.90	12.18	9.73	9.67	1.10
C22	肝脏	Liver	237	12.65	19.50	15.91	15.44	1.67
C23-C24	胆囊及其他	Gallbladder	14	0.75	1.15	0.90	0.92	0.09
C25	胰腺	Pancreas	25	1.33	2.06	1.76	1.73	0.26
C32	喉	Larynx	19	1.01	1.56	1.20	1.18	0.09
C33-C34	气管，支气管，肺	Trachea, Bronchus & Lung	395	21.09	32.50	26.67	26.50	3.24
C37-C38	其他的胸腔器官	Other thoracic organs	5	0.27	0.41	0.46	0.42	0.05
C40-C41	骨	Bone	11	0.59	0.91	0.81	0.85	0.10
C43	皮肤的黑色素瘤	Melanoma of skin	1	0.05	0.08	0.04	0.06	0.00
C50	乳房	Breast	31	1.66	5.46	4.45	4.25	0.45
C53	子宫颈	Cervix	33	1.76	5.81	4.60	4.49	0.59
C54-55	子宫体及子宫部位不明	Corpus Uterus & Unspectified	14	0.75	2.47	1.87	1.84	0.21
C56	卵巢	Ovary	15	0.80	2.64	1.97	1.92	0.22
C61	前列腺	Prostate	12	0.64	1.85	1.70	1.60	0.13
C62	睾丸	Testis	0	0.00	0.00	0.00	0.00	0.00
C64-66，68	肾及泌尿系统不明	Kidney & Unspecified Urinary Organs	7	0.37	0.58	0.49	0.51	0.09
C67	膀胱	Bladder	9	0.48	0.74	0.59	0.61	0.09
C70-C72; D32-33;D42-43	脑，神经系统	Brain & Central Nervous System	43	2.30	3.54	3.25	3.69	0.33
C73	甲状腺	Thyroid	7	0.37	0.58	0.46	0.44	0.03
C81-85,88,90,96	淋巴瘤	Lymphoma	36	1.92	2.96	2.51	2.50	0.33
C91-C95; D45-47	白血病	Leukaemia	37	1.98	3.04	2.87	3.21	0.24
Other	其他	Other	90	4.81	7.41	6.16	6.27	0.74
ALL	所有部位合计	All sites	1873	100.00	154.13	126.82	126.25	14.58
ALLbC44	所有部位除外 C44	All sites except C44	1854	98.99	152.56	125.68	125.02	14.46

附表 2-19　2019 年晋江市恶性肿瘤发病主要指标
Appendix Table 2-19　Cancer incidence in Jinjiang, 2019

ICD10	部位 Site		发病数 Cases	构成 Freq. （%）	粗率 Crude rate （1/10⁵）	中标率 ASR China （1/10⁵）	世标率 ASR world （1/10⁵）	累积率 Cum.rate （0~74，%）
C00-10, C12-14	口腔和咽喉（除外鼻咽）	Oral Cavity & Pharynx but Nasopharynx	80	2.07	6.74	4.93	5.10	0.63
C11	鼻咽	Nasopharynx	94	2.43	7.92	6.52	5.85	0.58
C15	食管	Esophagus	213	5.52	17.94	12.65	13.03	1.70
C16	胃	Stomach	251	6.50	21.14	15.71	15.69	2.07
C18-21	结直肠肛门	Colon, Rectum & Anus	457	11.84	38.48	28.55	28.39	3.70
C22	肝脏	Liver	335	8.68	28.21	21.02	20.52	2.42
C23-C24	胆囊及其他	Gallbladder	31	0.80	2.61	1.91	1.95	0.25
C25	胰腺	Pancreas	43	1.11	3.62	2.60	2.69	0.38
C32	喉	Larynx	38	0.98	3.20	2.36	2.37	0.30
C33-C34	气管，支气管，肺	Trachea, Bronchus & Lung	684	17.72	57.60	42.47	42.34	5.44
C37-C38	其他的胸腔器官	Other thoracic organs	5	0.13	0.42	0.34	0.36	0.02
C40-C41	骨	Bone	8	0.21	0.67	0.70	0.62	0.05
C43	皮肤的黑色素瘤	Melanoma of skin	3	0.08	0.25	0.19	0.19	0.03
C50	乳房	Breast	251	6.55	43.22	33.97	30.29	2.97
C53	子宫颈	Cervix	153	3.96	26.34	19.17	18.46	2.00
C54-55	子宫体及子宫部位不明	Corpus Uterus & Unspectified	63	1.63	10.85	8.00	7.57	0.79
C56	卵巢	Ovary	35	0.91	6.03	4.63	4.30	0.48
C61	前列腺	Prostate	71	1.84	11.70	9.58	9.34	1.25
C62	睾丸	Testis	4	0.10	0.66	0.66	0.52	0.03
C64-66，68	肾及泌尿系统不明	Kidney & Unspecified Urinary Organs	78	2.02	6.57	5.19	5.17	0.64
C67	膀胱	Bladder	68	1.76	5.73	4.18	4.12	0.55
C70-C72; D32-33;D42-43	脑，神经系统	Brain & Central Nervous System	98	2.54	8.25	6.87	6.52	0.71
C73	甲状腺	Thyroid	349	9.04	29.39	25.79	22.30	2.12
C81-85, 88,90,96	淋巴瘤	Lymphoma	85	2.20	7.16	5.72	5.38	0.62
C91-C95; D45-47	白血病	Leukaemia	59	1.53	4.97	4.73	5.27	0.41
Other	其他	Other	303	7.85	25.52	19.30	19.44	2.09
ALL	所有部位合计	All sites	3861	100.00	325.13	250.26	243.00	28.52
ALLbC44	所有部位除外 C44	All sites except C44	3827	99.12	322.27	248.32	241.06	28.28

附表 2-20　2019 年晋江市恶性肿瘤死亡主要指标

Appendix Table 2-20　Cancer mortality in Jinjiang, 2019

ICD10	部位 Site		死亡数 Deaths	构成 Freq. （%）	粗率 Crude rate （1/10⁵）	中标率 ASR China （1/10⁵）	世标率 ASR world （1/10⁵）	累积率 Cum.rate （0~74，%）
C00-10, C12-14	口腔和咽喉（除外鼻咽）	Oral Cavity & Pharynx but Nasopharynx	50	2.34	4.21	3.01	3.09	0.39
C11	鼻咽	Nasopharynx	38	1.78	3.20	2.40	2.34	0.26
C15	食管	Esophagus	211	9.86	17.77	12.23	12.31	1.35
C16	胃	Stomach	183	8.56	15.41	11.14	10.80	1.35
C18-21	结直肠肛门	Colon, Rectum & Anus	189	8.84	15.92	11.63	11.22	1.28
C22	肝脏	Liver	345	16.13	29.05	21.72	20.97	2.52
C23-C24	胆囊及其他	Gallbladder	22	1.03	1.85	1.24	1.27	0.17
C25	胰腺	Pancreas	57	2.66	4.80	3.35	3.32	0.39
C32	喉	Larynx	20	0.94	1.68	1.26	1.26	0.15
C33-C34	气管，支气管，肺	Trachea, Bronchus & Lung	556	25.99	46.82	33.66	33.36	4.18
C37-C38	其他的胸腔器官	Other thoracic organs	8	0.37	0.67	0.47	0.55	0.05
C40-C41	骨	Bone	8	0.37	0.67	0.50	0.47	0.06
C43	皮肤的黑色素瘤	Melanoma of skin	2	0.09	0.17	0.13	0.12	0.01
C50	乳房	Breast	45	2.15	7.75	5.65	5.36	0.58
C53	子宫颈	Cervix	36	1.68	6.20	4.40	4.25	0.51
C54-55	子宫体及子宫部位不明	Corpus Uterus & Unspectified	18	0.84	3.10	2.16	2.09	0.24
C56	卵巢	Ovary	16	0.75	2.75	1.81	1.80	0.23
C61	前列腺	Prostate	21	0.98	3.46	2.47	2.47	0.18
C62	睾丸	Testis	0	0.00	0.00	0.00	0.00	0.00
C64-66, 68	肾及泌尿系统不明	Kidney & Unspecified Urinary Organs	22	1.03	1.85	1.30	1.35	0.19
C67	膀胱	Bladder	19	0.89	1.60	1.13	1.01	0.07
C70-C72; D32-33; D42-43	脑，神经系统	Brain & Central Nervous System	49	2.29	4.13	3.21	3.16	0.36
C73	甲状腺	Thyroid	3	0.14	0.25	0.18	0.18	0.02
C81-85, 88,90,96	淋巴瘤	Lymphoma	53	2.48	4.46	3.41	3.26	0.43
C91-C95; D45-47	白血病	Leukaemia	39	1.82	3.28	2.84	2.88	0.27
Other	其他	Other	128	5.98	10.78	7.76	7.90	0.90
ALL	所有部位合计	All sites	2139	100.00	180.12	130.97	128.94	15.30
ALLbC44	所有部位除外 C44	All sites except C44	2136	99.86	179.87	130.86	128.80	15.29

附表 2-21　2019 年芗城区恶性肿瘤发病主要指标
Appendix Table 2-21　Cancer incidence in Xiangcheng, 2019

ICD10	部位 Site		发病数 Cases	构成 Freq. （%）	粗率 Crude rate （1/10⁵）	中标率 ASR China （1/10⁵）	世标率 ASR world （1/10⁵）	累积率 Cum.rate （0~74，%）
C00-10, C12-14	口腔和咽喉（除外鼻咽）	Oral Cavity & Pharynx but Nasopharynx	22	1.37	4.66	3.31	3.12	0.41
C11	鼻咽	Nasopharynx	22	1.37	4.66	3.68	3.26	0.37
C15	食管	Esophagus	40	2.49	8.47	4.48	4.57	0.51
C16	胃	Stomach	96	5.98	20.33	11.79	11.66	1.51
C18-21	结直肠肛门	Colon, Rectum & Anus	209	13.01	44.26	25.51	24.79	3.09
C22	肝脏	Liver	112	6.97	23.72	14.11	13.65	1.47
C23-C24	胆囊及其他	Gallbladder	6	0.37	1.27	0.59	0.60	0.04
C25	胰腺	Pancreas	13	0.81	2.75	1.60	1.55	0.19
C32	喉	Larynx	9	0.56	1.91	1.13	1.11	0.16
C33-C34	气管，支气管，肺	Trachea, Bronchus & Lung	278	17.31	58.87	34.19	34.12	4.47
C37-C38	其他的胸腔器官	Other thoracic organs	4	0.25	0.85	0.58	0.55	0.06
C40-C41	骨	Bone	4	0.25	0.85	0.74	0.68	0.05
C43	皮肤的黑色素瘤	Melanoma of skin	1	0.06	0.21	0.17	0.16	0.01
C50	乳房	Breast	147	9.28	61.09	43.12	39.73	4.08
C53	子宫颈	Cervix	51	3.18	21.19	15.06	13.55	1.48
C54-55	子宫体及子宫部位不明	Corpus Uterus & Unspectified	36	2.24	14.96	9.20	9.14	1.12
C56	卵巢	Ovary	21	1.31	8.73	5.96	5.93	0.60
C61	前列腺	Prostate	47	2.93	20.29	11.08	10.75	1.29
C62	睾丸	Testis	1	0.06	0.43	0.33	0.29	0.02
C64-66，68	肾及泌尿系统不明	Kidney & Unspecified Urinary Organs	31	1.93	6.56	3.81	3.80	0.43
C67	膀胱	Bladder	30	1.87	6.35	3.55	3.63	0.43
C70-C72; D32-33;D42-43	脑，神经系统	Brain & Central Nervous System	64	3.99	13.55	10.51	9.99	0.99
C73	甲状腺	Thyroid	192	11.96	40.66	35.85	31.09	2.81
C81-85, 88,90,96	淋巴瘤	Lymphoma	44	2.74	9.32	5.84	5.64	0.70
C91-C95; D45-47	白血病	Leukaemia	34	2.12	7.20	6.13	5.98	0.55
Other	其他	Other	90	5.60	19.06	11.56	11.57	1.33
ALL	所有部位合计	All sites	1606	100.00	340.07	223.00	212.28	23.96
ALLbC44	所有部位除外 C44	All sites except C44	1592	99.13	337.10	221.60	210.80	23.83

附表 2-22　2019 年芗城区恶性肿瘤死亡主要指标
Appendix Table 2-22　Cancer mortality in Xiangcheng, 2019

ICD10	部位	Site	死亡数 Deaths	构成 Freq. (%)	粗率 Crude rate (1/10⁵)	中标率 ASR China (1/10⁵)	世标率 ASR world (1/10⁵)	累积率 Cum.rate (0~74, %)
C00-10, C12-14	口腔和咽喉（除外鼻咽）	Oral Cavity & Pharynx but Nasopharynx	16	1.77	3.39	1.83	1.81	0.19
C11	鼻咽	Nasopharynx	17	1.88	3.60	2.06	2.04	0.24
C15	食管	Esophagus	48	5.32	10.16	5.46	5.66	0.74
C16	胃	Stomach	77	8.53	16.30	8.75	8.51	0.90
C18-21	结直肠肛门	Colon, Rectum & Anus	101	11.18	21.39	11.09	11.02	1.21
C22	肝脏	Liver	115	12.74	24.35	14.83	14.12	1.66
C23-C24	胆囊及其他	Gallbladder	12	1.33	2.54	1.09	1.19	0.10
C25	胰腺	Pancreas	19	2.10	4.02	2.13	2.23	0.24
C32	喉	Larynx	4	0.44	0.85	0.59	0.49	0.03
C33-C34	气管，支气管，肺	Trachea, Bronchus & Lung	266	29.46	56.32	31.65	31.57	3.97
C37-C38	其他的胸腔器官	Other thoracic organs	2	0.22	0.42	0.47	0.44	0.03
C40-C41	骨	Bone	5	0.55	1.06	0.61	0.58	0.06
C43	皮肤的黑色素瘤	Melanoma of skin	3	0.33	0.64	0.38	0.39	0.06
C50	乳房	Breast	28	3.21	11.64	7.30	6.89	0.80
C53	子宫颈	Cervix	12	1.33	4.99	3.44	3.09	0.34
C54-55	子宫体及子宫部位不明	Corpus Uterus & Unspectified	5	0.55	2.08	1.23	1.17	0.14
C56	卵巢	Ovary	6	0.66	2.49	1.47	1.56	0.18
C61	前列腺	Prostate	12	1.33	5.18	2.23	2.23	0.18
C62	睾丸	Testis	1	0.11	0.43	0.25	0.27	0.05
C64-66，68	肾及泌尿系统不明	Kidney & Unspecified Urinary Organs	9	1.00	1.91	0.98	0.90	0.08
C67	膀胱	Bladder	5	0.55	1.06	0.37	0.43	0.03
C70-C72; D32-33;D42-43	脑，神经系统	Brain & Central Nervous System	18	1.99	3.81	3.16	2.96	0.26
C73	甲状腺	Thyroid	4	0.44	0.85	0.48	0.52	0.09
C81-85, 88,90,96	淋巴瘤	Lymphoma	28	3.10	5.93	3.44	3.42	0.43
C91-C95; D45-47	白血病	Leukaemia	16	1.77	3.39	2.85	2.79	0.32
Other	其他	Other	73	8.08	15.46	8.90	9.21	1.16
ALL	所有部位合计	All sites	903	100.00	191.21	109.30	108.08	12.69
ALLbC44	所有部位除外 C44	All sites except C44	900	99.67	190.57	109.04	107.79	12.68

附表 2-23　2019 年长泰县恶性肿瘤发病主要指标

Appendix Table 2-23　Cancer incidence in Changtai, 2019

ICD10	部位 Site		发病数 Cases	构成 Freq. （%）	粗率 Crude rate （1/10⁵）	中标率 ASR China （1/10⁵）	世标率 ASR world （1/10⁵）	累积率 Cum.rate （0~74，%）
C00-10, C12-14	口腔和咽喉（除外鼻咽）	Oral Cavity & Pharynx but Nasopharynx	7	1.22	3.30	2.58	2.42	0.30
C11	鼻咽	Nasopharynx	7	1.22	3.30	2.12	1.99	0.23
C15	食管	Esophagus	31	5.39	14.61	7.76	8.31	1.02
C16	胃	Stomach	46	8.00	21.68	12.18	12.50	1.78
C18-21	结直肠肛门	Colon, Rectum & Anus	60	10.43	28.28	17.79	17.39	2.43
C22	肝脏	Liver	55	9.57	25.92	17.91	17.41	1.76
C23-C24	胆囊及其他	Gallbladder	8	1.39	3.77	2.20	2.19	0.21
C25	胰腺	Pancreas	8	1.39	3.77	2.30	2.00	0.17
C32	喉	Larynx	5	0.87	2.36	1.26	1.31	0.09
C33-C34	气管，支气管，肺	Trachea, Bronchus & Lung	130	22.61	61.27	35.36	34.78	4.31
C37-C38	其他的胸腔器官	Other thoracic organs	2	0.35	0.94	0.76	0.71	0.06
C40-C41	骨	Bone	1	0.17	0.47	0.19	0.21	0.03
C43	皮肤的黑色素瘤	Melanoma of skin	0	0.00	0.00	0.00	0.00	0.00
C50	乳房	Breast	30	5.22	28.70	24.22	21.88	2.13
C53	子宫颈	Cervix	15	2.61	14.35	11.18	10.12	1.09
C54-55	子宫体及子宫部位不明	Corpus Uterus & Unspectified	18	3.13	17.22	10.71	10.38	1.04
C56	卵巢	Ovary	8	1.39	7.65	6.16	5.99	0.70
C61	前列腺	Prostate	6	1.04	5.57	3.25	3.56	0.57
C62	睾丸	Testis	1	0.17	0.93	1.87	1.58	0.10
C64-66, 68	肾及泌尿系统不明	Kidney & Unspecified Urinary Organs	9	1.57	4.24	2.33	2.37	0.28
C67	膀胱	Bladder	16	2.78	7.54	5.33	5.20	0.57
C70-C72; D32-33;D42-43	脑，神经系统	Brain & Central Nervous System	17	2.96	8.01	6.54	6.01	0.62
C73	甲状腺	Thyroid	39	6.78	18.38	15.94	14.03	1.26
C81-85, 88,90,96	淋巴瘤	Lymphoma	13	2.26	6.13	4.09	4.10	0.53
C91-C95; D45-47	白血病	Leukaemia	14	2.43	6.60	5.27	4.82	0.58
Other	其他	Other	29	5.04	13.67	8.83	8.45	0.92
ALL	所有部位合计	All sites	575	100.00	270.99	179.40	172.86	19.95
ALLbC44	所有部位除外 C44	All sites except C44	571	99.30	269.11	178.32	171.59	19.78

附表 2-24　2019 年长泰县恶性肿瘤死亡主要指标

Appendix Table 2-24　Cancer mortality in Changtai, 2019

ICD10	部位 Site		发病数 Cases	构成 Freq.（%）	粗率 Crude rate（1/10⁵）	中标率 ASR China（1/10⁵）	世标率 ASR world（1/10⁵）	累积率 Cum.rate（0~74，%）
C00-10, C12-14	口腔和咽喉（除外鼻咽）	Oral Cavity & Pharynx but Nasopharynx	2	0.56	0.94	0.53	0.49	0.05
C11	鼻咽	Nasopharynx	8	2.23	3.77	2.85	2.54	0.29
C15	食管	Esophagus	34	9.50	16.02	8.61	8.75	1.15
C16	胃	Stomach	40	11.17	18.85	10.63	10.21	1.15
C18-21	结直肠肛门	Colon, Rectum & Anus	33	9.22	15.55	8.81	9.07	1.10
C22	肝脏	Liver	51	14.25	24.04	16.32	15.94	1.53
C23-C24	胆囊及其他	Gallbladder	4	1.12	1.89	1.73	1.58	0.18
C25	胰腺	Pancreas	6	1.68	2.83	1.46	1.32	0.12
C32	喉	Larynx	2	0.56	0.94	0.46	0.61	0.04
C33-C34	气管，支气管，肺	Trachea, Bronchus & Lung	99	27.65	46.66	26.48	26.36	3.00
C37-C38	其他的胸腔器官	Other thoracic organs	0	0.00	0.00	0.00	0.00	0.00
C40-C41	骨	Bone	2	0.56	0.94	0.47	0.42	0.03
C43	皮肤的黑色素瘤	Melanoma of skin	1	0.28	0.47	0.27	0.21	0.00
C50	乳房	Breast	6	1.68	5.74	4.75	4.50	0.52
C53	子宫颈	Cervix	2	0.56	1.91	1.51	1.37	0.12
C54-55	子宫体及子宫部位不明	Corpus Uterus & Unspectified	5	1.40	4.78	2.64	2.78	0.44
C56	卵巢	Ovary	4	1.12	3.83	2.06	2.35	0.32
C61	前列腺	Prostate	5	1.40	4.64	2.41	2.33	0.05
C62	睾丸	Testis	0	0.00	0.00	0.00	0.00	0.00
C64-66, 68	肾及泌尿系统不明	Kidney & Unspecified Urinary Organs	3	0.84	1.41	0.74	0.82	0.11
C67	膀胱	Bladder	3	0.84	1.41	0.94	0.99	0.08
C70-C72; D32-33;D42-43	脑，神经系统	Brain & Central Nervous System	5	1.40	2.36	1.49	1.35	0.18
C73	甲状腺	Thyroid	0	0.00	0.00	0.00	0.00	0.00
C81-85, 88,90,96	淋巴瘤	Lymphoma	10	2.79	4.71	2.90	2.93	0.34
C91-C95; D45-47	白血病	Leukaemia	6	1.68	2.83	1.81	1.77	0.18
Other	其他	Other	27	7.54	12.72	8.01	8.19	0.75
ALL	所有部位合计	All sites	358	100.00	168.72	101.08	100.09	11.02
ALLbC44	所有部位除外 C44	All sites except C44	355	99.16	167.31	100.56	99.29	11.02

附表 2-25　2019 年南靖县恶性肿瘤发病主要指标

Appendix Table 2-25　Cancer incidence in Nanjing, 2019

ICD10	部位 Site		发病数 Cases	构成 Freq. （%）	粗率 Crude rate （1/10⁵）	中标率 ASR China （1/10⁵）	世标率 ASR world （1/10⁵）	累积率 Cum.rate （0~74，%）
C00-10,C12-14	口腔和咽喉（除外鼻咽）	Oral Cavity & Pharynx but Nasopharynx	13	1.55	3.60	2.18	2.17	0.29
C11	鼻咽	Nasopharynx	19	2.26	5.26	3.61	3.23	0.32
C15	食管	Esophagus	29	3.45	8.03	4.36	4.68	0.63
C16	胃	Stomach	50	5.95	13.84	8.31	8.12	0.92
C18-21	结直肠肛门	Colon, Rectum & Anus	118	14.03	32.65	19.29	18.82	2.25
C22	肝脏	Liver	53	6.30	14.67	9.02	8.73	0.96
C23-C24	胆囊及其他	Gallbladder	3	0.36	0.83	0.48	0.46	0.05
C25	胰腺	Pancreas	10	1.19	2.77	1.52	1.56	0.21
C32	喉	Larynx	9	1.07	2.49	1.47	1.55	0.20
C33-C34	气管，支气管，肺	Trachea, Bronchus & Lung	158	18.79	43.72	26.09	26.54	3.49
C37-C38	其他的胸腔器官	Other thoracic organs	1	0.12	0.28	0.19	0.17	0.01
C40-C41	骨	Bone	1	0.12	0.28	0.14	0.17	0.02
C43	皮肤的黑色素瘤	Melanoma of skin	0	0.00	0.00	0.00	0.00	0.00
C50	乳房	Breast	60	7.25	34.00	24.79	22.15	2.19
C53	子宫颈	Cervix	26	3.09	14.73	9.28	9.20	1.11
C54-55	子宫体及子宫部位不明	Corpus Uterus & Unspectified	16	1.90	9.07	5.12	4.97	0.50
C56	卵巢	Ovary	10	1.19	5.67	4.52	4.58	0.52
C61	前列腺	Prostate	28	3.33	15.14	8.30	8.91	1.17
C62	睾丸	Testis	2	0.24	1.08	1.56	2.31	0.11
C64-66, 68	肾及泌尿系统不明	Kidney & Unspecified Urinary Organs	12	1.43	3.32	2.13	2.05	0.21
C67	膀胱	Bladder	23	2.73	6.36	3.55	3.48	0.39
C70-C72; D32-33;D42-43	脑，神经系统	Brain & Central Nervous System	29	3.45	8.03	5.99	5.75	0.69
C73	甲状腺	Thyroid	85	10.11	23.52	19.90	16.99	1.55
C81-85, 88,90,96	淋巴瘤	Lymphoma	25	2.97	6.92	4.90	4.46	0.48
C91-C95; D45-47	白血病	Leukaemia	10	1.19	2.77	2.05	2.28	0.19
Other	其他	Other	50	5.95	13.84	9.80	9.24	1.21
ALL	所有部位合计	All sites	841	100.00	232.73	151.43	146.20	16.89
ALLbC44	所有部位除外 C44	All sites except C44	838	99.64	231.90	150.89	145.76	16.87

附表 2-26　2019 年南靖县恶性肿瘤死亡主要指标
Appendix Table 2-26　Cancer mortality in Nanjing, 2019

ICD10	部位 Site		死亡数 Deaths	构成 Freq. （%）	粗率 Crude rate （1/10⁵）	中标率 ASR China （1/10⁵）	世标率 ASR world （1/10⁵）	累积率 Cum.rate （0 ~74，%）
C00-10, C12-14	口腔和咽喉（除外鼻咽）	Oral Cavity & Pharynx but Nasopharynx	5	0.93	1.38	0.59	0.64	0.04
C11	鼻咽	Nasopharynx	13	2.41	3.60	2.14	2.06	0.24
C15	食管	Esophagus	23	4.26	6.36	3.27	3.48	0.45
C16	胃	Stomach	43	7.96	11.90	7.05	6.70	0.70
C18-21	结直肠肛门	Colon, Rectum & Anus	68	12.59	18.82	10.08	10.08	1.18
C22	肝脏	Liver	71	13.15	19.65	11.16	10.83	1.26
C23-C24	胆囊及其他	Gallbladder	3	0.56	0.83	0.44	0.39	0.03
C25	胰腺	Pancreas	14	2.59	3.87	2.40	2.37	0.34
C32	喉	Larynx	3	0.56	0.83	0.36	0.42	0.01
C33-C34	气管，支气管，肺	Trachea, Bronchus & Lung	165	30.56	45.66	25.33	25.41	3.36
C37-C38	其他的胸腔器官	Other thoracic organs	1	0.19	0.28	0.15	0.16	0.02
C40-C41	骨	Bone	6	1.11	1.66	1.17	1.27	0.11
C43	皮肤的黑色素瘤	Melanoma of skin	1	0.19	0.28	0.16	0.17	0.03
C50	乳房	Breast	10	1.85	5.67	3.38	3.28	0.44
C53	子宫颈	Cervix	6	1.11	3.40	2.12	2.15	0.25
C54-55	子宫体及子宫部位不明	Corpus Uterus & Unspectified	1	0.19	0.57	0.30	0.32	0.04
C56	卵巢	Ovary	2	0.37	1.13	0.70	0.71	0.14
C61	前列腺	Prostate	11	2.04	5.95	3.46	3.67	0.46
C62	睾丸	Testis	1	0.19	0.54	0.80	0.68	0.04
C64-66, 68	肾及泌尿系统不明	Kidney & Unspecified Urinary Organs	5	0.93	1.38	0.92	0.88	0.14
C67	膀胱	Bladder	5	0.93	1.38	0.74	0.68	0.05
C70-C72; D32-33;D42-43	脑，神经系统	Brain & Central Nervous System	10	1.85	2.77	1.96	1.87	0.24
C73	甲状腺	Thyroid	3	0.56	0.83	0.60	0.51	0.02
C81-85, 88,90,96	淋巴瘤	Lymphoma	12	2.22	3.32	1.73	1.71	0.16
C91-C95; D45-47	白血病	Leukaemia	14	2.59	3.87	2.64	2.36	0.19
Other	其他	Other	44	8.15	12.18	6.92	6.93	0.95
ALL	所有部位合计	All sites	540	100.00	149.44	85.09	84.17	10.19
ALLbC44	所有部位除外 C44	All sites except C44	537	99.44	148.61	84.78	83.87	10.19

附表 2-27　2019 年平和县恶性肿瘤发病主要指标
Appendix Table 2-27　Cancer incidence in Pinghe, 2019

ICD10	部位 Site	发病数 Cases	构成 Freq. （%）	粗率 Crude rate （1/10^5）	中标率 ASR China （1/10^5）	世标率 ASR world （1/10^5）	累积率 Cum.rate （0~74，%）
C00–10, C12–14	口腔和咽喉（除外鼻咽）Oral Cavity & Pharynx but Nasopharynx	15	1.11	2.41	1.70	1.70	0.19
C11	鼻咽 Nasopharynx	46	3.40	7.40	6.47	5.90	0.58
C15	食管 Esophagus	136	10.04	21.88	14.52	14.96	2.10
C16	胃 Stomach	158	11.67	25.42	17.10	16.70	2.17
C18–21	结直肠肛门 Colon, Rectum & Anus	167	12.33	26.86	18.42	18.32	2.37
C22	肝脏 Liver	64	4.73	10.29	7.63	7.19	0.86
C23–C24	胆囊及其他 Gallbladder	8	0.59	1.29	0.82	0.85	0.09
C25	胰腺 Pancreas	12	0.89	1.93	1.36	1.26	0.14
C32	喉 Larynx	11	0.81	1.77	1.20	1.18	0.16
C33–C34	气管，支气管，肺 Trachea, Bronchus & Lung	213	15.73	34.26	23.73	23.50	3.07
C37–C38	其他的胸腔器官 Other thoracic organs	6	0.44	0.97	0.64	0.85	0.08
C40–C41	骨 Bone	4	0.30	0.64	0.55	0.52	0.04
C43	皮肤的黑色素瘤 Melanoma of skin	2	0.15	0.32	0.21	0.19	0.01
C50	乳房 Breast	73	5.47	25.12	19.11	17.76	1.94
C53	子宫颈 Cervix	59	4.36	20.30	15.47	14.41	1.51
C54–55	子宫体及子宫部位不明 Corpus Uterus & Unspectified	27	1.99	9.29	6.41	6.28	0.69
C56	卵巢 Ovary	15	1.11	5.16	3.45	3.36	0.37
C61	前列腺 Prostate	25	1.85	7.55	5.30	5.13	0.56
C62	睾丸 Testis	1	0.07	0.30	0.30	0.28	0.02
C64–66, 68	肾及泌尿系统不明 Kidney & Unspecified Urinary Organs	14	1.03	2.25	1.67	1.65	0.18
C67	膀胱 Bladder	19	1.40	3.06	2.38	2.19	0.30
C70–C72; D32–33;D42–43	脑，神经系统 Brain & Central Nervous System	39	2.88	6.27	5.20	5.34	0.47
C73	甲状腺 Thyroid	89	6.57	14.32	13.07	11.28	1.04
C81–85, 88,90,96	淋巴瘤 Lymphoma	25	1.85	4.02	3.26	3.07	0.43
C91–C95; D45–47	白血病 Leukaemia	27	1.99	4.34	3.85	3.85	0.31
Other	其他 Other	98	7.24	15.76	11.25	11.64	1.33
ALL	所有部位合计 All sites	1354	100.00	217.80	159.11	154.91	18.41
ALLbC44	所有部位除外 C44 All sites except C44	1335	98.60	214.74	157.26	153.10	18.23

附表 2-28　2019 年平和县恶性肿瘤死亡主要指标
Appendix Table 2-28　Cancer mortality in Pinghe, 2019

ICD10	部位 Site	死亡数 Deaths	构成 Freq. （%）	粗率 Crude rate （1/10⁵）	中标率 ASR China （1/10⁵）	世标率 ASR world （1/10⁵）	累积率 Cum.rate （0~74,%）
C00-10, C12-14	口腔和咽喉（除外鼻咽）	Oral Cavity & Pharynx but Nasopharynx	4	0.41	0.64	0.39	0.40	0.06
C11	鼻咽	Nasopharynx	16	1.65	2.57	1.64	1.66	0.20
C15	食管	Esophagus	135	13.93	21.72	13.69	13.67	1.68
C16	胃	Stomach	160	16.51	25.74	15.83	15.94	1.86
C18-21	结直肠肛门	Colon, Rectum & Anus	71	7.33	11.42	7.28	7.30	0.91
C22	肝脏	Liver	79	8.15	12.71	9.24	8.77	1.03
C23-C24	胆囊及其他	Gallbladder	3	0.31	0.48	0.32	0.28	0.03
C25	胰腺	Pancreas	16	1.65	2.57	1.67	1.62	0.20
C32	喉	Larynx	6	0.62	0.97	0.65	0.67	0.11
C33-C34	气管,支气管,肺	Trachea, Bronchus & Lung	282	29.10	45.36	30.26	29.62	3.78
C37-C38	其他的胸腔器官	Other thoracic organs	3	0.31	0.48	0.47	0.39	0.04
C40-C41	骨	Bone	6	0.62	0.97	0.71	0.65	0.05
C43	皮肤的黑色素瘤	Melanoma of skin	1	0.10	0.16	0.14	0.13	0.03
C50	乳房	Breast	19	1.96	6.54	4.69	4.52	0.51
C53	子宫颈	Cervix	21	2.17	7.23	4.73	4.73	0.55
C54-55	子宫体及子宫部位不明	Corpus Uterus & Unspectified	4	0.41	1.38	0.87	0.79	0.05
C56	卵巢	Ovary	7	0.72	2.41	1.81	1.93	0.19
C61	前列腺	Prostate	8	0.83	2.42	1.55	1.52	0.10
C62	睾丸	Testis	1	0.10	0.30	0.37	0.25	0.02
C64-66, 68	肾及泌尿系统不明	Kidney & Unspecified Urinary Organs	7	0.72	1.13	0.71	0.65	0.05
C67	膀胱	Bladder	6	0.62	0.97	0.64	0.59	0.08
C70-C72; D32-33;D42-43	脑,神经系统	Brain & Central Nervous System	22	2.27	3.54	2.67	2.73	0.33
C73	甲状腺	Thyroid	0	0.00	0.00	0.00	0.00	0.00
C81-85, 88,90,96	淋巴瘤	Lymphoma	16	1.65	2.57	1.99	1.71	0.21
C91-C95; D45-47	白血病	Leukaemia	30	3.10	4.83	4.16	3.84	0.28
Other	其他	Other	46	4.75	7.40	5.42	5.39	0.71
ALL	所有部位合计	All sites	969	100.00	155.87	104.63	102.62	12.33
ALLbC44	所有部位除外 C44	All sites except C44	965	99.59	155.23	104.24	102.26	12.30

附表 2-29　2019 年新罗区恶性肿瘤发病主要指标
Appendix Table 2-29　Cancer incidence in Xinluo, 2019

ICD10	部位	Site	发病数 Cases	构成 Freq. （%）	粗率 Crude rate （1/10⁵）	中标率 ASR China （1/10⁵）	世标率 ASR world （1/10⁵）	累积率 Cum.rate （0~74，%）
C00-10, C12-14	口腔和咽喉（除外鼻咽）	Oral Cavity & Pharynx but Nasopharynx	20	0.98	3.68	2.46	2.59	0.33
C11	鼻咽	Nasopharynx	32	1.57	5.89	4.28	4.02	0.49
C15	食管	Esophagus	49	2.40	9.02	5.72	5.62	0.77
C16	胃	Stomach	136	6.66	25.03	15.85	15.70	1.92
C18-21	结直肠肛门	Colon, Rectum & Anus	278	13.61	51.17	32.16	31.74	3.66
C22	肝脏	Liver	109	5.34	20.06	13.57	12.96	1.43
C23-C24	胆囊及其他	Gallbladder	18	0.88	3.31	2.21	2.09	0.31
C25	胰腺	Pancreas	37	1.81	6.81	3.99	3.99	0.49
C32	喉	Larynx	7	0.34	1.29	0.76	0.76	0.10
C33-C34	气管，支气管，肺	Trachea, Bronchus & Lung	434	21.25	79.89	52.69	51.31	6.16
C37-C38	其他的胸腔器官	Other thoracic organs	6	0.29	1.10	0.77	0.71	0.09
C40-C41	骨	Bone	5	0.24	0.92	0.48	0.57	0.07
C43	皮肤的黑色素瘤	Melanoma of skin	4	0.20	0.74	0.59	0.51	0.05
C50	乳房	Breast	146	7.25	53.76	39.92	36.43	3.84
C53	子宫颈	Cervix	67	3.28	24.67	17.28	16.56	1.88
C54-55	子宫体及子宫部位不明	Corpus Uterus & Unspectified	26	1.27	9.57	6.62	6.73	0.77
C56	卵巢	Ovary	20	0.98	7.36	6.31	6.09	0.55
C61	前列腺	Prostate	87	4.26	32.02	18.12	18.03	1.95
C62	睾丸	Testis	4	0.20	1.47	2.85	2.95	0.17
C64-66, 68	肾及泌尿系统不明	Kidney & Unspecified Urinary Organs	39	1.91	7.18	5.11	4.50	0.43
C67	膀胱	Bladder	36	1.76	6.63	3.74	3.82	0.41
C70-C72; D32-33;D42-43	脑，神经系统	Brain & Central Nervous System	48	2.35	8.84	7.00	6.58	0.84
C73	甲状腺	Thyroid	252	12.34	46.39	40.80	35.45	3.17
C81-85, 88,90,96	淋巴瘤	Lymphoma	43	2.11	7.92	5.64	5.17	0.54
C91-C95; D45-47	白血病	Leukaemia	22	1.08	4.05	3.27	3.30	0.33
Other	其他	Other	115	5.63	21.17	13.66	13.74	1.41
ALL	所有部位合计	All sites	2042	100.00	375.89	260.43	248.44	27.60
ALLbC44	所有部位除外 C44	All sites except C44	2017	98.78	371.29	257.77	245.72	27.33

附表 2-30　2019 年新罗区恶性肿瘤死亡主要指标
Appendix Table 2-30　Cancer mortality in Xinluo, 2019

ICD10	部位	Site	死亡数 Deaths	构成 Freq. (%)	粗率 Crude rate (1/10⁵)	中标率 ASR China (1/10⁵)	世标率 ASR world (1/10⁵)	累积率 Cum.rate (0~74, %)
C00-10, C12-14	口腔和咽喉（除外鼻咽）	Oral Cavity & Pharynx but Nasopharynx	11	1.42	2.02	1.22	1.20	0.14
C11	鼻咽	Nasopharynx	12	1.55	2.21	1.34	1.40	0.17
C15	食管	Esophagus	26	3.35	4.79	2.81	2.69	0.31
C16	胃	Stomach	75	9.66	13.81	7.92	7.77	0.74
C18-21	结直肠肛门	Colon, Rectum & Anus	97	12.50	17.86	10.78	10.59	1.22
C22	肝脏	Liver	86	11.08	15.83	10.33	10.12	1.13
C23-C24	胆囊及其他	Gallbladder	9	1.16	1.66	1.11	1.15	0.19
C25	胰腺	Pancreas	24	3.09	4.42	2.64	2.77	0.38
C32	喉	Larynx	7	0.90	1.29	0.72	0.64	0.08
C33-C34	气管，支气管，肺	Trachea, Bronchus & Lung	230	29.64	42.34	25.04	24.63	2.88
C37-C38	其他的胸腔器官	Other thoracic organs	4	0.52	0.74	0.36	0.33	0.02
C40-C41	骨	Bone	5	0.64	0.92	0.52	0.56	0.05
C43	皮肤的黑色素瘤	Melanoma of skin	4	0.52	0.74	0.43	0.43	0.04
C50	乳房	Breast	19	2.45	7.00	4.82	4.37	0.45
C53	子宫颈	Cervix	14	1.80	5.16	3.10	3.11	0.34
C54-55	子宫体及子宫部位不明	Corpus Uterus & Unspectified	3	0.39	1.10	0.72	0.66	0.05
C56	卵巢	Ovary	9	1.16	3.31	2.25	2.05	0.23
C61	前列腺	Prostate	16	2.06	5.89	2.53	3.17	0.10
C62	睾丸	Testis	0	0.00	0.00	0.00	0.00	0.00
C64-66，68	肾及泌尿系统不明	Kidney & Unspecified Urinary Organs	17	2.19	3.13	1.69	1.75	0.18
C67	膀胱	Bladder	8	1.03	1.47	0.83	0.86	0.13
C70-C72;D32-33;D42-43	脑，神经系统	Brain & Central Nervous System	20	2.58	3.68	2.57	2.57	0.30
C73	甲状腺	Thyroid	4	0.52	0.74	0.46	0.48	0.10
C81-85,88,90,96	淋巴瘤	Lymphoma	15	1.93	2.76	1.71	1.60	0.16
C91-C95;D45-47	白血病	Leukaemia	13	1.68	2.39	1.72	1.71	0.21
Other	其他	Other	48	6.19	8.84	5.68	5.64	0.59
ALL	所有部位合计	All sites	776	100.00	142.85	86.56	85.44	9.61
ALLbC44	所有部位除外 C44	All sites except C44	774	99.74	142.48	86.44	85.30	9.61

附表 2-31　2019 年永定区恶性肿瘤发病主要指标

Appendix Table 2-31　Cancer incidence in Yongding, 2019

ICD10	部位 Site		发病数 Cases	构成 Freq. （%）	粗率 Crude rate （1/10⁵）	中标率 ASR China （1/10⁵）	世标率 ASR world （1/10⁵）	累积率 Cum.rate （0~74，%）
C00-10,C12-14	口腔和咽喉（除外鼻咽）	Oral Cavity & Pharynx but Nasopharynx	22	1.54	4.49	3.30	3.26	0.39
C11	鼻咽	Nasopharynx	29	2.03	5.92	5.26	5.17	0.56
C15	食管	Esophagus	48	3.36	9.80	7.80	8.04	1.06
C16	胃	Stomach	84	5.88	17.15	13.41	12.94	1.35
C18-21	结直肠肛门	Colon, Rectum & Anus	224	15.68	45.74	35.14	34.69	4.11
C22	肝脏	Liver	137	9.59	27.98	22.55	22.29	2.48
C23-C24	胆囊及其他	Gallbladder	12	0.84	2.45	1.78	1.88	0.25
C25	胰腺	Pancreas	21	1.47	4.29	3.32	3.10	0.26
C32	喉	Larynx	9	0.63	1.84	1.54	1.62	0.27
C33-C34	气管，支气管，肺	Trachea, Bronchus & Lung	319	22.32	65.14	50.26	50.33	5.96
C37-C38	其他的胸腔器官	Other thoracic organs	5	0.35	1.02	0.77	0.82	0.11
C40-C41	骨	Bone	4	0.28	0.82	0.82	0.66	0.07
C43	皮肤的黑色素瘤	Melanoma of skin	4	0.28	0.82	0.61	0.64	0.09
C50	乳房	Breast	67	4.69	28.03	22.93	20.83	2.00
C53	子宫颈	Cervix	44	3.08	18.41	15.09	14.17	1.47
C54-55	子宫体及子宫部位不明	Corpus Uterus & Unspectified	29	2.03	12.13	9.73	9.11	0.94
C56	卵巢	Ovary	15	1.05	6.28	5.18	4.97	0.55
C61	前列腺	Prostate	28	1.96	11.17	8.72	8.54	0.62
C62	睾丸	Testis	0	0.00	0.00	0.00	0.00	0.00
C64-66，68	肾及泌尿系统不明	Kidney & Unspecified Urinary Organs	15	1.05	3.06	2.47	2.13	0.21
C67	膀胱	Bladder	20	1.40	4.08	3.24	3.27	0.53
C70-C72; D32-33;D42-43	脑，神经系统	Brain & Central Nervous System	44	3.08	8.99	7.69	7.46	0.77
C73	甲状腺	Thyroid	133	9.31	27.16	24.89	21.21	1.91
C81-85, 88,90,96	淋巴瘤	Lymphoma	24	1.68	4.90	3.84	4.07	0.50
C91-C95; D45-47	白血病	Leukaemia	26	1.82	5.31	4.89	5.18	0.45
Other	其他	Other	66	4.62	13.48	10.38	10.30	1.09
ALL	所有部位合计	All sites	1429	100.00	291.81	234.18	227.31	25.17
ALLbC44	所有部位除外 C44	All sites except C44	1407	98.46	287.32	230.78	223.82	24.80

附表 2-32　2019 年永定区恶性肿瘤死亡主要指标

Appendix Table 2-32　Cancer mortality in Yongding, 2019

ICD10	部位	Site	死亡数 Deaths	构成 Freq.（%）	粗率 Crude rate（1/10⁵）	中标率 ASR China（1/10⁵）	世标率 ASR world（1/10⁵）	累积率 Cum.rate（0~74，%）
C00-10, C12-14	口腔和咽喉（除外鼻咽）	Oral Cavity & Pharynx but Nasopharynx	14	1.78	2.86	2.31	2.41	0.31
C11	鼻咽	Nasopharynx	23	2.92	4.70	3.83	3.74	0.37
C15	食管	Esophagus	42	5.33	8.58	6.76	7.14	1.00
C16	胃	Stomach	62	7.87	12.66	9.67	9.54	0.96
C18-21	结直肠肛门	Colon, Rectum & Anus	107	13.58	21.85	16.52	16.38	1.79
C22	肝脏	Liver	115	14.59	23.48	18.62	18.46	2.02
C23-C24	胆囊及其他	Gallbladder	9	1.14	1.84	1.54	1.67	0.25
C25	胰腺	Pancreas	17	2.16	3.47	2.51	2.43	0.18
C32	喉	Larynx	4	0.51	0.82	0.63	0.67	0.08
C33-C34	气管，支气管，肺	Trachea, Bronchus & Lung	212	26.90	43.29	32.98	33.24	3.86
C37-C38	其他的胸腔器官	Other thoracic organs	4	0.51	0.82	0.56	0.64	0.08
C40-C41	骨	Bone	4	0.51	0.82	0.67	0.59	0.03
C43	皮肤的黑色素瘤	Melanoma of skin	2	0.25	0.41	0.36	0.36	0.07
C50	乳房	Breast	15	1.90	6.28	5.20	4.47	0.48
C53	子宫颈	Cervix	12	1.52	5.02	4.61	4.08	0.54
C54-55	子宫体及子宫部位不明	Corpus Uterus & Unspectified	8	1.02	3.35	2.61	2.64	0.35
C56	卵巢	Ovary	5	0.63	2.09	1.57	1.50	0.17
C61	前列腺	Prostate	14	1.78	5.58	4.40	4.84	0.41
C62	睾丸	Testis	0	0.00	0.00	0.00	0.00	0.00
C64-66，68	肾及泌尿系统不明	Kidney & Unspecified Urinary Organs	14	1.78	2.86	2.36	2.18	0.19
C67	膀胱	Bladder	13	1.65	2.65	1.84	1.96	0.12
C70-C72; D32-33;D42-43	脑，神经系统	Brain & Central Nervous System	22	2.79	4.49	3.76	4.03	0.34
C73	甲状腺	Thyroid	2	0.25	0.41	0.26	0.29	0.00
C81-85, 88,90,96	淋巴瘤	Lymphoma	14	1.78	2.86	2.24	2.31	0.25
C91-C95; D45-47	白血病	Leukaemia	18	2.28	3.68	3.18	3.18	0.30
Other	其他	Other	36	4.57	7.35	5.62	5.74	0.49
ALL	所有部位合计	All sites	788	100.00	160.91	125.14	125.42	13.65
ALLbC44	所有部位除外 C44	All sites except C44	786	99.75	160.51	124.84	125.12	13.63

附表 2-33　2019 年上杭县恶性肿瘤发病主要指标

Appendix Table 2-33　Cancer incidence in Shanghang, 2019

ICD10	部位 Site	发病数 Cases	构成 Freq.（%）	粗率 Crude rate（1/10⁵）	中标率 ASR China（1/10⁵）	世标率 ASR world（1/10⁵）	累积率 Cum.rate（0~74，%）
C00-10, C12-14	口腔和咽喉（除外鼻咽） Oral Cavity & Pharynx but Nasopharynx	19	1.30	3.60	2.49	2.45	0.23
C11	鼻咽 Nasopharynx	35	2.39	6.63	5.68	4.95	0.54
C15	食管 Esophagus	69	4.71	13.07	8.64	9.04	1.21
C16	胃 Stomach	108	7.37	20.46	13.86	13.35	1.75
C18-21	结直肠肛门 Colon, Rectum & Anus	214	14.60	40.53	26.45	26.07	3.16
C22	肝脏 Liver	123	8.39	23.30	16.20	15.85	1.99
C23-C24	胆囊及其他 Gallbladder	16	1.09	3.03	1.97	1.89	0.23
C25	胰腺 Pancreas	12	0.82	2.27	1.66	1.67	0.29
C32	喉 Larynx	6	0.41	1.14	0.71	0.69	0.09
C33-C34	气管，支气管，肺 Trachea, Bronchus & Lung	267	18.21	50.57	33.19	32.72	3.90
C37-C38	其他的胸腔器官 Other thoracic organs	6	0.41	1.14	0.75	0.71	0.07
C40-C41	骨 Bone	7	0.48	1.33	0.89	0.88	0.09
C43	皮肤的黑色素瘤 Melanoma of skin	3	0.20	0.57	0.45	0.45	0.06
C50	乳房 Breast	81	5.59	31.65	24.04	21.50	2.18
C53	子宫颈 Cervix	49	3.34	19.14	13.85	12.55	1.24
C54-55	子宫体及子宫部位不明 Corpus Uterus & Unspectified	29	1.98	11.33	7.11	7.12	0.82
C56	卵巢 Ovary	13	0.89	5.08	4.31	3.91	0.34
C61	前列腺 Prostate	38	2.59	13.97	8.75	8.26	0.75
C62	睾丸 Testis	1	0.07	0.37	0.22	0.21	0.02
C64-66，68	肾及泌尿系统不明 Kidney & Unspecified Urinary Organs	24	1.64	4.55	3.46	3.31	0.41
C67	膀胱 Bladder	30	2.05	5.68	3.41	3.53	0.36
C70-C72; D32-33;D42-43	脑，神经系统 Brain & Central Nervous System	48	3.27	9.09	7.34	7.25	0.66
C73	甲状腺 Thyroid	109	7.44	20.65	18.96	16.30	1.46
C81-85, 88,90,96	淋巴瘤 Lymphoma	30	2.05	5.68	3.96	4.01	0.55
C91-C95; D45-47	白血病 Leukaemia	29	1.98	5.49	4.85	4.59	0.44
Other	其他 Other	99	6.75	18.75	13.42	12.43	1.29
ALL	所有部位合计 All sites	1466	100.00	277.67	196.94	188.44	21.48
ALLbC44	所有部位除外 C44 All sites except C44	1443	98.43	273.31	194.51	186.20	21.32

附表 2-34　2019 年上杭县恶性肿瘤死亡主要指标

Appendix Table 2-34　Cancer mortality in Shanghang, 2019

ICD10	部位 Site		发病数 Cases	构成 Freq. （%）	粗率 Crude rate （1/10⁵）	中标率 ASR China （1/10⁵）	世标率 ASR world （1/10⁵）	累积率 Cum.rate （0~74，%）
C00-10, C12-14	口腔和咽喉（除外鼻咽）	Oral Cavity & Pharynx but Nasopharynx	17	2.15	3.22	2.20	2.26	0.34
C11	鼻咽	Nasopharynx	15	1.90	2.84	1.86	1.84	0.24
C15	食管	Esophagus	74	9.37	14.02	8.37	8.67	0.99
C16	胃	Stomach	77	9.75	14.58	9.27	9.02	1.04
C18-21	结直肠肛门	Colon, Rectum & Anus	87	11.01	16.48	9.07	9.22	0.97
C22	肝脏	Liver	114	14.43	21.59	14.15	13.96	1.64
C23-C24	胆囊及其他	Gallbladder	14	1.77	2.65	1.55	1.57	0.18
C25	胰腺	Pancreas	13	1.65	2.46	1.49	1.54	0.20
C32	喉	Larynx	9	1.14	1.70	1.13	1.16	0.15
C33-C34	气管，支气管，肺	Trachea, Bronchus & Lung	203	25.70	38.45	24.31	23.64	2.89
C37-C38	其他的胸腔器官	Other thoracic organs	3	0.38	0.57	0.32	0.37	0.05
C40-C41	骨	Bone	3	0.38	0.57	0.40	0.46	0.06
C43	皮肤的黑色素瘤	Melanoma of skin	1	0.13	0.19	0.13	0.14	0.02
C50	乳房	Breast	9	1.14	3.52	2.44	2.06	0.19
C53	子宫颈	Cervix	9	1.14	3.52	2.20	2.19	0.25
C54-55	子宫体及子宫部位不明	Corpus Uterus & Unspectified	7	0.89	2.73	1.48	1.38	0.16
C56	卵巢	Ovary	3	0.38	1.17	0.55	0.57	0.05
C61	前列腺	Prostate	9	1.14	3.31	1.91	1.98	0.14
C62	睾丸	Testis	0	0.00	0.00	0.00	0.00	0.00
C64-66, 68	肾及泌尿系统不明	Kidney & Unspecified Urinary Organs	8	1.01	1.52	1.00	0.98	0.09
C67	膀胱	Bladder	10	1.27	1.89	0.95	0.96	0.09
C70-C72; D32-33;D42-43	脑，神经系统	Brain & Central Nervous System	23	2.91	4.36	3.20	3.21	0.31
C73	甲状腺	Thyroid	0	0.00	0.00	0.00	0.00	0.00
C81-85,88,90,96	淋巴瘤	Lymphoma	15	1.90	2.84	2.06	2.03	0.32
C91-C95; D45-47	白血病	Leukaemia	27	3.42	5.11	4.08	3.98	0.43
Other	其他	Other	40	5.06	7.58	5.56	5.45	0.63
ALL	所有部位合计	All sites	790	100.00	149.63	95.30	94.46	11.05
ALLbC44	所有部位除外 C44	All sites except C44	788	99.75	149.25	95.12	94.23	11.03

附表 2-35　2019 年永安市恶性肿瘤发病主要指标
Appendix Table 2-35　Cancer incidence in Yong'an, 2019

ICD10	部位 Site		发病数 Cases	构成 Freq. (%)	粗率 Crude rate (1/10⁵)	中标率 ASR China (1/10⁵)	世标率 ASR world (1/10⁵)	累积率 Cum.rate (0~74, %)
C00-10,12-14	口腔和咽喉（除外鼻咽）	Oral Cavity & Pharynx but Nasopharynx	17	1.60	5.15	2.81	2.87	0.41
C11	鼻咽	Nasopharynx	18	1.70	5.45	3.76	3.56	0.36
C15	食管	Esophagus	35	3.30	10.59	5.82	6.07	0.75
C16	胃	Stomach	80	7.54	24.21	14.17	13.62	1.74
C18-21	结直肠肛门	Colon, Rectum & Anus	161	15.17	48.73	28.02	26.86	3.20
C22	肝脏	Liver	89	8.39	26.94	16.36	15.74	1.78
C23-C24	胆囊及其他	Gallbladder	13	1.23	3.93	2.42	2.29	0.24
C25	胰腺	Pancreas	16	1.51	4.84	2.24	2.14	0.17
C32	喉	Larynx	5	0.47	1.51	0.91	0.96	0.14
C33-C34	气管，支气管，肺	Trachea, Bronchus & Lung	183	17.25	55.39	31.03	30.90	3.90
C37-C38	其他的胸腔器官	Other thoracic organs	4	0.38	1.21	0.67	0.74	0.07
C40-C41	骨	Bone	2	0.19	0.61	0.74	0.72	0.06
C43	皮肤的黑色素瘤	Melanoma of skin	2	0.19	0.61	0.38	0.41	0.07
C50	乳房	Breast	76	7.26	47.22	32.03	29.27	2.88
C53	子宫颈	Cervix	40	3.77	24.86	16.20	14.98	1.63
C54-55	子宫体及子宫部位不明	Corpus Uterus & Unspectified	25	2.36	15.53	9.62	8.80	1.01
C56	卵巢	Ovary	15	1.41	9.32	6.05	6.21	0.81
C61	前列腺	Prostate	30	2.83	17.70	9.33	9.57	0.92
C62	睾丸	Testis	2	0.19	1.18	1.36	1.05	0.09
C64-66, 68	肾及泌尿系统不明	Kidney & Unspecified Urinary Organs	16	1.51	4.84	2.90	2.94	0.39
C67	膀胱	Bladder	14	1.32	4.24	2.42	2.43	0.29
C70-C72; D32-33;D42-43	脑，神经系统	Brain & Central Nervous System	29	2.73	8.78	5.19	5.29	0.52
C73	甲状腺	Thyroid	74	6.97	22.40	19.57	16.40	1.48
C81-85,88,90,96	淋巴瘤	Lymphoma	30	2.83	9.08	5.77	5.46	0.64
C91-C95;D45-47	白血病	Leukaemia	24	2.26	7.26	4.91	5.20	0.42
Other	其他	Other	60	5.66	18.16	11.61	11.39	0.98
ALL	所有部位合计	All sites	1061	100.00	321.12	198.84	190.75	21.29
ALLbC44	所有部位除外 C44	All sites except C44	1048	98.77	317.19	196.53	188.12	21.06

附表 2-36　2019 年永安市恶性肿瘤死亡主要指标

Appendix Table 2-36　Cancer mortality in Yong'an, 2019

ICD10	部位 Site		死亡数 Deaths	构成 Freq. （%）	粗率 Crude rate （1/10⁵）	中标率 ASR China （1/10⁵）	世标率 ASR world （1/10⁵）	累积率 Cum.rate （0~74，%）
C00-10, C12-14	口腔和咽喉（除外鼻咽）	Oral Cavity & Pharynx but Nasopharynx	5	0.87	1.51	0.75	0.73	0.07
C11	鼻咽	Nasopharynx	12	2.09	3.63	2.40	2.30	0.29
C15	食管	Esophagus	20	3.49	6.05	3.09	3.16	0.36
C16	胃	Stomach	62	10.82	18.76	9.29	8.99	0.87
C18-21	结直肠肛门	Colon, Rectum & Anus	89	15.53	26.94	14.73	14.02	1.44
C22	肝脏	Liver	72	12.57	21.79	12.70	12.52	1.41
C23-C24	胆囊及其他	Gallbladder	10	1.75	3.03	1.36	1.31	0.14
C25	胰腺	Pancreas	14	2.44	4.24	2.00	1.88	0.16
C32	喉	Larynx	5	0.87	1.51	0.81	0.85	0.12
C33-C34	气管，支气管，肺	Trachea, Bronchus & Lung	148	25.83	44.79	23.32	22.88	2.65
C37-C38	其他的胸腔器官	Other thoracic organs	2	0.35	0.61	0.59	0.66	0.03
C40-C41	骨	Bone	3	0.52	0.91	0.57	0.61	0.10
C43	皮肤的黑色素瘤	Melanoma of skin	1	0.17	0.30	0.20	0.19	0.05
C50	乳房	Breast	16	2.79	9.94	5.54	4.93	0.54
C53	子宫颈	Cervix	21	3.66	13.05	6.33	6.07	0.60
C54-55	子宫体及子宫部位不明	Corpus Uterus & Unspectified	6	1.05	3.73	2.07	1.99	0.33
C56	卵巢	Ovary	2	0.35	1.24	0.67	0.74	0.08
C61	前列腺	Prostate	15	2.62	8.85	3.32	3.66	0.07
C62	睾丸	Testis	0	0.00	0.00	0.00	0.00	0.00
C64-66，68	肾及泌尿系统不明	Kidney & Unspecified Urinary Organs	5	0.87	1.51	0.91	0.96	0.16
C67	膀胱	Bladder	5	0.87	1.51	0.69	0.64	0.04
C70-C72; D32-33; D42-43	脑，神经系统	Brain & Central Nervous System	10	1.75	3.03	1.55	1.65	0.21
C73	甲状腺	Thyroid	1	0.17	0.30	0.22	0.19	0.02
C81-85,88,90,96	淋巴瘤	Lymphoma	9	1.57	2.72	1.65	1.95	0.20
C91-C95;D45-47	白血病	Leukaemia	11	1.92	3.33	2.32	2.71	0.27
Other	其他	Other	29	5.06	8.78	4.25	4.05	0.33
ALL	所有部位合计	All sites	573	100.00	173.42	92.28	90.84	9.72
ALLbC44	所有部位除外 C44	All sites except C44	569	99.30	172.21	91.80	90.32	9.71

附表 2-37　　2019 年宁化县恶性肿瘤发病主要指标

Appendix Table 2-37　　Cancer incidence in Ninghua, 2019

ICD10	部位 Site	发病数 Cases	构成 Freq. （%）	粗率 Crude rate （1/10⁵）	中标率 ASR China （1/10⁵）	世标率 ASR world （1/10⁵）	累积率 Cum.rate （0~74，%）
C00-10, C12-14	口腔和咽喉（除外鼻咽） Oral Cavity & Pharynx but Nasopharynx	19	2.15	5.05	3.25	3.37	0.44
C11	鼻咽 Nasopharynx	31	3.51	8.24	5.84	5.44	0.63
C15	食管 Esophagus	59	6.67	15.68	9.21	9.65	1.13
C16	胃 Stomach	79	8.94	20.99	13.87	13.95	1.86
C18-21	结直肠肛门 Colon, Rectum & Anus	85	9.62	22.58	14.03	14.11	1.70
C22	肝脏 Liver	84	9.50	22.32	14.43	14.14	1.82
C23-C24	胆囊及其他 Gallbladder	17	1.92	4.52	3.05	3.04	0.44
C25	胰腺 Pancreas	24	2.71	6.38	3.86	3.75	0.50
C32	喉 Larynx	8	0.90	2.13	1.47	1.44	0.19
C33-C34	气管，支气管，肺 Trachea, Bronchus & Lung	183	20.70	48.62	31.77	31.06	4.01
C37-C38	其他的胸腔器官 Other thoracic organs	3	0.34	0.80	0.61	0.63	0.08
C40-C41	骨 Bone	4	0.45	1.06	0.80	0.81	0.05
C43	皮肤的黑色素瘤 Melanoma of skin	2	0.23	0.53	0.18	0.20	0.00
C50	乳房 Breast	36	4.07	20.12	15.80	14.16	1.38
C53	子宫颈 Cervix	36	4.07	20.12	12.61	12.59	1.46
C54-55	子宫体及子宫部位不明 Corpus Uterus & Unspectified	27	3.05	15.09	8.55	8.81	0.96
C56	卵巢 Ovary	13	1.47	7.27	5.56	5.59	0.55
C61	前列腺 Prostate	12	1.36	6.08	3.40	3.64	0.32
C62	睾丸 Testis	2	0.23	1.01	1.60	1.47	0.09
C64-66，68	肾及泌尿系统不明 Kidney & Unspecified Urinary Organs	16	1.81	4.25	3.25	2.88	0.35
C67	膀胱 Bladder	12	1.36	3.19	2.24	2.05	0.19
C70-C72; D32-33; D42-43	脑，神经系统 Brain & Central Nervous System	18	2.04	4.78	3.99	4.01	0.37
C73	甲状腺 Thyroid	28	3.17	7.44	5.85	5.41	0.51
C81-85,88,90,96	淋巴瘤 Lymphoma	12	1.36	3.19	2.26	2.14	0.33
C91-C95;D45-47	白血病 Leukaemia	9	1.02	2.39	1.91	1.61	0.20
Other	其他 Other	65	7.35	17.27	11.01	10.97	1.10
ALL	所有部位合计 All sites	884	100.00	234.86	156.20	153.41	18.25
ALLbC44	所有部位除外 C44 All sites except C44	873	98.76	231.94	154.34	151.65	18.12

附表 2-38　2019 年宁化县恶性肿瘤死亡主要指标
Appendix Table 2-38　Cancer mortality in Ninghua, 2019

ICD10	部位 Site		死亡数 Deaths	构成 Freq. （%）	粗率 Crude rate （1/10⁵）	中标率 ASR China （1/10⁵）	世标率 ASR world （1/10⁵）	累积率 Cum.rate （0~74，%）
C00-10, C12-14	口腔和咽喉（除外鼻咽）	Oral Cavity & Pharynx but Nasopharynx	6	0.99	1.59	1.01	0.97	0.11
C11	鼻咽	Nasopharynx	14	2.30	3.72	2.30	2.30	0.26
C15	食管	Esophagus	42	6.90	11.16	6.33	6.41	0.78
C16	胃	Stomach	72	11.82	19.13	11.25	11.00	1.25
C18-21	结直肠肛门	Colon, Rectum & Anus	55	9.03	14.61	9.51	8.88	0.99
C22	肝脏	Liver	90	14.78	23.91	15.90	15.20	1.84
C23-C24	胆囊及其他	Gallbladder	8	1.31	2.13	1.33	1.31	0.21
C25	胰腺	Pancreas	24	3.94	6.38	3.92	3.79	0.49
C32	喉	Larynx	5	0.82	1.33	0.88	0.90	0.10
C33-C34	气管，支气管，肺	Trachea, Bronchus & Lung	160	26.27	42.51	25.65	25.53	3.06
C37-C38	其他的胸腔器官	Other thoracic organs	1	0.16	0.27	0.18	0.19	0.03
C40-C41	骨	Bone	2	0.33	0.53	0.71	0.64	0.04
C43	皮肤的黑色素瘤	Melanoma of skin	1	0.16	0.27	0.16	0.17	0.02
C50	乳房	Breast	6	0.99	3.35	2.11	2.27	0.28
C53	子宫颈	Cervix	15	2.46	8.38	4.79	4.84	0.65
C54-55	子宫体及子宫部位不明	Corpus Uterus & Unspectified	8	1.31	4.47	2.31	2.01	0.13
C56	卵巢	Ovary	8	1.31	4.47	2.88	2.89	0.40
C61	前列腺	Prostate	10	1.64	5.06	2.84	2.86	0.16
C62	睾丸	Testis	0	0.00	0.00	0.00	0.00	0.00
C64-66，68	肾及泌尿系统不明	Kidney & Unspecified Urinary Organs	3	0.49	0.80	0.47	0.51	0.10
C67	膀胱	Bladder	7	1.15	1.86	0.91	1.03	0.13
C70-C72; D32-33;D42-43	脑，神经系统	Brain & Central Nervous System	11	1.81	2.92	2.52	2.62	0.25
C73	甲状腺	Thyroid	1	0.16	0.27	0.18	0.19	0.03
C81-85, 88,90,96	淋巴瘤	Lymphoma	9	1.48	2.39	1.63	1.64	0.28
C91-C95; D45-47	白血病	Leukaemia	5	0.82	1.33	1.43	1.57	0.11
Other	其他	Other	46	7.55	12.22	7.28	6.99	0.83
ALL	所有部位合计	All sites	609	100.00	161.80	101.00	99.22	11.72
ALLbC44	所有部位除外 C44	All sites except C44	606	99.51	161.00	100.60	98.76	11.67

附表 2-39　2019 年大田县恶性肿瘤发病主要指标
Appendix Table 2-39　Cancer incidence in Datian, 2019

ICD10	部位 Site		发病数 Cases	构成 Freq. （%）	粗率 Crude rate （1/10⁵）	中标率 ASR China （1/10⁵）	世标率 ASR world （1/10⁵）	累积率 Cum.rate （0~74，%）
C00-10, C12-14	口腔和咽喉（除外鼻咽）	Oral Cavity & Pharynx but Nasopharynx	16	1.60	3.85	3.22	2.96	0.42
C11	鼻咽	Nasopharynx	23	2.31	5.53	4.90	4.37	0.54
C15	食管	Esophagus	34	3.41	8.17	5.90	5.97	0.66
C16	胃	Stomach	107	10.73	25.72	19.95	19.33	2.48
C18-21	结直肠肛门	Colon, Rectum & Anus	138	13.84	33.17	25.33	25.42	2.93
C22	肝脏	Liver	75	7.52	18.03	14.17	13.96	1.62
C23-C24	胆囊及其他	Gallbladder	12	1.20	2.88	2.03	1.97	0.16
C25	胰腺	Pancreas	18	1.81	4.33	3.20	3.08	0.38
C32	喉	Larynx	5	0.50	1.20	0.98	1.02	0.16
C33-C34	气管，支气管，肺	Trachea, Bronchus & Lung	171	17.15	41.11	31.34	31.61	4.02
C37-C38	其他的胸腔器官	Other thoracic organs	0	0.00	0.00	0.00	0.00	0.00
C40-C41	骨	Bone	6	0.60	1.44	1.11	1.14	0.14
C43	皮肤的黑色素瘤	Melanoma of skin	3	0.30	0.72	0.54	0.48	0.07
C50	乳房	Breast	56	5.62	29.49	24.93	21.40	1.91
C53	子宫颈	Cervix	59	5.92	31.07	23.54	23.23	2.85
C54-55	子宫体及子宫部位不明	Corpus Uterus & Unspectified	20	2.01	10.53	7.04	6.89	0.77
C56	卵巢	Ovary	14	1.40	7.37	6.41	6.37	0.66
C61	前列腺	Prostate	20	2.01	8.85	7.01	7.06	1.03
C62	睾丸	Testis	0	0.00	0.00	0.00	0.00	0.00
C64-66, 68	肾及泌尿系统不明	Kidney & Unspecified Urinary Organs	13	1.30	3.13	2.55	2.73	0.37
C67	膀胱	Bladder	10	1.00	2.40	1.75	1.73	0.19
C70-C72; D32-33;D42-43	脑，神经系统	Brain & Central Nervous System	41	4.11	9.86	9.38	9.02	0.94
C73	甲状腺	Thyroid	56	5.62	13.46	12.44	10.22	0.90
C81-85, 88,90,96	淋巴瘤	Lymphoma	25	2.51	6.01	4.77	5.03	0.57
C91-C95; D45-47	白血病	Leukaemia	26	2.61	6.25	5.36	5.72	0.51
Other	其他	Other	49	4.91	11.78	9.76	9.67	1.16
ALL	所有部位合计	All sites	997	100.00	239.67	191.89	186.83	21.74
ALLbC44	所有部位除外 C44	All sites except C44	989	99.20	237.75	190.31	185.38	21.56

附表 2-40　　2019 年大田县恶性肿瘤死亡主要指标
Appendix Table 2-40　Cancer mortality in Datian, 2019

ICD10	部位 Site	死亡数 Deaths	构成 Freq. （%）	粗率 Crude rate （1/10⁵）	中标率 ASR China （1/10⁵）	世标率 ASR world （1/10⁵）	累积率 Cum.rate （0~74，%）
C00-10, C12-14	口腔和咽喉（除外鼻咽）	Oral Cavity & Pharynx but Nasopharynx	7	1.36	1.68	1.22	1.26	0.15
C11	鼻咽	Nasopharynx	9	1.75	2.16	1.74	1.74	0.23
C15	食管	Esophagus	26	5.05	6.25	4.48	4.54	0.56
C16	胃	Stomach	75	14.56	18.03	13.48	13.28	1.59
C18-21	结直肠肛门	Colon, Rectum & Anus	58	11.26	13.94	10.26	9.94	1.07
C22	肝脏	Liver	65	12.62	15.63	12.88	12.37	1.51
C23-C24	胆囊及其他	Gallbladder	4	0.78	0.96	0.63	0.65	0.05
C25	胰腺	Pancreas	15	2.91	3.61	2.63	2.68	0.29
C32	喉	Larynx	3	0.58	0.72	0.51	0.48	0.03
C33-C34	气管，支气管，肺	Trachea, Bronchus & Lung	122	23.69	29.33	22.30	22.73	2.90
C37-C38	其他的胸腔器官	Other thoracic organs	0	0.00	0.00	0.00	0.00	0.00
C40-C41	骨	Bone	7	1.36	1.68	1.29	1.36	0.20
C43	皮肤的黑色素瘤	Melanoma of skin	2	0.39	0.48	0.40	0.36	0.05
C50	乳房	Breast	5	0.97	2.63	2.09	1.72	0.11
C53	子宫颈	Cervix	29	5.63	15.27	10.64	10.97	1.44
C54-55	子宫体及子宫部位不明	Corpus Uterus & Unspectified	5	0.97	2.63	1.86	1.91	0.29
C56	卵巢	Ovary	5	0.97	2.63	2.00	2.00	0.34
C61	前列腺	Prostate	11	2.14	4.87	3.51	3.76	0.35
C62	睾丸	Testis	0	0.00	0.00	0.00	0.00	0.00
C64-66, 68	肾及泌尿系统不明	Kidney & Unspecified Urinary Organs	3	0.58	0.72	0.64	0.66	0.14
C67	膀胱	Bladder	5	0.97	1.20	0.72	0.75	0.05
C70-C72; D32-33; D42-43	脑，神经系统	Brain & Central Nervous System	9	1.75	2.16	2.47	2.21	0.16
C73	甲状腺	Thyroid	1	0.19	0.24	0.18	0.14	0.00
C81-85,88,90,96	淋巴瘤	Lymphoma	10	1.94	2.40	2.15	2.12	0.15
C91-C95; D45-47	白血病	Leukaemia	9	1.75	2.16	1.69	1.68	0.20
Other	其他	Other	30	5.83	7.21	5.73	5.83	0.75
ALL	所有部位合计	All sites	515	100.00	123.80	95.29	94.82	11.33
ALLbC44	所有部位除外 C44	All sites except C44	514	99.81	123.56	95.16	94.71	11.33

附表 2-41　2019 年建瓯市恶性肿瘤发病主要指标
Appendix Table 2-41　Cancer incidence in Jian'ou, 2019

ICD10	部位 Site		发病数 Cases	构成 Freq. （%）	粗率 Crude rate （1/10⁵）	中标率 ASR China （1/10⁵）	世标率 ASR world （1/10⁵）	累积率 Cum.rate （0~74，%）
C00-10, C12-14	口腔和咽喉（除外鼻咽）	Oral Cavity & Pharynx but Nasopharynx	15	0.90	2.72	2.19	2.04	0.19
C11	鼻咽	Nasopharynx	34	2.04	6.16	5.16	4.53	0.51
C15	食管	Esophagus	19	1.14	3.44	2.58	2.49	0.27
C16	胃	Stomach	156	9.35	28.25	23.10	23.29	3.04
C18-21	结直肠肛门	Colon, Rectum & Anus	258	15.46	46.72	37.13	36.89	4.60
C22	肝脏	Liver	163	9.77	29.52	24.15	23.84	2.93
C23-C24	胆囊及其他	Gallbladder	34	2.04	6.16	4.85	4.92	0.61
C25	胰腺	Pancreas	34	2.04	6.16	4.73	4.89	0.65
C32	喉	Larynx	10	0.60	1.81	1.50	1.57	0.21
C33-C34	气管，支气管，肺	Trachea, Bronchus & Lung	347	20.79	62.84	51.24	52.33	6.77
C37-C38	其他的胸腔器官	Other thoracic organs	3	0.18	0.54	0.46	0.48	0.10
C40-C41	骨	Bone	6	0.36	1.09	1.01	1.13	0.13
C43	皮肤的黑色素瘤	Melanoma of skin	4	0.24	0.72	0.62	0.47	0.03
C50	乳房	Breast	127	7.61	47.47	39.19	37.27	4.19
C53	子宫颈	Cervix	57	3.42	21.31	17.67	17.56	2.00
C54-55	子宫体及子宫部位不明	Corpus Uterus & Unspectified	29	1.74	10.84	8.66	9.32	1.21
C56	卵巢	Ovary	17	1.02	6.35	5.66	5.94	0.72
C61	前列腺	Prostate	34	2.04	11.94	9.14	9.04	0.90
C62	睾丸	Testis	0	0.00	0.00	0.00	0.00	0.00
C64-66，68	肾及泌尿系统不明	Kidney & Unspecified Urinary Organs	20	1.20	3.62	2.91	3.13	0.41
C67	膀胱	Bladder	18	1.08	3.26	2.56	2.49	0.27
C70-C72; D32-33;D42-43	脑，神经系统	Brain & Central Nervous System	47	2.82	8.51	6.81	6.59	0.74
C73	甲状腺	Thyroid	93	5.57	16.84	15.02	13.52	1.31
C81-85, 88,90,96	淋巴瘤	Lymphoma	44	2.64	7.97	6.71	6.63	0.80
C91-C95;D45-47	白血病	Leukaemia	22	1.32	3.98	4.05	4.45	0.46
Other	其他	Other	78	4.67	14.13	12.34	12.20	1.43
ALL	所有部位合计	All sites	1669	100.00	302.26	248.18	246.24	29.83
ALLbC44	所有部位除外 C44	All sites except C44	1658	99.34	300.27	246.63	244.77	29.73

附表 2-42　2019 年建瓯市恶性肿瘤死亡主要指标
Appendix Table 2-42　Cancer mortality in Jian'ou, 2019

ICD10	部位 Site	死亡数 Deaths	构成 Freq. （%）	粗率 Crude rate （1/10^5）	中标率 ASR China （1/10^5）	世标率 ASR world （1/10^5）	累积率 Cum.rate （0~74，%）
C00-10, C12-14	口腔和咽喉（除外鼻咽）	Oral Cavity & Pharynx but Nasopharynx	4	0.39	0.72	0.52	0.55	0.05
C11	鼻咽	Nasopharynx	19	1.83	3.44	2.71	2.81	0.41
C15	食管	Esophagus	21	2.03	3.80	3.02	2.87	0.36
C16	胃	Stomach	126	12.16	22.82	17.60	17.68	2.03
C18-21	结直肠肛门	Colon, Rectum & Anus	147	14.19	26.62	20.04	19.92	2.24
C22	肝脏	Liver	143	13.80	25.90	20.71	20.73	2.59
C23-C24	胆囊及其他	Gallbladder	26	2.51	4.71	3.91	3.99	0.57
C25	胰腺	Pancreas	29	2.80	5.25	3.87	3.91	0.49
C32	喉	Larynx	5	0.48	0.91	0.80	0.82	0.10
C33-C34	气管，支气管，肺	Trachea, Bronchus & Lung	262	25.29	47.45	38.13	38.83	4.81
C37-C38	其他的胸腔器官	Other thoracic organs	1	0.10	0.18	0.14	0.13	0.01
C40-C41	骨	Bone	7	0.68	1.27	1.01	1.03	0.12
C43	皮肤的黑色素瘤	Melanoma of skin	1	0.10	0.18	0.19	0.20	0.03
C50	乳房	Breast	25	2.41	9.34	7.06	7.09	0.78
C53	子宫颈	Cervix	20	1.93	7.48	5.98	5.89	0.77
C54-55	子宫体及子宫部位不明	Corpus Uterus & Unspectified	10	0.97	3.74	3.19	3.45	0.46
C56	卵巢	Ovary	16	1.54	5.98	5.10	5.36	0.71
C61	前列腺	Prostate	13	1.25	4.57	3.46	3.39	0.32
C62	睾丸	Testis	0	0.00	0.00	0.00	0.00	0.00
C64-66，68	肾及泌尿系统不明	Kidney & Unspecified Urinary Organs	9	0.87	1.63	1.15	1.27	0.19
C67	膀胱	Bladder	8	0.77	1.45	0.93	0.91	0.02
C70-C72; D32-33; D42-43	脑，神经系统	Brain & Central Nervous System	38	3.67	6.88	5.54	5.21	0.61
C73	甲状腺	Thyroid	2	0.19	0.36	0.28	0.32	0.04
C81-85,88,90,96	淋巴瘤	Lymphoma	24	2.32	4.35	3.71	3.82	0.50
C91-C95;D45-47	白血病	Leukaemia	17	1.64	3.08	2.78	2.73	0.41
Other	其他	Other	63	6.08	11.41	9.39	9.35	1.12
ALL	所有部位合计	All sites	1036	100.00	187.62	148.43	149.27	18.20
ALLbC44	所有部位除外 C44	All sites except C44	1029	99.32	186.35	147.58	148.52	18.15

附表 2-43　2019 年延平区恶性肿瘤发病主要指标
Appendix Table 2-43　Cancer incidence in Yanping, 2019

ICD10	部位 Site		发病数 Cases	构成 Freq. （%）	粗率 Crude rate （1/10⁵）	中标率 ASR China （1/10⁵）	世标率 ASR world （1/10⁵）	累积率 Cum.rate （0~74, %）
C00-10, C12-14	口腔和咽喉（除外鼻咽）	Oral Cavity & Pharynx but Nasopharynx	25	1.34	5.01	2.79	2.75	0.30
C11	鼻咽	Nasopharynx	22	1.18	4.41	3.04	2.78	0.33
C15	食管	Esophagus	28	1.51	5.61	3.23	3.23	0.42
C16	胃	Stomach	129	6.94	25.85	14.46	14.53	1.90
C18-21	结直肠肛门	Colon, Rectum & Anus	259	13.93	51.91	28.52	28.17	3.55
C22	肝脏	Liver	156	8.39	31.27	18.98	18.43	1.99
C23-C24	胆囊及其他	Gallbladder	25	1.34	5.01	2.83	2.81	0.37
C25	胰腺	Pancreas	22	1.18	4.41	2.35	2.43	0.35
C32	喉	Larynx	14	0.75	2.81	1.57	1.58	0.20
C33-C34	气管，支气管,肺	Trachea, Bronchus & Lung	256	13.77	51.31	27.99	27.85	3.52
C37-C38	其他的胸腔器官	Other thoracic organs	6	0.32	1.20	0.88	0.87	0.10
C40-C41	骨	Bone	7	0.38	1.40	1.31	1.08	0.08
C43	皮肤的黑色素瘤	Melanoma of skin	3	0.16	0.60	0.43	0.41	0.04
C50	乳房	Breast	147	7.91	60.44	39.65	36.37	3.70
C53	子宫颈	Cervix	41	2.21	16.86	10.97	10.17	1.34
C54-55	子宫体及子宫部位不明	Corpus Uterus & Unspectified	19	1.02	7.81	4.35	4.33	0.59
C56	卵巢	Ovary	19	1.02	7.81	5.20	5.09	0.59
C61	前列腺	Prostate	47	2.53	18.38	9.99	9.26	0.84
C62	睾丸	Testis	1	0.05	0.39	0.64	0.70	0.04
C64-66, 68	肾及泌尿系统不明	Kidney & Unspecified Urinary Organs	31	1.67	6.21	3.76	3.45	0.44
C67	膀胱	Bladder	31	1.67	6.21	3.34	3.36	0.42
C70-C72;D32-33; D42-43	脑，神经系统	Brain & Central Nervous System	77	4.14	15.43	10.26	9.93	1.00
C73	甲状腺	Thyroid	293	15.76	58.72	52.15	43.74	4.07
C81-85,88,90,96	淋巴瘤	Lymphoma	57	3.07	11.42	7.40	7.42	0.80
C91-C95; D45-47	白血病	Leukaemia	39	2.10	7.82	5.40	5.44	0.49
Other	其他	Other	105	5.65	21.04	12.80	12.80	1.48
ALL	所有部位合计	All sites	1859	100.00	372.58	238.48	225.66	25.38
ALLbC44	所有部位除外 C44	All sites except C44	1853	99.68	371.38	237.79	224.98	25.30

附表 2-44　2019 年延平区恶性肿瘤死亡主要指标

Appendix Table 2-44　Cancer mortality in Yanping, 2019

ICD10	部位 Site		死亡数 Deaths	构成 Freq. （%）	粗率 Crude rate （1/10^5）	中标率 ASR China （1/10^5）	世标率 ASR world （1/10^5）	累积率 Cum.rate （0~74，%）
C00-10, C12-14	口腔和咽喉（除外鼻咽）	Oral Cavity & Pharynx but Nasopharynx	11	1.34	2.20	1.07	1.12	0.17
C11	鼻咽	Nasopharynx	23	2.81	4.61	2.98	2.83	0.33
C15	食管	Esophagus	31	3.79	6.21	3.32	3.31	0.49
C16	胃	Stomach	94	11.49	18.84	9.14	8.97	0.95
C18-21	结直肠肛门	Colon, Rectum & Anus	108	13.20	21.65	10.98	10.90	1.19
C22	肝脏	Liver	135	16.50	27.06	15.30	14.94	1.84
C23-C24	胆囊及其他	Gallbladder	20	2.44	4.01	2.04	2.00	0.23
C25	胰腺	Pancreas	29	3.55	5.81	3.03	3.03	0.35
C32	喉	Larynx	1	0.12	0.20	0.10	0.11	0.01
C33-C34	气管，支气管，肺	Trachea, Bronchus & Lung	165	20.17	33.07	17.42	17.24	2.21
C37-C38	其他的胸腔器官	Other thoracic organs	2	0.24	0.40	0.22	0.27	0.03
C40-C41	骨	Bone	9	1.10	1.80	1.01	0.92	0.04
C43	皮肤的黑色素瘤	Melanoma of skin	2	0.24	0.40	0.23	0.21	0.02
C50	乳房	Breast	13	1.59	5.35	3.01	2.93	0.28
C53	子宫颈	Cervix	8	0.98	3.29	1.56	1.63	0.22
C54-55	子宫体及子宫部位不明	Corpus Uterus & Unspectified	9	1.10	3.70	1.59	1.65	0.18
C56	卵巢	Ovary	11	1.34	4.52	2.54	2.49	0.31
C61	前列腺	Prostate	13	1.59	5.08	2.40	2.46	0.28
C62	睾丸	Testis	0	0.00	0.00	0.00	0.00	0.00
C64-66, 68	肾及泌尿系统不明	Kidney & Unspecified Urinary Organs	3	0.37	0.60	0.31	0.25	0.01
C67	膀胱	Bladder	6	0.73	1.20	0.57	0.59	0.08
C70-C72; D32-33; D42-43	脑，神经系统	Brain & Central Nervous System	19	2.32	3.81	2.26	2.20	0.32
C73	甲状腺	Thyroid	1	0.12	0.20	0.12	0.12	0.03
C81-85,88,90,96	淋巴瘤	Lymphoma	32	3.91	6.41	3.57	3.60	0.38
C91-C95; D45-47	白血病	Leukaemia	23	2.81	4.61	2.47	2.46	0.22
Other	其他	Other	50	6.11	10.02	5.20	5.27	0.66
ALL	所有部位合计	All sites	818	100.00	163.94	86.86	85.89	10.22
ALLbC44	所有部位除外 C44	All sites except C44	818	100.00	163.94	86.86	85.89	10.22

附表 2-45　2019 年浦城县恶性肿瘤发病主要指标

Appendix Table 2-45　Cancer incidence in Pucheng, 2019

ICD10	部位 Site		发病数 Cases	构成 Freq. （%）	粗率 Crude rate （1/10^5）	中标率 ASR China （1/10^5）	世标率 ASR world （1/10^5）	累积率 Cum.rate （0~74，%）
C00-10, C12-14	口腔和咽喉（除外鼻咽）	Oral Cavity & Pharynx but Nasopharynx	8	0.70	1.87	1.04	1.01	0.11
C11	鼻咽	Nasopharynx	16	1.40	3.74	2.92	2.53	0.25
C15	食管	Esophagus	19	1.66	4.44	2.47	2.46	0.30
C16	胃	Stomach	94	8.22	21.98	12.75	12.16	1.46
C18-21	结直肠肛门	Colon, Rectum & Anus	172	15.03	40.21	23.78	23.10	2.79
C22	肝脏	Liver	104	9.09	24.32	15.47	14.54	1.61
C23-C24	胆囊及其他	Gallbladder	22	1.92	5.14	2.91	2.84	0.32
C25	胰腺	Pancreas	23	2.01	5.38	3.00	3.06	0.37
C32	喉	Larynx	4	0.35	0.94	0.48	0.51	0.06
C33-C34	气管，支气管，肺	Trachea, Bronchus & Lung	250	21.85	58.45	33.39	33.46	4.35
C37-C38	其他的胸腔器官	Other thoracic organs	4	0.35	0.94	0.55	0.55	0.08
C40-C41	骨	Bone	9	0.79	2.10	1.53	2.18	0.18
C43	皮肤的黑色素瘤	Melanoma of skin	0	0.00	0.00	0.00	0.00	0.00
C50	乳房	Breast	63	5.51	30.41	20.78	19.04	1.89
C53	子宫颈	Cervix	31	2.71	14.96	9.45	8.88	1.14
C54-55	子宫体及子宫部位不明	Corpus Uterus & Unspectified	20	1.75	9.65	5.43	5.36	0.58
C56	卵巢	Ovary	13	1.14	6.27	5.18	5.24	0.62
C61	前列腺	Prostate	31	2.71	14.06	7.59	7.17	0.81
C62	睾丸	Testis	1	0.09	0.45	0.28	0.22	0.00
C64-66，68	肾及泌尿系统不明	Kidney & Unspecified Urinary Organs	26	2.27	6.08	3.40	3.29	0.38
C67	膀胱	Bladder	29	2.53	6.78	3.60	3.57	0.39
C70-C72; D32-33;D42-43	脑，神经系统	Brain & Central Nervous System	41	3.58	9.59	7.00	6.39	0.66
C73	甲状腺	Thyroid	49	4.28	11.46	11.90	9.58	0.88
C81-85,88,90,96	淋巴瘤	Lymphoma	23	2.01	5.38	4.30	3.76	0.36
C91-C95;D45-47	白血病	Leukaemia	23	2.01	5.38	4.59	4.58	0.35
Other	其他	Other	69	6.03	16.13	9.49	9.64	0.95
ALL	所有部位合计	All sites	1144	100.00	267.47	168.41	161.66	18.32
ALLbC44	所有部位除外 C44	All sites except C44	1140	99.65	266.54	167.91	161.14	18.27

附表 2-46　2019 年浦城县恶性肿瘤死亡主要指标

Appendix Table 2-46　Cancer mortality in Pucheng, 2019

ICD10	部位 Site	死亡数 Deaths	构成 Freq. （%）	粗率 Crude rate （1/10^5）	中标率 ASR China （1/10^5）	世标率 ASR world （1/10^5）	累积率 Cum.rate （0~74,%）
C00-10, C12-14	口腔和咽喉（除外鼻咽）	Oral Cavity & Pharynx but Nasopharynx	2	0.33	0.47	0.27	0.23	0.01
C11	鼻咽 Nasopharynx	5	0.82	1.17	0.68	0.65	0.05
C15	食管 Esophagus	20	3.27	4.68	2.38	2.29	0.21
C16	胃 Stomach	66	10.78	15.43	8.26	7.90	0.93
C18-21	结直肠肛门 Colon, Rectum & Anus	69	11.27	16.13	8.21	8.14	0.90
C22	肝脏 Liver	100	16.34	23.38	13.46	13.16	1.61
C23-C24	胆囊及其他 Gallbladder	16	2.61	3.74	2.14	2.04	0.19
C25	胰腺 Pancreas	9	1.47	2.10	1.26	1.31	0.18
C32	喉 Larynx	5	0.82	1.17	0.67	0.61	0.09
C33-C34	气管，支气管，肺 Trachea, Bronchus & Lung	172	28.10	40.21	22.01	22.22	2.97
C37-C38	其他的胸腔器官 Other thoracic organs	1	0.16	0.23	0.15	0.15	0.04
C40-C41	骨 Bone	5	0.82	1.17	0.59	0.56	0.05
C43	皮肤的黑色素瘤 Melanoma of skin	1	0.16	0.23	0.13	0.16	0.02
C50	乳房 Breast	25	4.08	12.07	7.17	7.41	0.96
C53	子宫颈 Cervix	4	0.65	1.93	1.12	1.23	0.20
C54-55	子宫体及子宫部位不明 Corpus Uterus & Unspectified	4	0.65	1.93	1.47	1.28	0.16
C56	卵巢 Ovary	6	0.98	2.90	1.52	1.54	0.18
C61	前列腺 Prostate	11	1.80	4.99	2.39	2.27	0.27
C62	睾丸 Testis	1	0.16	0.45	0.28	0.22	0.00
C64-66，68	肾及泌尿系统不明 Kidney & Unspecified Urinary Organs	4	0.65	0.94	0.45	0.46	0.03
C67	膀胱 Bladder	10	1.63	2.34	1.03	1.06	0.03
C70-C72; D32-33; D42-43	脑，神经系统 Brain & Central Nervous System	18	2.94	4.21	2.65	2.51	0.32
C73	甲状腺 Thyroid	1	0.16	0.23	0.15	0.12	0.00
C81-85,88,90,96	淋巴瘤 Lymphoma	9	1.47	2.10	1.09	1.08	0.15
C91-C95; D45-47	白血病 Leukaemia	19	3.10	4.44	2.82	2.69	0.25
Other	其他 Other	29	4.74	6.78	3.48	3.53	0.42
ALL	所有部位合计 All sites	612	100.00	143.09	78.70	77.70	9.32
ALLbC44	所有部位除外 C44 All sites except C44	608	99.35	142.15	78.31	77.32	9.28

附表 2-47　2019 年蕉城区恶性肿瘤发病主要指标

Appendix Table 2-47　Cancer incidence in Jiaocheng, 2019

ICD10	部位 Site		发病数 Cases	构成 Freq. （%）	粗率 Crude rate （1/10^5）	中标率 ASR China （1/10^5）	世标率 ASR world （1/10^5）	累积率 Cum.rate （0~74，%）
C00-10, C12-14	口腔和咽喉（除外鼻咽）	Oral Cavity & Pharynx but Nasopharynx	20	1.55	4.29	3.14	3.03	0.36
C11	鼻咽	Nasopharynx	20	1.55	4.29	3.62	3.27	0.33
C15	食管	Esophagus	23	1.78	4.93	3.46	3.63	0.50
C16	胃	Stomach	58	4.49	12.43	8.95	8.63	1.12
C18-21	结直肠肛门	Colon, Rectum & Anus	129	9.99	27.65	19.09	19.37	2.48
C22	肝脏	Liver	78	6.04	16.72	12.24	11.90	1.47
C23-C24	胆囊及其他	Gallbladder	8	0.62	1.71	1.24	1.26	0.18
C25	胰腺	Pancreas	12	0.93	2.57	1.85	1.90	0.27
C32	喉	Larynx	4	0.31	0.86	0.60	0.63	0.10
C33-C34	气管，支气管，肺	Trachea, Bronchus & Lung	246	19.05	52.72	37.63	37.71	5.07
C37-C38	其他的胸腔器官	Other thoracic organs	5	0.39	1.07	1.02	1.06	0.10
C40-C41	骨	Bone	4	0.31	0.86	0.88	0.95	0.10
C43	皮肤的黑色素瘤	Melanoma of skin	2	0.15	0.43	0.30	0.33	0.05
C50	乳房	Breast	87	6.74	38.16	29.80	27.80	3.05
C53	子宫颈	Cervix	66	5.11	28.95	21.77	20.96	2.18
C54-55	子宫体及子宫部位不明	Corpus Uterus & Unspectified	10	0.77	4.39	3.29	3.13	0.30
C56	卵巢	Ovary	13	1.01	5.70	4.37	3.91	0.39
C61	前列腺	Prostate	12	0.93	5.03	3.16	3.13	0.39
C62	睾丸	Testis	2	0.15	0.84	0.64	0.98	0.05
C64-66, 68	肾及泌尿系统不明	Kidney & Unspecified Urinary Organs	23	1.78	4.93	3.56	3.47	0.41
C67	膀胱	Bladder	15	1.16	3.21	2.22	2.21	0.27
C70-C72; D32-33; D42-43	脑，神经系统	Brain & Central Nervous System	45	3.49	9.64	7.71	7.51	0.77
C73	甲状腺	Thyroid	267	20.68	57.23	50.47	44.34	4.05
C81-85,88,90,96	淋巴瘤	Lymphoma	54	4.18	11.57	8.83	8.51	0.97
C91-C95; D45-47	白血病	Leukaemia	29	2.25	6.22	5.92	6.52	0.49
Other	其他	Other	59	4.57	12.65	9.86	9.12	1.18
ALL	所有部位合计	All sites	1291	100.00	276.69	213.33	204.52	23.37
ALLbC44	所有部位除外 C44	All sites except C44	1282	99.30	274.77	211.95	203.23	23.24

附表 2-48　2019 年蕉城区恶性肿瘤死亡主要指标

Appendix Table 2-48　Cancer mortality in Jiaocheng, 2019

ICD10	部位 Site	死亡数 Deaths	构成 Freq. （%）	粗率 Crude rate （1/10⁵）	中标率 ASR China （1/10⁵）	世标率 ASR world （1/10⁵）	累积率 Cum.rate （0~74，%）
C00-10, C12-14	口腔和咽喉（除外鼻咽） Oral Cavity & Pharynx but Nasopharynx	16	2.30	3.43	2.35	2.43	0.26
C11	鼻咽 Nasopharynx	10	1.44	2.14	1.51	1.53	0.18
C15	食管 Esophagus	30	4.31	6.43	4.19	4.42	0.58
C16	胃 Stomach	61	8.76	13.07	8.69	8.24	0.91
C18-21	结直肠肛门 Colon, Rectum & Anus	60	8.62	12.86	8.41	8.45	1.04
C22	肝脏 Liver	78	11.21	16.72	11.92	11.30	1.23
C23-C24	胆囊及其他 Gallbladder	20	2.87	4.29	2.88	2.86	0.33
C25	胰腺 Pancreas	14	2.01	3.00	1.97	1.96	0.21
C32	喉 Larynx	7	1.01	1.50	1.09	1.10	0.18
C33-C34	气管，支气管，肺 Trachea, Bronchus & Lung	209	30.03	44.79	30.34	30.29	4.23
C37-C38	其他的胸腔器官 Other thoracic organs	3	0.43	0.64	0.45	0.43	0.04
C40-C41	骨 Bone	3	0.43	0.64	0.94	0.96	0.06
C43	皮肤的黑色素瘤 Melanoma of skin	3	0.43	0.64	0.45	0.49	0.07
C50	乳房 Breast	16	2.30	7.02	5.05	4.86	0.58
C53	子宫颈 Cervix	17	2.44	7.46	5.26	5.39	0.82
C54-55	子宫体及子宫部位不明 Corpus Uterus & Unspecified	4	0.57	1.75	1.07	1.12	0.11
C56	卵巢 Ovary	10	1.44	4.39	3.13	3.00	0.49
C61	前列腺 Prostate	8	1.15	3.35	1.50	1.62	0.08
C62	睾丸 Testis	0	0.00	0.00	0.00	0.00	0.00
C64-66, 68	肾及泌尿系统不明 Kidney & Unspecified Urinary Organs	9	1.29	1.93	1.22	1.23	0.14
C67	膀胱 Bladder	8	1.15	1.71	0.93	1.00	0.15
C70-C72; D32-33;D42-43	脑，神经系统 Brain & Central Nervous System	19	2.73	4.07	2.60	2.54	0.28
C73	甲状腺 Thyroid	4	0.57	0.86	0.48	0.58	0.06
C81-85,88,90,96	淋巴瘤 Lymphoma	28	4.02	6.00	4.51	4.11	0.44
C91-C95;D45-47	白血病 Leukaemia	19	2.73	4.07	3.34	3.37	0.23
Other	其他 Other	40	5.75	8.57	6.05	6.07	0.77
ALL	所有部位合计 All sites	696	100.00	149.17	102.02	101.01	12.37
ALLbC44	所有部位除外 C44 All sites except C44	692	99.43	148.31	101.52	100.57	12.35